Practical Approaches to Applied Research and Program Evaluation for Counselors

Practical Approaches to Applied Research and Program Evaluation for Counselors is a comprehensive textbook that presents master's-level counselors with the skills and knowledge they need to consume literature to inform practice, apply research methods to practice settings, and evaluate the effectiveness of counseling services.

Each chapter, aligned with 2024 Council for Accreditation of Counseling and Related Educational Programs (CACREP) standards, guides readers through study design and evaluation fundamentals that will help them understand existing research and link the characteristics of that evidence to their practice. Readers will also be supported in the development of studies to assess their own applied evaluation questions. Readers will learn the basics of research concepts as applied to evaluative tasks, the art of matching evaluative methods to questions, specific considerations for practice-based evaluative tasks, and practical statistical options matched to practice-based tasks.

Readers can also turn to the book's support material to access sample course outlines for implementation by instructors of 15-, 10- and 5-week courses, worksheets for practitioner and student planning exercises, spreadsheets with formulas for basic data analysis, a sample database, PowerPoint outlines, and discussion questions and activities aligned to each chapter.

Casey A. Barrio Minton, PhD, NCC, is a Professor of Counselor Education and Department Head of Counseling, Human Development, and Family Science at the University of Tennessee, Knoxville.

A. Stephen Lenz, PhD, LPC-S, is a Professor of Counselor Education and Coordinator of Counseling Programs at Texas A&M University—San Antonio.

Both authors are Past-Presidents of the Association for Assessment and Research in Counseling and Fellows of the American Counseling Association.

Practical Approaches to Applied Research and Program Evaluation for Counselors

Second Edition

Casey A. Barrio Minton and
A. Stephen Lenz

Routledge
Taylor & Francis Group
NEW YORK AND LONDON

Designed cover image: Getty Images

Second edition published 2026
by Routledge
605 Third Avenue, New York, NY 10158

and by Routledge
4 Park Square, Milton Park, Abingdon, Oxon, OX14 4RN

Routledge is an imprint of the Taylor & Francis Group, an informa business

First edition published by Routledge 2019

Library of Congress Cataloging-in-Publication Data
A catalog record for this book has been requested

ISBN: 978-1-032-95725-8 (hbk)
ISBN: 978-1-032-95721-0 (pbk)
ISBN: 978-1-003-58621-0 (ebk)

DOI: 10.4324/9781003586210

Typeset in Sabon
by Apex CoVantage, LLC

Access the Support Material: https://resourcecentre.routledge.com/books/9781032957258

To you. Thank you for your curiosity, energy, and spirit.
Our profession and communities need them all.

Contents

Preface

We began this book with a passion for research, a firm belief in the power of professional counselors to do good work, and a sense we needed to bridge a persistent gap between research and practice in our beloved profession. We were tired of seeing counseling students and master's-level counselors plugging through statistics and research coursework as a hurdle to jump over rather than a foundation on which to ensure ethical and effective practice. We nodded on the inside when students asked when they would ever need to hand-calculate a standard deviation or why they were learning one research method each week, knowing they would never implement a truly scientific study as an entry-level clinical mental health or school counselor.

We were inspired by life-changing, effective interventions and programs we have seen implemented in our communities and schools. Yet, we were concerned about the long-term viability of these programs in the face of budget cuts and ever-growing expectations to demonstrate effectiveness. We envisioned a world where master's-level counselors wrap together art and science by bringing pieces of what we know about research into their counseling practices and programs. We wanted to design a starting place for that conversion. So here we are.

In Part I, we highlight the importance of converging art and science in counseling practice. We center counseling practice through an exploration of processes for developing interventions and explicating goals, outcomes, and objectives in any activity. Next, we explore the matter of question–design fit and provide an overview of major research paradigms. With those foundations set, we introduce methodological and statistical concepts you will need to understand in order to navigate research literature, and we draw connections between those principles and evaluation activities you may find yourself doing in your own counseling practice. We explore ethical, legal, and cultural considerations that are relevant to the research or program evaluation process. Finally, Part I concludes with strategies for reading literature, searching for evidence, evaluating what you find, and using that literature to support counseling practice.

Part II includes coverage of various research designs with a special program evaluation spin. We worked to illustrate how you might pull from these designs to understand your own counseling programs and practices. We provided examples from our own clinical and educational experiences, and we worked to make these principles come alive as something that might matter to you. In each chapter, we provide resources for reviewing the literature and hallmarks of quality studies. We also provide you with templates for writing up results of your own projects.

Finally, we designed Part III to serve as a practical toolkit you will want to revisit time and again. We provide no-nonsense, direct advice for selecting assessment measures; managing and protecting data; and closing the loop by presenting results to partners, making changes, and sharing findings with other professionals.

If you work through these pieces systematically, you will have a framework for building strong counseling interventions and programs and designing evaluations to help you understand what is working and what needs to change. In so doing, you will enhance your ability to advocate for those you serve through the development of strong, evidence-based, culturally sustaining counseling services. Additionally, you will be able to use data to advocate for continued service and continually grow your potential.

Professional Acknowledgments

We are indebted to Zeming Wang for careful reading, editorial precision, and student-focused feedback on the draft of this edition. Your deep commitment to bridging research and practice and your vision of counseling as a transformative tool in our schools and communities touches each page of this book. This work is stronger because of you.

We have much respect for the Routledge family, especially Grace McDonnell. Your support and guidance have been a gift through this process.

PERSONAL ACKNOWLEDGEMENTS

To Leah, who continues to be my most beautiful, indispensable obstacle to completing any project and who fills every "lost" workday with joy and a spark of hope for a more perfect future.

To Joel, who has been unwavering in support of my professional development and personal wellness and who will proudly promote this book without ever opening the cover.

~ Casey

To Rachel and Hayes—you have painted this canvas with all the colors of love, home, laughter, and encouragement. You are proof that life can be perpetually giving.

~ Stephen

We had the distinctive honor of authoring this text. Our names are on the cover, and the chapters are nuanced with the tones of our writing styles. Yet, a great deal of acknowledgment and gratitude belongs to our mentors, colleagues, and students who have helped us forge these perspectives across our careers. To y'all, thank you.

Lastly, we send whole-hearted appreciation and gratitude for those students and counselors who are engaging applied research and evaluation projects in a quest to shape our communities for the better. Your creativity and energies are a gift. Thank you.

PART I
Establishing Foundations

CHAPTER 1

Where Research and Program Evaluation Meet Practice

This chapter introduces the importance of applied research and program evaluation in counseling with special attention to the importance of evidence-informed practice and scientist-practitioner models in a profession focused on abstract human relationships. We discuss the development of the accountability era and introduce evidence-based practice and hierarchies of evidence. We then illustrate the mutually informative relationship between research and program evaluation with counseling practice. The chapter concludes with an overview of this book, including strategies for optimizing learning.

BOX 1.1 CHAPTER LEARNING OUTCOMES

- Deepen understanding regarding the important role of research and program evaluation in ensuring ethical and effective practice
- Conceptualize hierarchies of evidence used to support evidence-based practices

PROFESSIONAL IDENTITY AND FOUNDATIONS

Professional counselors are charged with facilitating healing and optimal functioning for the most vulnerable of populations. Although the degree of focus may vary across professionals and specialized settings, there is widespread agreement that such relationships and processes must be grounded in both art and science. Certainly, the integration of science in practice involving complex human experiences and relationships is an art.

Research and program evaluation have been of longstanding interest in mental health professions. The earliest and most famous theorists—players such as Freud, Skinner, and Rogers—were scientists who developed and modified theories based on rigorous inquiry. As theorists began building silos of research, other scholars began considering common factors that cut across approaches in hopes they could help us

DOI: 10.4324/9781003586210-2

better understand how counseling works and, in turn, how counselors best engage the science of counseling. Consider this excerpt from over 60 years ago:

> The more we learn from our research, the more acutely aware we become of the limitations and inadequacies of our current theoretical formulations. Individual schools of counseling and psychotherapy cannot account for the multitude of variables which in all probability ultimately will constitute the process of psychotherapeutic personality change. However, these varied approaches have proved themselves to be of research value in the past. Any attempted formulations in the future should, therefore, leave themselves open to their potential contributions to research in the therapeutic process. Indeed, common elements, stemming from, yet cutting across these various theoretical approaches, have already demonstrated significant heuristic meaning.
>
> (Truax & Carkhuff, 1964, p. 860)

More recently, scholars concluded:

> Despite the field's love affair with technique, nearly a half century of empirical investigation has revealed that the effectiveness of psychotherapy resides not in the many variables that ostensibly distinguish one approach from another. Instead, the success of treatment is principally found in the factors that all approaches share in common.
>
> (Duncan et al., 2010, p. xxvii)

Research and program evaluation are foundational to the work of professional counselors. The American Counseling Association (2014) *Code of Ethics* requires counselors to work with clients to develop "counseling plans that offer reasonable promise of success" (p. 4) and counselor educators to "promote the use of techniques/procedures/modalities that are grounded in theory and/or have an empirical or scientific foundation" (p. 14). The standards also require that "counselors continually monitor their effectiveness as professionals and take steps to improve when necessary" (p. 9). These ethical responsibilities serve as the foundation for research and program evaluation as one of eight longstanding foundational curricular areas for master's students in programs accredited by the Council for Accreditation of Counseling and Related Educational Programs (CACREP).

A closer examination of CACREP 2024 *Standards* reveals the interconnected nature of research, program evaluation, and practice. Professional counselors understand that these tools are essential for delivering ethical and effective services. Research advances the counseling profession by informing practice and helping counselors identify the evidence base for counseling services (3.H.1, 3.H.2). This means counselors need to be familiar with a wide range of research designs (3.H.3), including practice-based and action research (3.H.4), and be able to understand statistical findings reported in studies related to their practice (3.H.5, 3.H.6). Counselors also use data and applied research principles to evaluate outcomes of their services (3.H.7). Program evaluation—including needs assessments, formative evaluations, and summative assessments—can support counselor decision-making and advocacy efforts (3.H.8). Throughout this process, counselors are responsible for upholding ethical and legal standards (3.H.10) as they ensure their program evaluation activities are both culturally sustaining and developmentally appropriate for those they serve (3.H.9, 3.H.11). Together, ethical codes and preparation standards reflect both the internal development of the counseling profession and external realities of practice in what some call the era of accountability.

BOX 1.2 ETHICAL RESPONSIBILITY TO ENSURE EFFECTIVE PRACTICE

Non-maleficence: Do no harm. Medical and mental health professionals alike recognize their responsibility to protect those they serve from intentional and unintentional harm. We are also guided by a number of other ethical principles. *Beneficence* refers to doing good or making a positive impact. It is not enough to exist in a neutral state of not doing harm. We must also do good.

From a philosophical and practical standpoint, we might argue that failure to do good may be harmful. At a most basic level, failure to do good wastes precious time, energy, and financial resources. More philosophically, failure to do good could send an unsavory message regarding a consumer's hope for the future and the value of the professions we hold dear.

If we agree that doing no harm is a necessary, but not sufficient, bar for practice, we must turn attention to how we know we are doing good. How do we know our programs and practices are having their intended effects? How do we understand opportunities to minimize potential for harm among our most vulnerable of clients? Whatever your theoretical or philosophical foundations, we hope you agree that the answer lies in developing an ability to evaluate our programs and practices in an effort to continually grow, improve, and reach toward our ethical striving to do good.

THE ERA OF ACCOUNTABILITY

Mental health professionals are under unprecedented expectations to work efficiently and effectively and to be transparent about both the process and outcome with a variety of partners. Our most important constituents are those we serve through prevention and early intervention programs as well as through individual, group, couple, or family counseling services. Engaging in counseling requires considerable resources, and most people do not engage in the process when things are going well. Consumers need to be able to trust that they are investing their time, money, and emotional reserves in ways that are likely to facilitate positive outcomes.

Consumers of mental health services are not our only *interest holders*—individuals and entities who have a legitimate direct or indirect interest in the success of research and program evaluation endeavors (Akl et al., 2024). Instead, it is imperative to see the activities and outcomes inherent within counseling research and evaluation as having implications across a broader ecology of interest holders (See Figure 1.1). While several frameworks have been identified in association with the allied mental health professions (Smith et al., 2021; Yamaguchi et al., 2022), in general, they tend to illustrate the importance of research and evaluation results for consumers, provider networks, regulatory bodies, payer networks, and society which includes supporting the greater public good. Professional counselors who work in agencies, schools, and other settings are accountable to parents or caregivers as well as supervisors, coworkers, administrators, staff, and referral partners.

Research and evaluation also have an interconnected relationship with regulatory bodies such as state licensing boards, accreditation entities, and ethics review committees that define and monitor the purview of related activities. Payer networks such as public funding sources (e.g., educational systems), public or private insurance (e.g., third-party payers), grant funders, and fourth-party payers such as Employee Assistance Programs are similarly interested in assuring quality of care and efficient use of resources. Finally, research and evaluation practices are often central to legislative appropriations as a mechanism to demonstrate advancements in science or practice and lessons learned that could be considered during future decision-making.

Multiple parties need to know that the "parts" of an greater intervention or program are working. A number of individuals often influence budget decisions regarding service authorization. Just as consumers want to know they are making a wise investment, interest holders are keen to understand the return on investments of funding, personnel, facilities, good faith, and hope. Although a full discussion of mental health reimbursement, accountability, and management systems is beyond the scope of this book (see Brown and Minami (2010) for a history), it is important to understand that our current focus on outcome management and accountability is rooted in a long

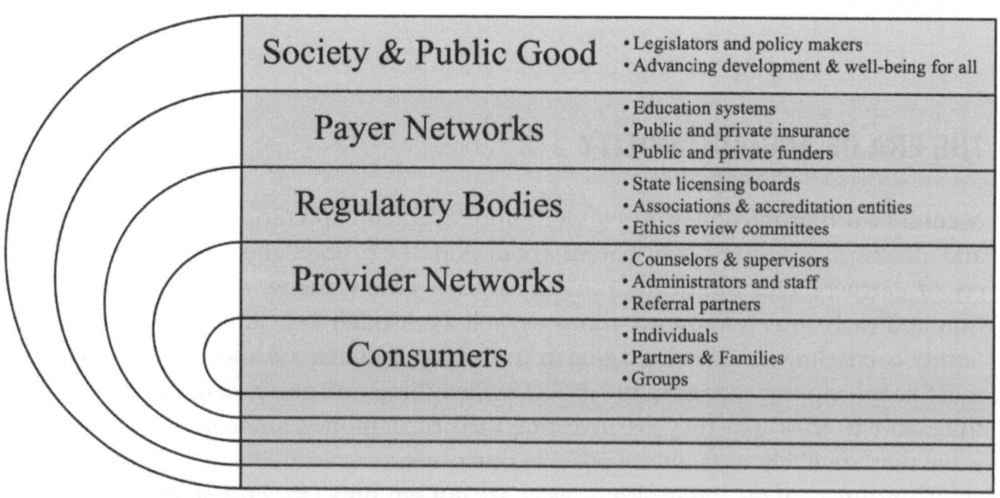

Figure 1.1 The Ecology of Research and Evaluation Interest Holders

history of exponentially expanding utilization of mental health services in which there was not always a focus on cost control or demonstrated effectiveness. This led to utilization review services in which payers authorized type and number of services based on pre-established sets of treatment guidelines and criteria. More recently, formal interest holding entities have shifted to requiring progress measurement and reporting of treatment outcomes as a condition of funding, continued payment, and reimbursement.

Accountability requirements bring both strengths and limitations. Certainly, they do not always neatly match to the complex richness of human experience or to our professional foundations in strengths, optimal development, and holistic wellness. Still, the take-home messages are clear: counselors must be able to (a) justify the selection of specific interventions or programs based on the current body of evidence, (b) articulate how we provide services with strong probability of success, and (c) demonstrate outcomes for individual clients and programs. As you learn about ways to identify and discuss research and evaluation findings, you will be poised to do just that. A great place to start is with a conversation about evidence-based practices (EBPs), evidence-supported treatments (ESTs), and hierarchies of evidence.

EVIDENCE-BASED PRACTICE, EVIDENCE-SUPPORTED TREATMENTS, AND HIERARCHIES OF EVIDENCE

As you have read already in this chapter, counselors are expected to integrate research and evaluation results to make decisions that inform our clinical practice. This has given rise to an alphabet soup of acronyms designed to help counselors and researchers determine just what that looks like. Evidence-based practice (EBP), sometimes referred to as evidence-informed practice, is the most recent focus of attention in mental health professions. EBP features "integration of the best available research within clinical expertise in the context of patient characteristics, culture, and preferences" (APA Presidential Task Force on Evidence-based Practice, 2006, p. 273).

By definition, EBP features acceptance of a broad array of research evidence and recognition that the strongest evidence bases are built upon a variety of different designs. In particular, EBP recognizes that "different research designs are better suited to address different types of questions" (APA Presidential Task Force on Evidence-based Practice, 2006, p. 274). Designs can include clinical observation, qualitative research, systematic case studies, single-case experimental designs, public health and ethnographic research, process-outcome studies, naturalistic studies of interventions, randomized controlled trials (RCT), and meta-analyses.

This approach lends itself to a valuing of *methodological pluralism* that views the best clues to inform EBP as lying in the overlapping convergence of findings across multiple approaches to research and evaluation in juxtaposition to those elements and outcomes that diverge from the center (See Figure 1.2). As noted by Lenz (2018) "through equitable valuing of various methods and meaningful integration of related findings, the best research evidence available will more closely represent interactions between counseling interventions and client experiences" (p. 2).

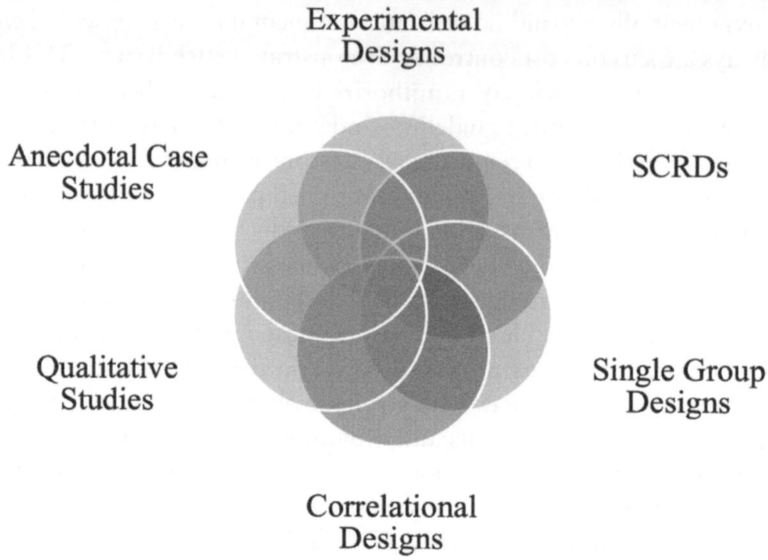

Figure 1.2 Visual Illustration of the Methodological Pluralism Associated with Evidence-Based Practice

However, it is widely accepted that certain research and evaluation designs are superior to other designs when answering specific questions. For example, well-designed RCTs offer superior evidence of intervention or program efficacy when compared to quasi-experimental or case study investigations. However, if one wants to understand experiences that lead a high percentage of clients to discontinue participation in an intervention, a qualitative design revealing insights into the related decision and motivational factors is well-suited for gathering data that can answer the question. We would likely also agree to put more weight on a meta-analysis synthesizing results of multiple well-designed studies than on any one individual study.

The definition of EBP also includes attention to client characteristics, culture, and preferences while also calling upon professionals to use clinical expertise and research findings. Clinical expertise is defined as

> (a) assessment, diagnostic judgment, systematic case formulation, and treatment planning; (b) clinical decision making, treatment implementation, and monitoring of patient progress; (c) interpersonal expertise; (d) continual self-reflection and acquisition of skills; (e) appropriate evaluation and use of research evidence in both basic and applied psychological science; (f) understanding the influence of individual and cultural differences on treatment; (g) seeking available resources (e.g., consultation, adjunctive or alternative services) as needed; and (h) having a cogent rationale for clinical strategies.
>
> (APA Presidential Task Force on Evidence-based Practice, 2006, p. 276)

More recently, the APA (2021) reaffirmed this conceptualization of EBP as a three-legged stool involving best available research; clinical expertise; and patient characteristics, culture, and preferences in their *Professional Practice Guidelines for Evidence-based Psychological Practice in Healthcare*. These updates reflect a deeper understanding of both the research informing practice and the complexities of clinical expertise and client characteristics, culture, and preferences (Melchert et al., 2024).

Long before the concept of EBP emerged, some groups worked to categorize best available research by creating lists or rankings of programs believed to be most appropriate or effective. These are often called empirically supported treatments (ESTs). In their foundational work on the topic, Chambless and Hollon (1998) defined ESTs as "clearly specified psychological treatments shown to be efficacious in controlled research with a delineated population" (p. 7). In addition, the authors developed criteria for determining therapeutic approaches as empirically supported. For example, those receiving interventions needed to be compared to another group, core practices and processes were required to be described in manuals, clear population and problem parameters were identified, as well as description of suitable outcome measures and rigorous data analysis. The evidence for ESTs is typically regarded as either very strong, strong, weak, or having insufficient evidence based on a collective review of individual research and evaluation studies (Tolin, 2020; Tolin et al., 2015).

The EST movement has indelibly influenced the way that mental health professionals value evidence. Consequently, a hierarchy of evidence has emerged that values highly controlled experimental designs and subsequent synthesis of their results (Rubin & Bellamy, 2022). Conceptualizations such as those in Figure 1.3 have proven useful in answering the fundamental questions *What works for whom? How? And under what circumstance?* with the result being numerous treatment packages available to counselors that often include screening criteria, assessment tools, treatment manuals, and therapist guides. However, we stress that such hierarchies are not indicative of the inherent value or practical utility of various research design. Instead, they

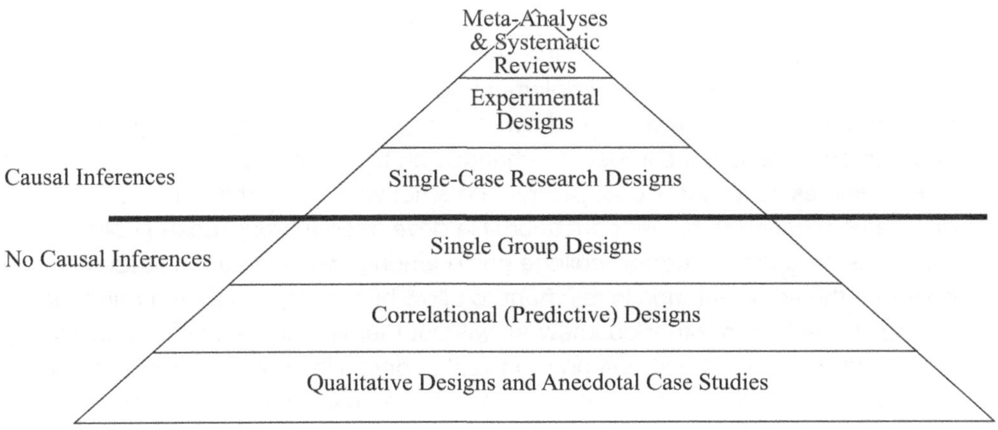

Figure 1.3 Hierarchy of Causal Evidence Associated with Evidence-Supported Treatments

provide a gradient for conceptualizing the ability of various approaches to research and evaluation to demonstrate defensible cause and effect relationships between interventions and observed outcomes.

Although the use of menu-like treatment lists may be attractive to some, this practice is not realistic for practice in a world where clients and their problems are complex and rarely fit neat boxes required for the most stringent of RCTs. Many professionals worry that a strict focus on lists of ESTs negates nuanced attention to client characteristics, culture, and preferences alongside clinical judgement as required for EBP. Others argued that synthesis across studies is more important than attention to individual studies, and yet others noted the likelihood of bias in systematic reviews (Littell, 2010). More recently, scholars proposed a both/and approach in which practitioners consider ESTs as one leg of a "three-legged stool" involving research evidence, client characteristics, and clinical expertise (Tolin, 2020; Tolin et al., 2015). They further proposed new strategies for evaluating and classifying the strength of evidence for specific approaches to treatment.

Counselors must be strong consumers of research when providing services and planning programs, and our responsibilities do not end at using research to inform practice. Counselors also need to be prepared to use research and program evaluation principles to evaluate their own programs and practices, advocate for program resources, and ensure ethical practice. Let's turn attention to three professional counselors who face program and practice evaluation questions critical to their work.

BOX 1.3 CASE STUDY

Maria is a clinical director for a small nonprofit agency that specializes in providing services for survivors of sexual assault. Her agency has been affected by reductions in funding at local, state, and federal levels. Historically, the agency has been able to offer services without time constraints. As funding shrinks and the wait list grows, Maria wonders whether the agency could serve consumers more effectively by implementing groups or imposing limits on the number of sessions. She wonders how she might find information to guide her decision and evaluate the impact of changes on those she serves.

Paul serves as a school counselor in a district where less than 30% of graduates proceed to higher education. He developed a group-based college readiness program to support college going among first-generation students; however, the administration is reluctant to allow him to implement it, noting that pulling students from other coursework will put them behind in this coursework and jeopardize the school's already-low test scores. He convinces the principal to allow him to implement a pilot program for one year, with renewal contingent on evidence that the program is achieving its aims without unanticipated consequences.

Irma works with a program that provides wraparound services for teenage mothers and their infant children. Most clients live in poverty, have low educational attainment, and have a history of trauma. The program is built upon several well-respected and researched practices related to trauma and parent–child attachment. Although the program has robust referrals and strong initial enrollment, Irma has become discouraged, as many mothers discontinue the program after just a few short months. She is confident the program works for those who persist, but she's not sure how to address the problem with attrition.

HOW TO USE THIS BOOK

The cases in this chapter represent common scenarios faced by master's level counselors. We designed this book to serve as a practical guidebook for people like them who are called upon to use scientific literature to inform practice and also demonstrate the effectiveness of their programs and practices. In the following chapters, we introduce the nuts and bolts of research concepts as related to applied research and program evaluation tasks, the art of matching methods to questions, specific considerations for a variety of practice-based tasks, and practical statistical options matched to these tasks.

This book is presented in three major sections. *Part I: Establishing Foundations* is designed to introduce applied research and program evaluation and provide a foundation overview of basic concepts that apply across evaluation tasks. This section will be essential for those who have not had previous coursework in research and program evaluation. For others, this section will serve as a quick review of concepts they will encounter in later parts of the text. Part I first grounds us in our greater goals by exploring processes for developing counseling interventions and mapping programs through logic models; Chapter 2 helps us specify what we are doing and why thus setting the stage for inquiry. This also includes an overview of approaches to scientific inquiry and program evaluation, including matching research designs to questions (Chapter 3). We then attend to methodological concepts (Chapter 4); measurement and statistical concepts (Chapter 5); and ethical, legal, and cultural considerations (Chapter 6) relevant to all forms of applied research and program evaluation. Part I concludes with an exploration of how counselors can utilize literature to support counseling practice (Chapter 7).

Part II: Using Research and Program Evaluation in Practice systematically walks through a variety of qualitative and quantitative designs that answer applied research and program evaluation questions. After attending to the use of surveys for needs assessment, process evaluations, and satisfaction surveys (Chapter 8), this section outlines a variety of methods for process and outcome evaluations (Chapters 9–13). The section concludes with an exploration of method for combining findings across studies

(Chapter 14). Each chapter attends to method and design considerations and has specific suggestions for data analysis and reporting relevant to your practice.

Building on foundations established in Parts I and II, Part III: *Putting Evaluation Practice into Motion* features some how-to guides filled with resources designed to meet the logistical and technical support needs of counselors in a variety of settings. Topics in this section include selecting assessment measures (Chapter 15), managing and protecting data (Chapter 16), and reporting and communicating with interest holders (Chapter 17).

All chapters open with an overview of major content and articulation of chapter learning outcomes. All chapters will also include a variety of features including

- *Case studies* designed to illustrate content and applied in real-life counseling settings including schools, clinical mental health agencies, hospitals, and non-profit organizations,
- *Practical checklists* to help you recognize quality indicators or key steps as have been addressed in the chapters, and
- *Sidebar discussions* to highlight ethical and cultural considerations.

Each chapter will end with a summary and a list of resources you may find helpful in applying or extending the material.

CHAPTER SUMMARY

This chapter highlighted the importance of applying research and program evaluation principles in practice. Counselors must be prepared to consume research and artfully combine the best available research with an understanding of client characteristics and clinical expertise. In addition to meeting ethical standards of practice, mental health professionals must use research and program evaluation to respond to calls for accountability from grant funders, third- and fourth-party payers, and key stakeholders.

RESOURCES

- American Psychological Association. (2018) Policy statement on evidence-based practice in psychology. www.apa.org/practice/guidelines/evidence-based-statement.aspx
- American Psychological Association. (2021a). Professional practice guidelines for evidence-based psychological practice in health care. www.apa.org/about/policy/psychological-practice-health-care.pdf
- British Association for Counselling & Psychotherapy
- *An introduction to counselling research (1/3): Why is research important?* www.youtube.com/watch?v=BbGPjOK5PFY
- *An introduction to counselling research (2/3): The relationship between research and practice.* www.youtube.com/watch?v=J8l20RMa_T0
- *An introduction to counselling research (3/3): How has research informed my practice.* www.youtube.com/watch?v=xhgw356fmjI

- Counselling Tutor, *The Importance & Purpose of Research in Counselling & Psychotherapy*. www.youtube.com/watch?v=OwfyYe0H9hQ
- McMorrow, S. (2017, March). What gets in the way? Examining the breakdown between research and practice in counseling. https://ctarchive.counseling.org/2017/03/gets-way-examining-breakdown-research-practice-counseling/
- Substance Abuse and Mental Health Services Administration, *Evidence-Based Practices Resource Center*. www.samhsa.gov/libraries/evidence-based-practices-resource-center

REFERENCES

Akl, E. A., Khabsa, J., Petkovic, J., Magwood, O., Lytvyn, L., Motilall, A., Campbell, P., Todhunter-Brown, A., Schünemann, H. J., Welch, V., Tugwell, P., & Concannon, T. W. (2024). "Interest-holders": A new term to replace "stakeholders" in the context of health research and policy. *Cochrane Evidence Synthesis and Methods*, *2*(11), e70007. https://doi.org/10.1002/cesm.70007

American Counseling Association. (2014). *Code of ethics*. www.counseling.org/ethics

American Psychological Association. (2021). Professional practice guidelines for evidence-based psychological practice in health care. www.apa.org/about/policy/psychological-practice-health-care.pdf

APA Presidential Task Force on Evidence-based Practice. (2006). Evidence based practice in psychology. *American Psychologist*, *61*(4), 271–285. https://doi.org/10.1037/0003-066X.61.4.271

Brown, G. S., & Minami, T. (2010). Outcomes management, reimbursement, and the future of psychotherapy. In B. L. Duncan, S. D. Miller, B. E. Wampold, & M. A. Hubble (Eds.), The heart & soul of change: Delivering what works in therapy (2nd ed., pp. 267–297). American Psychological Association.

Chambless, D. L., & Hollon, S. D. (1998). Defining empirically supported therapies. *Journal of Consulting and Clinical Psychology*, *66*(1), 7–18. https://doi.org/10.1037/0022-006X.66.1.7

Council for the Accreditation of Counseling and Related Educational Programs. (2024). 2024 standards. https://www.cacrep.org/for-programs/2024-cacrep-standards/

Duncan, B. L., Miller, S. D., Wampold, B. E., & Hubble, M. A. (2010). *The heart & soul of change: Delivering what works in therapy* (2nd ed.). American Psychological Association.

Lenz, A. S. (2018). Reconsidering the value assigned to counseling research paradigms and outcomes. *Counseling Outcome Research and Evaluation*, *9*(1), 1–4. https://doi.org/10.1080/21501378.2017.1423202

Littell, J. H. (2010). Evidence-based practice: Evidence or orthodoxy? In B. L. Duncan, S. D. Miller, B. E. Wampold, & M. A. Hubble (Eds.), *The heart & soul of change: Delivering what works in therapy* (2nd ed., pp. 167–198). American Psychological Association.

Melchert, T. P., Halfond, R. W., Hamdi, N. R., Bufka, L. F., Hollon, S. D., & Cuttler, M. J. (2024). Evidence-based practice in psychology: Context, guidelines, and action. *American Psychologist*, *79*(6), 824–837. https://doi.org/10.1037/amp0001253

Rubin, A., & Bellamy, J. (2022). *Practitioner's guide to using research for evidence-informed practice* (3rd ed.). Wiley.

Smith, P., Nicaise, P., Thunus, S., Neyens, I., Walker, C., & Lorant, V. (2021). Stakeholder coalitions and priorities around the policy goals of a nation-wide mental health care reform. *Administration and Policy in Mental Health and Mental Health Services Research*, *48*(4), 639–653. https://doi.org/10.1007/s10488-020-01100-8

Tolin, D. F. (2020). Advances in the identification of empirically supported psychological treatments. *Clinical Psychology: Science and Practice*, 27(4), Article e12356. https://doi.org/10.1111/cpsp.12356

Tolin, D. F., McKay, D., Forman, E. M., Klonsky, E. D., & Thombs, B. D. (2015). Empirically supported treatment: Recommendations for a new model. *Clinical Psychology: Science and Practice*, *22*(4), 317–338. https://doi.org/10.1111/cpsp.12122

Traux, C. B., & Carkuff, R. R. (1964). The old and the new: Theory and research in counseling and psychotherapy. *The Personnel and Guidance Journal*, *42*(9), 860–866. https://doi.org/10.1002/j.2164-4918.1964.tb04744.x

Yamaguchi, S., Abe, M., Kawaguchi, T., Igarashi, M., Shiozawa, T., Ogawa, M., Yasuma, N., Sato, S., Miyamoto, Y., & Fujii, C. (2022). Multiple stakeholders' perspectives on patient and public involvement in community mental health services research: A qualitative analysis. *Health Expectations*, *25*, 1844–1860. https://doi.org/ 10.1111/hex.13529

CHAPTER 2

Understanding Interventions, Programs, and Logic Models

We opened Chapter 1 by exploring where research and program evaluation intersect with counseling practice. This chapter builds on that foundation, guiding you in identifying and articulating elements of counseling work in ways that naturally lead to meaningful research and program evaluation questions. We begin by clarifying what we mean by counseling techniques, interventions, and programs. Then, we introduce key principles for developing quality programs and discuss the crucial concept of treatment fidelity.

After establishing these foundations, we present the logic model as a tool to describe how programs function and what they aim to achieve. We conclude with practical strategies for writing goals, objectives, and outcomes—three essential components you will encounter in a variety of counseling settings. You will need to be able to write these for individual client treatment plans, agency or school programs, and funding requests. These elements also serve as a foundation for evaluation planning. After all, being clear about what we are doing in counseling and what outcomes we expect lays the groundwork for asking meaningful research and evaluation questions.

BOX 2.1 CHAPTER LEARNING OUTCOMES

- Differentiate between counseling techniques, interventions, and programs
- Describe strategies for counseling program development
- Explain the critical role in treatment fidelity in evaluating the impact of interventions and programs
- Utilize a logic model to illustrate how a program is expected to work
- Understand characteristics of strong goals, objectives, and outcomes
- Develop measurable outcomes for counseling interventions and programs

COUNSELING TECHNIQUES, INTERVENTIONS, AND PROGRAMS

Before we dive into the heart of developing interventions and programs, we need to take a moment to make sure we are using common language to describe what we do and why we

DOI: 10.4324/9781003586210-3

do it. We can use cooking as a metaphor to explain how techniques, interventions, and programs work together. Think of techniques as ingredients in a recipe, interventions as a dish prepared using a specific recipe, and programs as a full-course meal of coordinated dishes.

Most counselors default to the world of interventions. Interventions are simply a purposeful approach to targeting a specific issue often through a series of engagements. The following list of counseling interventions will probably look quite familiar to you:

- Individual, trauma-focused cognitive behavioral therapy (TF-CBT)
- Individual, solution-focused brief therapy (SFBT)
- Emotion-focused therapy for couples (EFT)
- Acceptance and Commitment Therapy (ACT) group counseling for grief
- STAC bullying intervention program (2025) for middle schoolers

You might be thinking, "wait, that sounds like counseling." And, it is. Counseling *is* the intervention. You might also be confused because STAC has "program" in the name. However, STAC consists of a 90-minute classroom lesson and two 15-minute booster sessions. So, we will go ahead and call it an intervention despite the name. Counselors may evaluate effectiveness of our work with a singular client, couple, family, classroom, or group *or* we might evaluate the effectiveness of an intervention across multiple clients, couples, families, schools, or groups. Either way, we are focused on an intervention.

Counselors use a number of **techniques** to facilitate any given intervention. Techniques are simply specific, discrete skills used within any given intervention. At the most essential level, reflective listening is a technique, as are more advanced skills such as Socratic questioning or confrontation. Certainly, person-centered approaches to counseling lean very heavily on reflective listening. Techniques can also be specific to an intervention. TF-CBT, for example, includes a variety of techniques including psychoeducation, relaxation strategies, cognitive coping strategies, and ultimately the construction and processing of a trauma narrative (Cohen et al., 2013). Counselors operating from an EFT framework will utilize techniques to de-escalate negative cycles, help couples recognize defensive patterns or cycles, examine their beliefs about relationships, and intentionally break cycles (Greenberg & Goldman, 2018). In any of these examples, counselors might recommend homework between sessions. In any case, these are all micro-level techniques within an intervention. Although techniques might be the focus of more advanced research designs (e.g., effectiveness of TF-CBT with or without the trauma narrative), counselors rarely research or evaluate specific techniques in isolation.

This brings us to counseling **programs**. Counseling programs are coordinated sets of interventions designed for a distinct purpose. School counselors are responsible for developing comprehensive, developmental school counseling programs that meet the distinct needs of their schools and communities. These programs may include leaning on a multi-tiered systems of supports (MTSS) framework (Goodman-Scott et al., 2020). Within MTSS, counselors implement Tier 1 interventions for all students in the school (e.g., STAC). They may also engage in universal screening or other efforts to identify students who may benefit from more targeted Tier 2 interventions, perhaps offering evidence-informed small group interventions focused on emotion regulation or social skills. Finally, school counselors will identify those who would benefit from Tier 3 intensive interventions. Together, these activities comprise a program.

We also see counseling programs offered in community settings. For example, clients in an alternative to prison program for addiction-related offenses may receive medication-assisted therapy from a psychiatrist; participate in daily psychoeducation classes focused on life skills such as career development, financial management, healthy relationships, and coping strategies; engage in daily group counseling; and have weekly individual and family sessions with a counselor. Likewise, youth living in a therapeutic group home may engage in a program that includes milieu therapy (e.g., living in a safe, structured foster home); tutoring; medication management with a psychiatrist; biweekly group counseling with other residents; weekly individual counseling; and weekly parent consultation. Together, those services comprise a program. Just as counselors and researchers may investigate the effectiveness of interventions, they may investigate the effectiveness of programs. See Table 2.1 for an illustration of the differences between techniques, interventions, and programs.

TABLE 2.1 Comparing Counseling Techniques, Interventions, and Programs

Feature	Techniques	Interventions	Programs
Definition	Discrete, micro-level counseling skills or strategies	Purposeful approaches to address a specific concern, often over a series of sessions	Coordinated sets of interventions designed to address broad or complex client, school, or community needs
Scope	Moment-to-moment within a session	Session-level or short-term service targeting specific presenting concerns	Multilayered and sustained across clients, service types, and time
Examples	Reflective listening, Socratic questioning, confrontation, homework assignments	TF-CBT, EFT, solution-focused brief therapy, grief counseling groups, STAC bullying prevention intervention	Comprehensive school counseling program, therapeutic group home services, re-entry support programs
Evaluation Focus	Rarely evaluated in isolation	Commonly evaluated for effectiveness with specific populations or presenting issues	Evaluated for overall outcomes across service domains, populations, and time frames
Relation to Other Levels	Used within interventions to facilitate change	Comprised of multiple techniques tailored to a presenting concern	Comprised of multiple interventions targeting multiple needs or tiers of service

DEVELOPING INTERVENTIONS AND PROGRAMS

Now that we have clarified the differences between techniques, interventions, and programs, we are ready to explore what it means to develop interventions and programs. Developing an intervention or a program is a virtuous endeavor. Although you may be tempted to put together an experience-informed intervention or program, a more systematic approach has several benefits. A more systematic approach is more likely to address the problem of interest by targeting the intended goal and helping you to specify appropriate outcomes. Clearly defining processes and practices will promote procedural transparency that contributes to honest implementation across settings. This transparency helps to estimate positioning and potential impact within a socio-ecological context. Let's take a look at each of these essential activities.

Clarifying the Broader Problem

It is important to clarify the broader problem that your intervention or program is designed to address. When you view a presenting issue through a wide lens, you may be able to better understand an overarching problem a group of individuals or a community may be facing. For example, some communities may be facing economic or environmental challenges that may contribute to increased stress or health issues which adversely affect mental health and coping strategies. In other communities, broader problems may be represented by links between social factors such as high incarceration rates of individuals with mental health diagnoses and barriers to housing.

Identifying the Goal of Intervention or Program

Once we understand the broader problem, we are ready to establish general goals. Your identified goal should state what effect your intervention or program will have on the problem using a statement that specifies the problem or risk behavior of interest and the target population. For example, you may be interested in decreasing recidivism among individuals who have mental health diagnoses, decreasing the incidence of opioid-related deaths among individuals with chronic pain diagnoses, or reducing disproportionality in disciplinary referrals and suspensions in your school. This goal will provide you with a basis for specifying your target outcomes. We provide practical strategies for explicating goals in the second part of this chapter.

Specifying Objectives

Goals are achieved through meeting a series of objectives, and we can identify outcomes in several ways. Therefore, objectives should specify what success looks like and how goals will be achieved. In most cases, we will need multiple objectives to achieve a single goal. Objectives can be either process- or outcome-oriented. Process objectives are associated with the number and type of activities, services, or strategies inherent within an intervention or program. Outcome objectives depict the degree to which an intended effect was realized. In either case, best practice will be to characterize them using a SMART (specific, measurable, attainable, relevant, and time-referenced) strategy and pair them with an assessment or data point that depicts the degree to which you are meeting objectives. The second half of this chapter includes practical strategies for writing objectives for clients and programs.

Describing the Nature of an Intervention or Program

When we are ready to begin a new project, most of us like to jump immediately to what we will do and how we will do it. This step will be more meaningful if we make sure we understand the previous components as well. When designing programs, we will need to account for schools of thought that inform our frameworks; culturally responsive techniques, procedures, activities, and equipment; roles and activities; and considerations regarding optimal number and length of services. These foundation steps are critical for designing meaningful interventions and programs.

Determining Your Framework

Most interventions and programs are based on underlying theories of development and change, which serve as the foundational framework for desired change to occur. For example, Aaron Beck's cognitive behavioral therapy emerged as a reflection of the cognitive model of depression (Beck, 2020). Marsha Linehan's dialectical behavioral therapy was grounded in the biosocial theory (Linehan, 2015). Michael White's expression of narrative therapy was informed to some degree by Foucault's post-structural philosophy (White, 2007). All interventions and programs should start with a framework that helps us understand how and why they should work.

Identifying or Developing Culturally Responsive Techniques, Procedures, Activities, and Equipment

Once we have identified a framework, you can begin working to identify related component parts and processes. Although cognitive therapy, dialectical behavior therapy, and narrative therapy are disparate in their component parts and processes, they are similar in their representations of values inherent within their frameworks. You can include techniques, procedures, and activities that already have strong evidentiary support (evidence-informed practices) or those that are grounded in your practical experience (practice-based evidence). Regardless of what you select, all component parts and processes should be culturally responsive to your target population. Being culturally responsive includes consideration of use and access to required equipment or technology.

Defining Roles and Activities of Those Involved

This sounds intuitive, but you should work to clearly define the roles of all individuals who come into contact with your intervention or program. Four common clusters of individuals that warrant clarification include interventionists or service providers; participants, clients, students, or families; administrative supports; and researchers or evaluators.

Considering Dosage–Impact Interactions

Finally, you will want to consider what type of impact you expect from the dosage or amount of participant exposure to interventions or program content. For example, how many intervention hours would be needed to experience the therapeutic effect? Is there a percentage of eligible community members who would need to be served by a program to meet your goals? There are no steadfast guidelines for making these determinations, but they should be grounded in standards for reasonable practice. By ensuring enough exposure to salient components of an intervention or program, you increase chances for making a meaningful impact and achieving your goals.

Assuring Fidelity of Interventions and Programs

In the world of counseling interventions and programs, *fidelity* refers to the extent that the key elements believed to produce therapeutic change were included and delivered as intended. When interventions and programs are delivered with a strong degree of fidelity, the related research or evaluation activities may be considered a good test of their potential (Rubin & Bellamy, 2022). By contrast, the absence of such information makes it impossible to rule out deviations from the intended intervention (i.e., *therapeutic drift*) thereby reducing confidence in the relationship between interventions and outcomes.

Gearing et al. (2011) suggested four components of intervention fidelity for consideration. First, **design fidelity** refers to the degree that an intervention is grounded in a framework that logically connects therapeutic interventions and processes with the desired goals in ways that could be expected given the cultural, social, and personal characteristics of your intended population. Second, **training fidelity** is represented by the use of clear protocols to teach, practice, troubleshoot, and supervise the use of an intervention. Third, **delivery fidelity** accounts for activities that monitor the implementation of core intervention elements at the right time in the right amounts with the expected degree of competency. Finally, **treatment receipt fidelity** alludes to the degree that participants acquire the intended knowledge, skills, or capabilities as a function of their engagement with the intervention. Ideally, these features are described within treatment manuals, implementation protocols, and method sections within published studies.

From a research and evaluation perspective, the use of intervention and program fidelity procedures signals a commitment to rigor within the selected method. When fidelity practices are in place and demonstrate a high degree of adherence, consumers of the scientific literature can place a greater degree of confidence that any observed outcomes may be more closely aligned with intervention or program elements, rather than another factor (Power et al., 2022). From a practitioner's perspective, implementing interventions and programs with a strong degree of fidelity increases the odds that your clients may benefit from outcomes similar to the participants whose data is represented in the broader outcome literature. Stated another way, in the absence of practitioner fidelity when implementing evidence-based practices and evidence-supported treatments, the accuracy of client outcomes may be inaccurately attributed to the care received (Gearing et al., 2011). Thus, we encourage you to regard information and resources about fidelity as a signal of scientific rigor, but also a guide for your use of interventions and programs in your personal practice.

CONNECTING THE DOTS THROUGH LOGIC MODELING

Given the complexity of most interventions and programs, it can be helpful to create a logic model that connects the dots and portrays the relationships between the problem to be addressed, inputs (i.e. resources), therapeutic or programmatic activities, outputs, short-term outcomes, and long-term impacts. Figure 2.1 includes a template to help you get started in the logic modeling process. Note that some logic models include more nuances and distinctions. For example, they may include attention to assumptions and external factors that may both drive and influence a program.

These graphic models can be helpful in a number of ways. First, visual depictions of links can support the discovery of gaps in your reasoning, missing pieces, or mistakes in your planning. Second, this graphic can support discussions about your project with others. Third, the logic model can serve as a resource during your evaluation or study by helping you keep an eye on the big picture. Finally, by capturing the essence of your intervention or program, logic models can provide a safeguard against drifting away from the intended purpose and activities. Taken together, this simple graphic can support your team as you test the frontiers of what is helpful to participants, clients, students, and community members. Because practitioners often use logic models when communicating the need for programs and applying for funding, we have included links to some additional logic model resources at the end of this chapter.

Goals or Aims

Before jumping in to developing a logic model, it is important to clarify our overarching goal or aims as these aims drive the entire model. **Goals or aims** are broad statements that encompass an overall mission or purpose of a program. We write goals in ways that are general and often unifying. For example, a sexual assault center may have a goal to "enhance quality of life for survivors of sexual assault while creating societal change." Similarly, a school-based program may state a goal to "empower youth in social and emotional development." Goals help us understand the broader focus of an intervention or program, but they do not help us understand what that intervention or program will look like.

Inputs, Activities, and Objectives or Process Outcomes

You'll notice the logic model opens with a list of **resources or inputs**. Inputs are human and non-human resources needed to deliver a program. Inputs might include trained

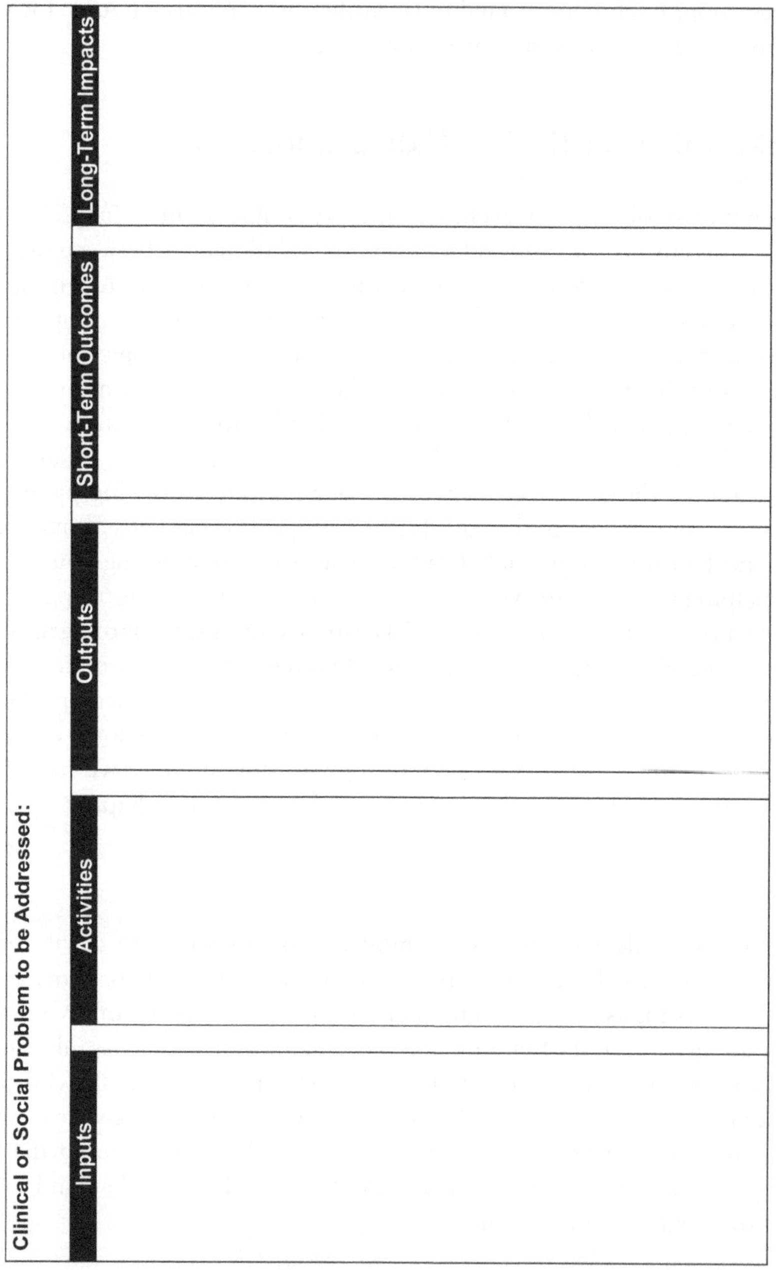

Figure 2.1 Template for a Logic Model

counselors as interventionists, food and copies for information and interest meetings, funding for advertising, funding for outcome measures, and specialized supplies for the counseling process (e.g., play or sandtray kits, manipulatives, workbooks). Next, **activities** include specific actions, services, or tasks we carry out using resources or inputs. Activities might include recruitment, administering pre- and post-tests, community information sessions, fidelity training and supervision for counselors, and number of sessions conducted. Then, **outputs** include the measurable, tangible products of activities.

Objectives are specific statements regarding activities and outputs that provide some level of detail regarding how one will go about realizing the goals or aims. Objectives are often related to intervention or program activities. Sometimes, objectives are known as **process outcomes**. Process outcomes often focus on what we do and who we reach. Taylor-Powell et al. (2003) provided the following examples of targets for process objectives or outcomes:

- Activities/What we do: conduct workshops or meetings; deliver services; develop products, curriculum, resources; training; provide counseling; assess; facilitate; partner; work with media.
- Outputs/Who we reach: participants, clients, agencies, decision-makers, consumers.

Process objectives or outcomes can also focus on quality assurance (Royse et al., 2015). Quality assurance process objectives may include access to services, adherence to intervention or curriculum, procedures, and consumer satisfaction. For example, the sexual assault center noted earlier may write objectives around timely hospital response, increased reporting and prosecution of sexual assault, and provision of trauma services with high evidence of fidelity. In all, they focus on what the counselor or organization will do to help reach the goal.

At the planning stage, outputs are the same as process objectives. These might include number of participants screened and recruited, number of information sessions conducted, number of sessions delivered, and number of participants who completed the program. The evaluation process will equip us with the tools to determine the degree to which we met our process outcomes.

Outcomes and Impacts

The next part of the logic model shifts to focusing on the results of our efforts and investments. **Outcomes** capture how life will be different for the client/student, family/system, organization, or community served as a result of engagement in the intervention or program. Outcomes zero in on what will be happening when the work is successful. Outcomes are our end goal. For example, we do not (or should not!) offer counseling services (a process) for the sheer sake of having a job. We offer counseling services so that people's lives improve in meaningful ways (an outcome). Consider the following potential foci of short, medium, and long-term outcomes (Taylor-Powell et al., 2003):

- Short-term learning: awareness, knowledge, attitudes, skills, opinions, aspirations, motivations.
- Medium-term action: behavior, practice, decision-making, policies, social action.
- Long-term conditions: social, economic, civic environmental.

Counselors often write outcomes as part of treatment planning with an individual, couple or group or broader program planning in schools and agencies. For example, we may focus in on developing self-regulation skills, reducing PTSD symptoms, enhancing social relationships, and increasing specific wellness behaviors. We may also write program-level outcomes. For example, we may note a percentage of participants who will demonstrate a certain level of knowledge, learn a skill, or change a status or diagnosis as a result of the program (short term) or ultimately earn a college degree (long term).

Operationalizing Objectives and Outcomes

There are a number of easily accessible online resources for writing quality objectives and outcomes. Many organizations have adopted the SMART acronym for writing objectives and outcomes. SMART stands for **S** pecific, **M** easurable, **A** chievable, **R** ealistic, and **T** ime-Bound. The Centers for Disease Control (2015) provided the following definitions of SMART:

- **Specific:** Concrete, detailed, and well defined so that you know where you are going and what to expect when you arrive.
- **Measurable:** Numbers and quantities provide a means of measurement and comparison.
- **Achievable:** Feasible and easy to put into action.
- **Realistic:** Considers constraints such as resources, personnel, cost, and time frame.
- **Time-Bound:** A time frame helps to set boundaries around the objective.

We can write SMART objectives for service providers and programs as a whole, and we can write SMART outcomes for individual clients/students, families, organizations, and programs. When writing objectives and outcomes, it is important to be clear, concise, and specific about the nature of the outcome. As much as possible, objectives and outcomes should be stated positively rather than negatively.

The University of Wisconsin-Madison (2025) offers a classic, open-access course and series of resources that is an excellent resource for anyone who is planning on developing and evaluating counseling and human services programs. The program suggests using the following formula to start writing outcome statements: **who/what (the target audience) + change/desired effect (action verb) + in what (expected results) + by when (date)**. Table 2.2 includes several examples of process and outcome objectives for the example in this chapter. See if you can identify which items are focused on the process of the agency and which are focused on outcomes for consumers. See also if you can identify whether these examples are short, medium, or long term in nature.

TABLE 2.2 Sample Outcome Statements

Who/What	Change/Desired effect	In what	By when
survivors of sexual assault	report decreased	trauma symptoms	after 12 sessions of TF-CBT
survivors of sexual assault	increase awareness	of community resources	following initial contact with advocate
agency counselors	increase certifications	trauma-focused cognitive behavioral counseling (TF-CBT)	at end of fiscal year
agency	increase timely	service provision	at end of fiscal year
partnering hospital	increase offer for	advocate accompaniment for Sexual Assault Nurse Examination	at end of fiscal year

Although the formula provided earlier may help you to begin to craft SMART goals, your goals will be incomplete without two additional components: targets and indicators. First, each statement should have a target. In most settings, it is not enough to note that something increased or decreased—we need to indicate the degree to which the knowledge, skill, or behavior is attained. In other words, we need to operationalize the change or desired effect so that it is measurable.

In Table 2.2, we note that agency counselors would increase certifications in TF-CBT by the end of the fiscal year. Perhaps we have a small agency, and we've decided 100% of counselors should hold the certification. We could simply rewrite the process objective to read "100% of agency counselors will be certified in TF-CBT by the end of the fiscal year." Other targets may be a bit more complicated to construct. For example, we note that sexual assault survivors would report decreased symptoms of PTSD. In order to make that outcome measurable, we first need to explore the assumption that clients seeking services at our center are experiencing PTSD symptoms and are experiencing them at such a level where we could anticipate a reduction in symptoms as a result of our program. Next, we must decide (a) what proportion of survivors should meet the target and (b) what constitutes a "decrease" in trauma symptoms. To set a realistic target, we have to consider what we know about the response to our intervention for our population *and* we need to know enough about measurement to understand what constitutes reliable change. In the end, we might decide that it is neither realistic nor achievable for 100% of clients to benefit from the program. However, we might decide that 70% of clients benefiting is a strong target. And we might explore our instrument to determine that a reduction of four points or more is considered clinically significant, reliable change. Thus, our new outcome might be "70% of sexual assault survivors will experience a clinically significant reduction (4 points or more) in trauma symptoms after 12 sessions of TF-CBT."

This last revision brings up the importance of specifying indicators in addition to targets. An indicator simply answers the question "how will we know?" As with the examples earlier, some indicators may be readily apparent and not need further specification. For example, completion of a certification in a specific program includes the indicator. For other outcomes, however, we will need to specify our data source. We can do this by adding "as evidenced by" to the end of our outcome. In the PTSD example, we might simply say "as evidenced by client report on the [instrument name]." Other data sources may include clinical records, school reports (e.g., end-of-year tests, attendance report), client self-report, or follow-up telephone calls or interviews.

BOX 2.2 CHECKLIST FOR QUALITY OBJECTIVES AND OUTCOMES

- Is the item an objective (process-oriented) or outcome (end goal for stakeholder)?
- If process-oriented, is the item focused on what the professional or organization will do to help the consumer reach the end goal?
- If outcome-oriented, is the item focused on what will be different for the consumer as a result of participating in an intervention or program?
- Is the objective/outcome intended to be short, medium, or long term in nature?
- Is the objective/outcome specific?
- Is the objective/outcome measurable?
- Is the objective/outcome achievable?
- Is the objective/outcome realistic?
- Is the objective/outcome time-bound?
- Is the target of the objective/outcome clearly identified?
- Is the indicator of the objective/outcome clearly identified?

BOX 2.3 CASE STUDY

Throughout this chapter, we provided the example of a multidisciplinary sexual assault center. Let's look at goals, objectives, and outcomes for a theoretical intervention program focused on adolescents.

- Goal—enhance quality of life for survivors of sexual assault and create societal change.
- Process objective—100% of agency mental health professionals will be certified in TF-CBT by the end of the fiscal year.
- Process objective—90% of adolescent sexual assault survivors will have the opportunity to be seen by a mental health professional within one week of initial contact with the agency.

- Process objective—partnering hospital will offer opportunity for advocate accompaniment during 90% of Sexual Assault Nurse Examinations as evidenced by record review at the end of the fiscal year.
- Process objective—80% of adolescent sexual assault survivors will report satisfaction with services received as evidenced by an average score of 4.5 or higher on the *Instrument Name*.
- Short-term outcome—70% of adolescent sexual assault survivors will report awareness of at least two community resources following initial contact with an advocate, as evidenced by survivor reports at one-week follow-up call.
- Short-term outcome—70% of adolescent sexual assault survivors will demonstrate at least two skills for identifying and regulating emotions as evidenced by clinician report at the end of four sessions
- Medium-term outcome—70% of adolescent sexual assault survivors will experience a clinically significant reduction (4 points or more) in trauma symptoms after 12 sessions of TF-CBT as evidenced by *Instrument Name*.

CHAPTER SUMMARY

This chapter identified and described fundamental aspects associated with program development, research, and evaluation. Our approach to program development is intended to support you in clarifying the broader problem, identifying the goal of the intervention or program, specifying the objectives, and describing the nature of interventions or activities. To connect the dots among your project features, we provided introductory guidance on using logic models.

In this chapter, we reviewed the importance of using goals, objectives, and outcomes to develop and evaluate interventions and programs. We attended to important distinctions between goals, objectives, and outcomes, and we provided tips for writing strong objectives and outcomes. Finally, we introduced a formula for writing objectives, and we reviewed the importance of ensuring objectives and outcomes were SMART with clear targets and indicators. The chapter concluded with a case study example of objectives and outcomes for an adolescent sexual assault intervention program.

RESOURCES

- Ingoldsby, E., Morrison, C., Ruben, J., Melz, H., & Cairone, K. (2020). Using logic models grounded in theory of change to support trauma-informed initiatives. Trauma-informed approaches: Connecting research, policy, and practice to build resilience in children and families (ASPE Issue Brief). Submitted to the Office of the Assistant Secretary for Planning and Evaluation (ASPE), U.S. Department of Health and Human Services (HHS). https://aspe.hhs.gov/sites/default/files/private/pdf/262051/trauma-informed-logic-models.pdf

- Kansas University Community Toolbox—Developing a Logic Model or Theory of Change, https://ctb.ku.edu/en/table-of-contents/overview/models-for-community-health-and-development/logic-model-development/main
- Designing Programs, University of Wisconsin-Extension. https://fyi.extension.wisc.edu/programdevelopment/designing-programs/

REFERENCES

Beck, J. S. (2020). *Cognitive therapy: Basics and beyond* (3rd ed.). Guilford.

Centers for Disease Control. (2015). CDC– Develop SMART objectives. www.cdc.gov/phcommunities/resourcekit/evaluate/smart_objectives.html

Cohen, J. A., Mannarino, A. P., & Deblinger, E. (2013). *Trauma-focused CBT for children and adolescents: Treatment applications*. Guilford.

Gearing, R. E., El-Bassel, N., Ghesquiere, A., Baldwin, S., Gillies, J., & Ngeow, E. (2011). Major ingredients of fidelity: A review and scientific guide to improving quality of intervention research implementation. *Clinical Psychology Review*, *31*(1), 79–88.

Goodman-Scott, E., Betters-Bubon, J., Olsen, J., & Donohue, P. (2020). Making MTSS work. American School Counselor Association.

Greenberg, L., S., & Goldman, R. N. (2018). *Clinical handbook of emotion-focused therapy*. American Psychological Association.

Linehan, M. M. (2015). *DBT skills training manual* (2nd ed). Guilford.

Power, N., Noble, L. A., Simmonds-Buckley, M., Kellett, S., Stockton, C., Firth, N., & Delgadillo, J. (2022). Associations between treatment adherence–competence–integrity (ACI) and adult psychotherapy outcomes: A systematic review and meta-analysis. *Journal of Consulting and Clinical Psychology*, *90*(5), 427.

Royse, D., Thyer, B. A., & Padgett, D. K. (2015). *Program evaluation: An introduction to an evidence-based approach* (6th ed.). Cengage.

Rubin, A., & Bellamy, J. (2022). *Practitioner's guide to using research for evidence-informed practice* (3rd ed.). Wiley.

STAC Bullying Intervention Program. (2025). www.boisestate.edu/healthsciences-counselored/stac/

Taylor-Powell, E., Jones, L., & Henert, E. (2003). *Enhancing program performance with logic models*. University of Wisconsin-Extension. www.uwex.edu/ces/lmcourse

The University of Wisconsin-Madison. (2025). *Enhancing program performance with logic models*. https://logicmodel.extension.wisc.edu/

White, M. (2007). *Maps of narrative practice*. Norton.

CHAPTER 3

Asking Questions and Informing Design Choices

Approaches to Scientific Inquiry and Program Evaluation

Let's be honest—when most of us were looking forward to starting our counseling programs, we were not *in it* for the research coursework. Assessment may have been less intimidating, but it may have been a hard pass, too. A quick survey of your colleagues will likely confirm that *science* and *systematic inquiry* are not terms most counselors use to characterize their interests. What if we told you that you were not giving yourself enough credit—that your existing skills are already grounded in the foundation for research and evaluation?

In your role as a counselor, you collect, manage, and analyze incredible amounts of data all day long. You challenge your clients and students with questions like "why do I feel this way?" "what can help me?" and "where do I go from here?" In response, you consider their unique context, generate hypotheses, and draw from your training to select and apply interventions. Then, you work alongside clients to collaboratively refine skills as they test them in the laboratories of their lives. You collaboratively assess what worked and didn't and adjust course accordingly. If an approach works, you ask the client to try it again. If it keeps working, you decide it has value for this client and maybe even others. If it does not work, you modify or scrap the first idea and take it from the top all over again.

Congratulations! You're already using the scientific method—gathering and applying data in systematic ways to support meaningful change. These data are incredibly valuable for individual progress. When examined across clients or programs, they offer insight into broader trends, service effectiveness, and community well-being. This chapter provides an overview of systems of inquiry for applied researchers and program evaluators. Together, this information will help you organize more specific approaches to answering the applied research and evaluation questions we present in Part II of this book.

When most people think about research, their mind jumps to the images of white coats, experiments, and maybe even a Pavlovian puppy or two. Surely, experimental designs have great value for advancing knowledge and informing best practices in counseling. However, there are a number of other types of designs that can be helpful additions to your toolkit. All of these designs contribute to the corpus of best available evidence (Lenz, 2018). With so many designs available, how can you determine which ones will meet your needs? The answer lies in the nature of your research question.

DOI: 10.4324/9781003586210-4

This chapter introduces you to the proposition that all methodological design options for applied research and program evaluation have the potential to be useful to counselors. Yet some designs are better suited to answer some questions than others. The value of one paradigm compared to another depends on the degree to which you can use results to support best practices in client care, demonstrate the impact of interventions, secure funding, or engage key stakeholders. We will explore the notion that each research paradigm or method has a specific form best suited to a particular function—a concept we refer to as question–design fit. To support this process, we provide a table linking research paradigms, evaluation questions, and types of information yielded. This chapter also includes a decision tree you can use to match your questions and setting characteristics with an appropriate approach to inquiry. This will prepare you to use Chapters 8 to 14 to develop strategies specific to the types of designs that best fit your questions.

BOX 3.1 CHAPTER LEARNING OUTCOMES

- Distinguish between types of research and program evaluation
- Describe differences and similarities between approaches to research and program evaluation
- Discuss key characteristics of quantitative, qualitative, and mixed-methods approaches to research
- Understand how research and evaluation questions shape the inquiries that advance the counseling profession
- Develop research questions for use with a variety of research and evaluation designs

A TALE OF TWO SCIENCES: RESEARCH AND PROGRAM EVALUATION

Research and program evaluation can serve as frameworks for answering questions about *what works?*, *for whom?*, *how?*, and *under what circumstances?* Although we tend to use similar methods for collecting and analyzing data during these activities, the two paradigms often share as many differences as they do similarities. In this section, we discuss the traditional model of the scientific method and its adaptation for applied research before reviewing some common approaches to program evaluation that can be used across settings.

The Scientific Method as a Fundamental Research Process

Research is the "systematic investigation, including research development, testing, and evaluation, designed to develop or contribute to generalizable knowledge" (U.S. Department of Health & Human Services, 2025, n.p.). In its most fundamental application, research supports efforts to *prove* the presence or influence of a phenomenon by progressing through a prescriptive set of stages referred to as the scientific method (See Figure 3.2). Through the scientific method, you will make observations, ask a question, review the literature, develop a hypothesis, test a hypothesis, analyze data, draw conclusions, and communicate results. Let's take a closer look at each of these activities.

Making Observations

Every research project launches from the nexus of our observations about the phenomena occurring within our unique socio-ecological context. Counselors note gaps in understanding regarding which client issues or characteristics are associated with certain activities, traits, or outcomes. We like to think of these as *curiosity stuck points*. Curiosity stuck points are things we know through personal experiences, work settings, and community spaces that leave us perpetually interested. When we encounter curiosity stuck points, we often sense that there is something that could be helpful to know.

Ask a Question

Once you have identified your curiosity stuck point, you can develop a question that specifies what you find so puzzling. Initially, these questions tend to be reflexive responses to your observations. As your project becomes more refined, your questions will become more specific. As you will learn later in this chapter, certain types of questions can prompt specific approaches to exploring answers.

Review the Literature

If you noticed something curious about a phenomenon, someone else has probably noticed this too. Therefore, it is important to gather relevant information and review literature to determine what is known, emerging, and unknown about your topic. Although subscriber databases are available for students, practicing professional counselors can lean on other sources such as non-academic books, repositories, and government reports. We provide specific strategies for using literature to support practice and inform inquiry in Chapter 7.

Develop a Research Question or Hypothesis

If your literature review has not resolved your curiosity, you will develop an educated guess about the nature of your phenomenon. This supposition should include operational terms that allow for testing of veracity. In research terms, it is known as a research question or hypothesis.

Test a Research Question or Hypothesis

Next, we explore research questions and test hypotheses for their veracity by implementing research designs that illuminate complex phenomena (in qualitative methods) or provide information consistent with or contrary to your supposition (in quantitative methods).

In many cases, researchers will begin under the assumption that their intervention is not effective or that no meaningful relationships exist across phenomena. This is referred to as a null hypothesis, indicated by the symbol $H_{0.}$ By contrast, the alternative hypothesis (H_a or H_1) is one wherein the interventions or relationships appeared meaningful enough to reject the null hypothesis. You will learn more about hypothesis testing in Chapter 5.

Analyze Data and Draw Conclusions

After a research design has been implemented, related data should be analyzed using techniques consistent with the standard for practice. Part II of this book will provide you with support to understand which analyses and interpretations will help you represent data accurately. With project-level data in hand, you can make comparisons to previous findings in the literature and connect these findings back to your local context. In the end, this will allow you to draw conclusions about the nature of outcomes and implications for practice in your setting.

Communicate Results

Although you could file findings away in a drawer somewhere or otherwise keep your wonderful findings all to yourself, we encourage you to share findings with stakeholders and others within our professional communities. After all, science is all about developing knowledge and understanding. It makes sense to share findings in multiple avenues to inform the future work of yourself and others. Chapter 17 is focused on practical strategies for reporting and sharing results with others.

Applied Research: A Practical Application for Counseling Professionals

The scientific method is a helpful strategy for generating knowledge. However, as mental health professionals, we are rarely concerned with knowledge in and of itself. Rather, we use knowledge as a means to support our clients and communities. An applied discipline such as counseling calls for an applied research base to inform practice. That is, we must venture beyond the theoretical, basic principles that define or prove the presence of a phenomenon. Applied research is intended to help us investigate, describe, and generate solutions to everyday issues that influence development and well-being across the lifespan.

We believe applied research is a practical alternative well suited for counselors. Whereas basic research scratches the itch of curiosity, applied research uses the scientific method to find a practical solution to an existing problem. Sometimes, applied research projects result in innovative practices or modification of existing practices. Through applied research, you can answer specific questions related to barriers on the local level where you, your family, friends, and fellow citizens work and live. Importantly, applied research is amenable to identifying outcomes that speak across intersections of culture and diversity, rather than to larger, less defined populations. Through the accumulation of applied research outcomes, it is possible to create changes with the potential to positively affect unique cross-sections of counselors and consumers alike.

Program Evaluation as a Science for Quality Improvement

So far, we have discussed the priorities of basic research for generating knowledge and applied research for addressing real-world problems at local and systemic levels. Both are wonderful, useful tools for any professional counselor's toolkit. However, neither approach is intended to be responsive to proximal needs nor immediate changes in contextual factors. Thus, program evaluation offers a systematic, yet flexible, strategy for monitoring programs and estimating their quality, worth, merit, and impact.

Program evaluation is "a systematic method for collecting, analyzing, and using data to examine the effectiveness and efficiency of programs and, as importantly, to contribute to continuous program improvement" (Centers for Disease Control and Prevention, 2018, n.p.). Like traditional research activities, program evaluation is systematic, grounded in prudent measurement practices, uses a variety of methods for inquiry, and emphasizes objectivity in reporting. Contrary to research, program evaluation is largely concerned with providing feedback about the degree to which program objectives are met, rather than increasing a body of generalizable knowledge. Whereas research relies upon a fixed series of procedures, program evaluations are also intended to be continuous and dynamic in response to ongoing feedback and real-world developments. To this point, program evaluation emphasizes external validity and real-world depictions of impact rather than internal validity and control. In short, whereas research projects are intended to *prove* something, program evaluations are implemented to *improve* something.

There are a number of helpful frameworks counselors can use to monitor, evaluate, and enhance their programs. These frameworks are not intended to be prescriptive. Rather, they are intended to provide a general scope of activities that will help you consider what makes most sense for you, your program, and those you serve. The Centers for Disease Control (Kidder et al., 2024) provided a tried-and-true framework for evaluating programs that is intended to reflect three cross-cutting actions, five evaluation standards, and six steps essential to any project (See Figure 3.1). The CDC's framework is intentionally non-prescriptive about activities in an effort to promote strategies that can be implemented in everyday practices across settings. Although the model depicts a circular process, each step is connected to and informed by all other components. Therefore, it is important to have a working understanding of framework components and their fit with the reason for your evaluation.

Standards across Evaluations

Cross-cutting actions are core principles and practices that should be evident throughout all aspects of a program evaluation. These include engaging interested parties collaboratively to foster shared ownership of the evaluation process and findings. Evaluations should also promote equitable opportunities for input, involvement, and outcomes related to program activities. Finally, rather than completing one-off summaries or reports, evaluators should emphasize continuous learning by using data to inform ongoing program improvement and maximize impact.

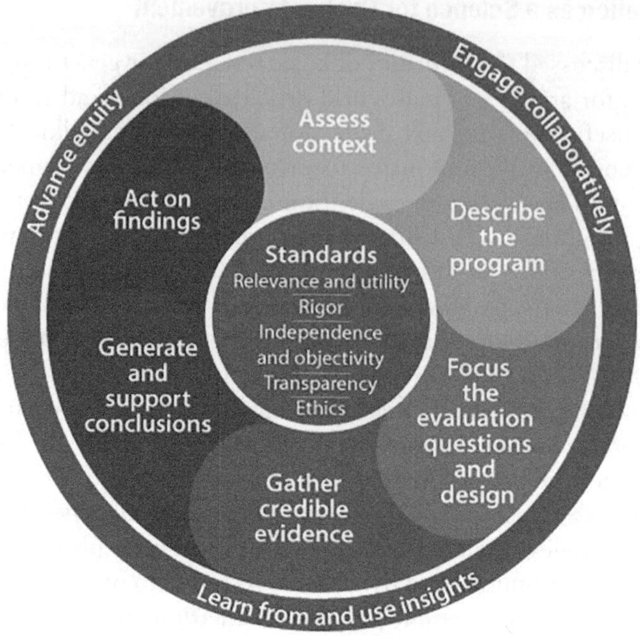

Figure 3.1 CDC Program Evaluation Framework

Source: Centers for Disease Control and Prevention (CDC). *CDC Program Evaluation Framework Action Guide* (2024).
Disclaimer: Use of this material does not imply endorsement by CDC, HHS, or the United States Government.
Note: This content is publicly available at no cost from the CDC website.

We should conduct all evaluation activities in a manner that promotes relevance and utility, rigor, independence and objectivity, transparency, and ethics. Relevance and utility refer to ensuring that the evaluation meets the information needs of partners in a timely and actionable way. This includes identifying key informants, defining a clear scope, selecting meaningful data, and presenting findings in a clear and accessible format. Rigorous approaches to design, planning, implementation, interpretation, and reporting position the findings to be met with confidence by stakeholders. Evaluations should also be completed independently and objectively without the undue influence of factors that affect the acceptability of findings among stakeholders, experts, and the public. Decisions about the evaluation purpose, objectives, design, and results should also be made transparent to stakeholders. Ethics standards promote adherence to conducting evaluations in legal, ethical ways that preserve the well-being of program users (see Chapter 6). Accuracy references efforts to collect, analyze, interpret, report, and represent findings in an even-handed, unbiased manner.

Step 1: Assess the Context

All evaluations should begin with an assessment of key contextual characteristics that promote the likelihood of a meaningful and representative evaluation process and outcome. These characteristics include an evaluability assessment to determine the plausibility and readiness for evaluation given a clearly defined program structure, openness to the process, availability of data, and adequacy of resources. Evaluators also need to consider the person- and organization-level context, such as program participants, employees, local residents who may be interested in or affected by evaluation findings. These individuals can provide valuable insights into acceptance or reticence about program activities. Finally, clearly defining the program's key features and the environment in which services are delivered provides essential context for an evaluation.

Step 2: Describe the Program

A description of your program will provide readers with a reference point that will serve as the foundation of all subsequent activities. Program descriptions should be clear, logical depictions of fundamental components such as need, expected effects, related activities, available resources, stage of program development, and contextual layers surrounding the program. As noted earlier in this chapter, you can depict these program components within a logic model.

Step 3: Focus the Evaluation Questions and Design

Based on engagement with stakeholders and description of the program, you can develop evaluation questions that will help in the development and implementation of an evaluation design that includes target processes, outcomes, and goals of interest. During this step, it can be helpful to consider the purpose for evaluation, how information will be used, which questions you intend to answer, methods that suit your questions, and activities required to promote evaluation fidelity while protecting participants' rights. Some evaluation designs focus on activities early in a program's life cycle to assess feasibility and appropriateness (i.e., formative evaluation) or implementation and efficiency (i.e., process evaluation) whereas others are focused on outcomes, impacts, and economic influences. Part II of this book focuses on several methods that may be helpful for focusing the evaluation design.

Step 4: Gather Credible Evidence

You are surrounded by tons of data every day when evaluating a program. However, you must ensure that the data you are gathering is related to your purpose and questions so that it will have a degree of credibility among your stakeholders. This involves collecting data using multiple sources that are reasonable, reliable, and valid. It also involves collecting data that are readily understood, practical for making statements about usefulness, and lend themselves to being plainly spoken and visually illustrated.

Step 5: Generate and Support Conclusions

The use of evaluation evidence culminates in a set of conclusions that represent links between program activities and indicators of success. These are often noted by comparisons of findings to agreed upon standards that provide a justification for your conclusions related to program merit, worth, and significance.

Step 6. Act on the Findings

Every evaluation should improve a program in some meaningful way and promote culturally-informed use. Therefore, we must gather and disseminate findings in ways that inform decision-making and support action. Because those invested in your services likely range from local to broader levels, it is important to cast a wide net when sharing findings. Common targets for evaluation reports or summaries include program informational pages, advisory boards, local news outlets, professional publications, and policymakers. Chapter 17 focuses on practical strategies for ensuring the use of data and sharing lessons learned.

SOURCING AND DEVELOPING QUALITY RESEARCH AND EVALUATION QUESTIONS

The questions we ask one another tend to be reflexive and general in nature. However, questions that serve as the foundation of scientific inquiries involving trends, phenomena, life events, and relationships warrant greater intention and thoughtful consideration. Research and evaluation questions tend to be sourced from some common venues (Mattick et al., 2018). In some cases, they are provided to you by others, such as community members, funders, or the mission of a research team. Other times, they may be indicated by gaps in the scientific literature, emerging data trends, aspects of a theory, or developments in counseling practice. In any of these scenarios, questions often begin with a smaller, more local scope of interest that magnifies over time to larger, more generalizable populations (Mattick et al., 2018). With these considerations in mind, you can ask yourself which source is calling you to action. It is plausible that the answer may be "many of them" or "I am not sure." That's okay. With investment of time, effort, and acumen, a clearer picture will emerge.

Remember, the first steps of the scientific method (i.e., making an observation) and program evaluation cycles (i.e., assessing the context) are no small feats. Even the best, most well-intentioned professionals can get caught up wondering how to crack the code that unlocks quality research questions. There are some common characteristics of all research questions that range from promising to pitfall. A research question can be a valuable guide or an unintentional departure, so getting a good start to your project is imperative. With a solid question in place, your project is more likely to stay on track and yield relevant information.

Generally speaking, promising characteristics of research and evaluation questions include being relevant to your target audience, original in contribution to an applied knowledge base, and ethical in intention. Strong research questions are clear and concise, yet inclusive of information pertinent to your project. By contrast, questions that lend themselves to nonspecific, categorical responses (yes or no) or do not include vital details can be troublesome. In any case, taking the time to develop a well-articulated research or evaluation question is recommended over not asking a question at all or developing questions at the end of the research or evaluation process. Doing so will assure that the purpose of your inquiry is clear. Fortunately, most general research and evaluation questions share some essential ingredients and there are a number of frameworks available to support your success.

FRAMEWORKS FOR DEVELOPING RESEARCH AND EVALUATION QUESTIONS

Once you have a general depiction of your applied research or evaluation question, it is time to make sure it contains the functional features that will guide your project. Three strategies for shaping research and evaluation questions include the PICO, SPIDER, and VISTA frameworks. Each of these is a simple acronym to reference the chief elements that will support your inquiries.

PICO Framework

The PICO framework (Schardt et al., 2007) is helpful for questions associated with evaluating clinical and educational interventions. PICO questions include information about **P** articipants/ Patient problems, **I** ntervention, **C** omparison, and **O** utcome. For example, someone may ask the question: "Is there a statistically significant difference in relationship satisfaction (**O** utcome) among partners experiencing distress following separation due to military deployment (**P** articipants/ Patient problems) who complete a 12-week integrative couples therapy intervention (**I** ntervention) when compared to psychoeducation (**C** omparison)?"

SPIDER Framework

The SPIDER framework (Cooke et al., 2012) accommodates questions that tend to be more qualitative in nature, rather than focused on quantitative estimation of improvement and estimation. SPIDER questions contain details about the **S** ample, **P** henomenon of **I** nterest, **D** esign, **E** valuation, and **R** esearch type. For example, someone may ask the question: "What experiences (**E** valuation) do couples (**S** ample) describe (**D** esign) as being salient when completing a 12-week integrative couples therapy intervention (**P** henomenon of **I** nterest) following distress associated with military deployment?" In this example, the qualitative nature of the research type (**R**) is inferred by the other content.

VISTA Framework

We developed the VISTA framework to support questions associated with relationships between variables and events, rather than interventions or qualitative phenomena. VISTA questions feature information about **V** ariables of **I** nterest, **S** ample, **T** ime, and **A** im. For example, someone may ask: "To what degree do attachment styles (**V** ariable of **I** nterest) predict (**A** im) treatment progress (**V** ariables of **I** nterest) among couples (**S** ample) completing a 12-week integrative couples therapy intervention following military deployment (**T** ime)?"

These frameworks can provide a useful guide for conceptualizing functional components needed to address your larger problem under investigation. Deciding upon which framework suits your project will require some critical thinking about the nature of your inquiry. With this information in hand, you will be ready to pair your research or evaluation question to a methodological paradigm that facilitates your inquiry.

BOX 3.2 CHECKLIST FOR QUALITY RESEARCH AND EVALUATION QUESTIONS

- Questions are derived from sources such as stakeholders, funders, journal publication priorities, or the mission of a research team
- Questions are relevant to the problem at hand
- Questions are original
- Questions are ethical in intent
- Questions are inclusive of relevant content as reflected in the PICO, SPIDER, or VISTA frameworks

A CADRE OF METHODOLOGICAL APPROACHES

Tools: Quantitative, Qualitative, and Mixed Methods

Certain types of questions can only be answered with certain types of data. Therefore, you will need to identify and leverage the applied research or evaluation approach best suited to yield the type of information you require (see Figure 3.2). Methodolog-

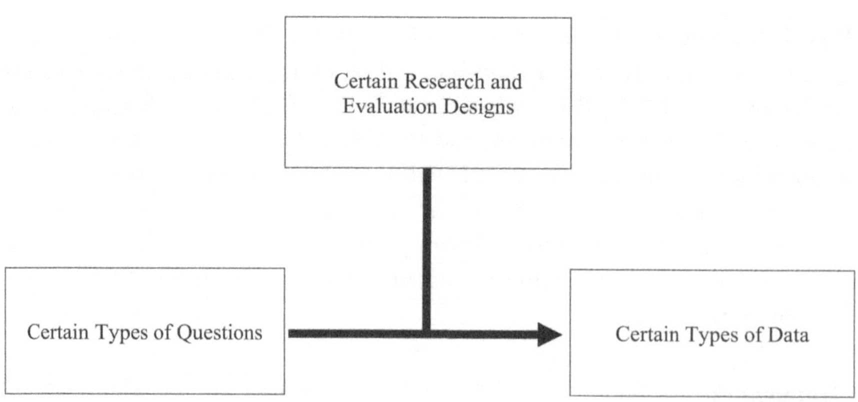

Figure 3.2 Relationships between Research Questions, Designs, and Type of Data Yielded

ical approaches can be broadly divided into two primary categories: quantitative and qualitative. Each approach is informed by different epistemological assumptions and uses distinct tools and designs. Quantitative approaches focus on numerical data, statistical analysis, and testing hypotheses to explain and predict phenomena. By contrast, qualitative approaches emphasize language, context, and meaning-making, aiming to understand how individuals experience and construct reality. Selecting the appropriate approach depends on your research goals, the nature of the question, and the type of insight you hope to achieve. Table 3.1 includes an overview of the characteristics of quantitative and qualitative research.

Mixed methods research and evaluation designs offers a third major approach to research. Mixed methods combine quantitative and qualitative approaches to take advantage of the strengths of each that is greater than the whole of its parts. By using quantitative data and qualitative insights together, researchers can better understand complex questions than they could with just one type of data. This

TABLE 3.1 Characteristics of Quantitative and Qualitative Approaches to Research

Characteristic	Quantitative	Qualitative
Purpose	Explains phenomena using numerical data	Explains phenomena in the form of natural language and expression
Data approach	Relies on mathematical and statistical methods	Relies on representation of patterns, themes, meanings, and insights
Theoretical focus	Tests theories and related hypotheses	Builds, explores, and refines theories rather than tests them
Data collection methods	Observations, surveys, instrumentation, and other quantifiable methods	Observations, interviews, focus groups, document analysis, and audio-visual materials
Epistemological orientation	Objectivist epistemology	Constructivist epistemology
Aim	To develop universally representative explanations for social behavior	To understand how social and psychological experiences are created and assigned meaning
Representation of reality	Articulation of causal and predictive relationships among isolated variables	Socially constructed and dynamic representation of reality
Common terms	Value-free, logical, reductionistic, deterministic	Value-laden, flexible, holistic, context sensitive
Examples	Experiments, surveys, correlational studies	Phenomenology, grounded theory, narrative analyses

approach supports triangulation, where different types of data are used to confirm and enrich findings. Mixed methods also reflect the idea of dialectical pluralism—that no single way of knowing is best, and that different perspectives can contribute valuable insights. Timing and structure are important in mixed methods designs. In sequential explanatory designs, researchers begin with quantitative data and follow up with qualitative data to help explain the results. In sequential exploratory designs, the process is reversed: qualitative data informs the design of the quantitative phase. In convergent designs, both types of data are collected and analyzed at the same time to create a fuller picture of the question. See Wester and McKibben (2019) for a fuller exploration of mixed methods approaches to counseling research.

Frameworks: Community-Based Participatory Research and Action Research

Whereas quantitative, qualitative, and mixed methods describe tools researchers and evaluators use to collect and analyze data, it is also important to consider the frameworks that guide how and why research is conducted in counseling settings. These frameworks influence the counselor's role in the research process, the degree of collaboration with clients or communities, and the intended use of findings. For example, action research and community-based participatory research (CBPR) are especially relevant because they align with our core professional values such as empowerment, advocacy, and social justice. These approaches emphasize working alongside clients, schools, or communities to identify concerns, co-create solutions, and apply findings in practical ways that improve services. Bringing together these research tools and guiding frameworks allows professional counselors to initiate inquiries in ways that advance practice and live out philosophical commitments.

PAIRING RESEARCH AND EVALUATION QUESTIONS TO METHODOLOGICAL APPROACHES

The onus of pairing questions to the most appropriate methodological approach for inquiry is yours. It can be tempting to start a project with the design in mind and attempt to reverse-engineer the questions from there. Who doesn't want to check meta-analysis off their bucket list, right? Instead, it is imperative to begin with a well-developed question. With a strong question established, you will be able to launch into your project with a strong foundation.

Table 3.2 includes a summary of the types of research designs you will learn about in Part II. For each design, we provide a brief overview of the types of questions the design can help answer, and we illustrate this connection with sample applied research and program evaluation questions. Because the matter of question–design fit is so important, we begin each chapter in Part II of this text with a more detailed overview of situations in which the design is most appropriate.

TABLE 3.2 Examples of Question–Design Fit

Type of design	Purposes	Example questions
Descriptive survey	Understanding and meeting program and policy needs (e.g., needs assessment), evaluating programs throughout outcome and satisfaction surveys, or understanding characteristics of a group of interest	What is the level of relationship satisfaction among partners following military deployment? To what degree do couples experiencing distress associated with military deployment report satisfaction with a 12-week integrative couples therapy intervention?
Predictive	Demonstrating simple links between two variables, testing hypotheses about clusters of variables that predict a phenomenon, or predicting the likelihood of an event happening	To what degree do attachment styles predict treatment progress among couples completing a 12-week integrative couples therapy intervention following military deployment?
Single case	Evaluating change within an individual; understanding the efficacy of an individual, establishing preliminary support for novel practices, or assessing applications of treatments with low incidence or understudied groups	What is the course of treatment response for a 12-week integrative couples therapy intervention for increasing relationship satisfaction following military deployment?
Single groups	Demonstrating the course or magnitude of treatment effect over time for a single group of individuals; measuring improvement in association with an intervention/ program, relating improvement to participant with intervention/ program characteristics, or understanding readiness for more complex evaluations	Do participants report statistically significant increases in relationship satisfaction following a 12-week integrative couples therapy intervention delivered in a family services setting?
Between-groups methods	Estimating performance of an intervention compared to nothing; understanding performance of an intervention compared to one or more existing standards or interventions; or understanding interactions between interventions, outcomes, and other important variables	Is there a statistically significant difference in relationship satisfaction among partners experiencing distress following separation due to military deployment who complete a 12-week integrative couples therapy intervention when compared to couples who receive the existing psychoeducation packet?

(*Continued*)

TABLE 3.2 (Continued)

Type of design	Purposes	Example questions
Qualitative	Answering "how" and "why" questions related to lived experiences; providing a starting point for needs assessment, understanding common experiences, or giving context of quantitative findings	What experiences do couples describe as being salient when completing a 12-week integrative couples therapy intervention following distress associated with military deployment?
Meta-analysis	Combining findings across studies or sites into a single estimate of effectiveness; understanding mean effect associated with an intervention/program, relationships of participant and study characteristics associated with mean effect, or predicting future effects for similar studies	What is the mean treatment effect of a 12-week integrative couples therapy intervention when compared to alternative psychoeducational approaches?

CHAPTER SUMMARY

This chapter opened with an exploration of the scientific method and its implementation in applied research paradigms, a practical alternative for counselors and other helping professionals. After introducing program evaluation as a strategy for counselors interested in improving programming, we provided a framework you may find helpful for situating these activities. Next, we introduced basic tools and frameworks for carrying out applied research and program evaluation designs. This chapter concluded with an exploration of the art and science of developing research and evaluation questions aligned to the nature of your question.

RESOURCES

- Agee, J. (2009). Developing qualitative research questions: A reflective process. *International Journal of Qualitative Studies in Education*, 22, 431–447. https://doi.org/10.1080/09518390902736512
- Alkin, M. C., Vo, A. T., & Christie, C. A. (2024). *Evaluation essentials from A to Z* (3rd ed.). Guilford.
- Centers for Disease Control. (2024). *CDC program evaluation framework action guide*. www.cdc.gov/evaluation/php/evaluation-framework-action-guide/index.html
- Centers for Disease Control. *Developing Evaluation Questions*. www.cdc.gov/evaluation/php/evaluation-framework-action-guide/step-3-focus-the-evaluation-questions-and-design.html
- Flamez, B. N., Lenz, A. S., Balkin, R. S., & Smith, R. L. (2017). Creating the problem statement, purpose statement, and research questions. In B. N. Flamez, A. S. Lenz, R. S.

Balkin, & R. L. Smith (Eds.), *A counselor's guide to the dissertation process: Where to start and how to finish* (pp. 111–122). American Counseling Association.

- Spikard, J. (2017). *Research basics: Design to data analysis in six steps*. Sage.
- Tully, M. P. (2014). Research: Articulating questions, generating hypotheses, and choosing study designs. *The Canadian Journal of Hospital Pharmacy*, *67*, 31–34.

REFERENCES

Centers for Disease Control and Prevention. (2018). www.cdc.gov

Cooke, A., Smith, D., & Booth, A. (2012). Beyond PICO: The SPIDER tool for qualitative evidence synthesis. *Qualitative Health Research*, *22*(10), 1435–1443. https://doi.org/10.1177/1049732312452938

Kidder D. P., Fierro, L. A., Luna, E., et al. (2024), CDC program evaluation framework. *Morbidity and Mortality Weekly Report*, *73*(No. RR-6), 1–37. http://dx.doi.org/10.15585/mmwr.rr7306a1

Lenz, A. S. (2018). Reconsidering the value assigned to counseling research paradigms and outcomes. *Counseling Outcome Research and Evaluation*, *9*(1), 1–4. https://doi.org/10.1080/21501378.2017.1423202

Mattick, K., Johnston, J., & de la Croix, A. (2018). How to . . . write a good research question. *The Clinical Teacher*, *15*, 104–108.

Office for Human Research Protections. (2024). 45 C.F.R. § 46.102: Definitions. Electronic Code of Federal Regulations. www.ecfr.gov/current/title-45/subtitle-A/subchapter-A/part-46/subpart-A/section-46.102

Schardt, C., Adams, M. B., Owens, T., Keitz, S., & Fontelo, P. (2007). Utilization of the PICO framework to improve searching PubMed for clinical questions. *BMC Medical Informatics & Decision Making*, *7*(16). https://doi.org/10.1186/1472-6947-7-16

Wester, K., & McKibben, B. (2019). Integrating mixed methods approaches in counseling research. *Counseling Outcome Research and Evaluation*, *10*(1). https://doi-org/10.1080/21501378.2018.1531239

CHAPTER 4

Navigating Methodological Concepts

This chapter includes an overview of concepts and terms most often used across different types of research and program evaluation methodologies. By understanding these concepts, you will be better able to make sense of the research you read, and you'll have a foundation on which to design evaluations of counseling practices and programs as discussed in Part II of this book. In particular, we attend to theory, concepts, constructs, and variables; populations and samples; instruments; interventions; and types of validity and trustworthiness in research and program evaluation design. Each concept will include definitions, illustrations, and examples to support application to your interests. We also include brief discussion regarding why these nuts-and-bolts elements matter when designing evaluations or reviewing the research literature. We include a checklist to help you understand and critique a methods section of an article.

BOX 4.1 CHAPTER LEARNING OUTCOMES

- Understand definitions of common methodological concepts such as theory, constructs, variables, population, samples, instruments, interventions, validity, and trustworthiness
- Identify methodological concepts when reviewing research
- Apply methodological concepts to program evaluation design

THEORY, CONCEPTS, CONSTRUCTS, AND VARIABLES

Theory

All research and program evaluation should begin with **theory** in mind. Merriam-Webster (2025) offers six definitions of theory. Broadly speaking, *theory* refers to a structured set of ideas that explains or organizes phenomena. It can describe a guiding framework for action or policy, a set of assumptions proposed for study or argument, or a collection of principles that offer a coherent view of a field. In some contexts,

DOI: 10.4324/9781003586210-5

theory also denotes abstract or conceptual thinking about the relationships among facts, concepts, or practices within a discipline.

Within the social and behavioral sciences, a theory is "a set of interrelated concepts, definitions, and propositions that explains or predicts events or situations by specifying relations among variables" (Office of Behavioral & Social Sciences Research, n.d., p. 4). In other words, a theory helps us understand why something happens or how something works. In the world of counselors, this often equates to illustrating the pathways toward and away from optimal development and well-being.

Counseling and psychology scholars often combine philosophy, observation, and research to create theories to explain experiences. For example, Joiner (2009) developed the Interpersonal Theory of Suicide to explain how individuals come to be at risk for suicide and engage in suicidal behavior. Joiner proposed that thwarted belongingness and perceived burdensomeness combine to create suicide ideation; further, acquired capability moves people to overcome the fear of death and act on thoughts of suicide. In addition to explaining experiences, some theories explain and guide the counseling process. For example, Rogers (1961) based his Person-Centered Theory on a proposition that humans possess a self-actualizing tendency that is activated within relationships in which six necessary and sufficient conditions exist: therapist–client psychological contact, client incongruence, therapist congruence or genuineness, unconditional positive regard, empathic understanding, and client perception of the conditions. Lent et al. (1994) drew from research and previous theoretical work to propose a Social Cognitive Career Theory (SCCT) in which learning experiences inform self-efficacy and outcome expectations, which inform interests, goals, and actions; the theory includes a number of complex relationships between each of these ideas. Although these examples of theories in mental health professions are overly simplified, they highlight the presence of theory in guiding the way we think about human experience and the counseling process.

Theories play a number of roles within research and program evaluation. First, some researchers develop studies to test or evaluate components of a theory, assertions within a theory, or the nature of relationships proposed within a theory. A systematic review of 66 studies focused on Joiner's theory showed that there is the strongest support for the influence of perceived burdensomeness on suicide ideation (Ma et al., 2016). Other researchers may conduct studies to refine an existing theory or develop a new theory. For example, in an investigation using SCCT as a framework, researchers found several new types of outcome expectations they believed helped explain the underrepresentation of women and people of color in science, technology, engineering, and math (STEM) occupations (Shoffner et al., 2015). Still other researchers may use theory to justify a specific research project. For example, researchers may use Rogers' (1961) work to justify exploration regarding factors that influence perceptions of unconditional positive regard in counseling relationships. Finally, professional counselors may use theory to inform the design of interventions or programs using the strategies discussed in Chapter 2. For example, counselors who work with individuals at risk of suicide may develop an intervention aimed at reducing perceived burdensomeness and, theoretically, the risk of suicide. Regardless of whether one is working to build a theory, evaluate a theory, or use theory to inform practice, theories are often explained in terms of concepts, constructs, and variables.

Concepts and Constructs

There are subtle but important distinctions between concepts and constructs. "A **concept** is an expression of an abstraction formed from the generalization of particulars" (Kerlinger & Lee, 2000, p. 59). By definition, concepts are abstract and cannot be observed. For example, Rogers' (1961) self-actualizing tendency is an abstract concept embedded within a theory.

"A **construct** is a concept that has been formulated so that it can be used in science. It is used in theoretical schemes. It is defined so it can be observed and measured" (Kerlinger & Lee, 2000, p. 59). Constructs are abstract and often subjective in nature. Researchers develop constructs as representations within theories to allow them to move toward measuring that which cannot be seen. For example, Joiner (2009) proposed clear definitions of the three main constructs he believed lead to suicidal behavior: thwarted belongingness, perceived burdensomeness, and acquired capability. Each construct has an **operational definition** that describes the component parts to guide researchers toward developing ways of measuring constructs as variables. Such *operationalization* is imperative to help researchers and practitioners have a common understanding of constructs within the broader context of leveraging our understanding of human development to support helpful counseling practice.

Variables

A **variable** "is a property that can take on different values. It is a symbol to which values are assigned" (Kerlinger & Lee, 2000, p. 59). Variables can be simple or complex, and there are often many ways of assigning values to variables. For example, one way to assign value to the construct of gender identity is to ask participants to self-identify as man, woman, or non-binary/non-confirming. This may result in three different values assigned to the variable. Another way to assign value to the construct of gender would be to administer a survey instrument designed to assess identification with traits associated with gender identity. This may result in hundreds of different values assigned to the variable. Similarly, researchers interested in Joiner's (2009) theory may develop or locate instruments aligned with constructs of thwarted belongingness, perceived burdensomeness, and acquired capability. In essence, when constructs are measured in a way that allows a value to be assigned to them, they become variables. In Chapter 5, we further explore the process of assigning value to variables, including different types and levels of data that may serve as variables and considerations related to the validity and reliability of test scores.

Dozens of different types of variables are included in research and program evaluation designs. At the most basic level, the two most important types are **independent variables (IVs)** and **dependent variables (DVs)**. IVs are determined by nature or manipulated by researchers. You may wish to think of IVs coming first in a research equation. For example, demographic variables such as gender identity, race, ethnicity, or age are givens in that they are not manipulated by researchers; researchers often investigate the degree to which these independent variables **predict** or influence other variables. IVs can also be constructs believed to come first within a theory. For example, researchers interested in Rogers' theory may measure therapeutic relationship as an IV because the relationship is believed to occur first and result in change. Finally, IVs can be **manipulated** by researchers as part of **treatment** groups. For example, someone may wish to know whether group counseling intervention is as effective as individual intervention. In this case, the type of treatment is the IV and should be clearly operationalized so that the reader understands just what was included in the treatment.

Dependent variables (DVs) are believed to result from or depend upon the IVs. They come second in the research equation. In other words, IVs cause, influence, or predict DVs. Using the examples stated earlier, researchers may examine how gender, race/ethnicity, and age (IVs) predict perceived burdensomeness (DV). Those interested in Rogers' (1961) theory may investigate the degree to which client perception of high versus low ratings of the therapeutic relationship (IV) influences reduction in symptoms of depression (DV). Finally, the evaluators who wished to compare the effectiveness of group compared to individual counseling (IV) may assess the impact on overall functioning (DV). In program evaluations or nonexperimental designs, DVs may also be referred to as **outcome variables**.

Although you can always expect to see IVs and DVs in quantitative designs, you will also encounter a number of other types of variables. **Control variables** are things held constant within a research study so they do not influence relationships between other variables. For example, school counselors who are conducting a school-based intervention focused on anxiety may control for the impact of standardized testing by making sure all interventions and assessments are completed at the same time of year and well in advance of testing season. **Confounding variables** sometimes referred to as ***extraneous variables*** are unexpected influences that unintentionally change or obscure relationships between variables. For example, school counselors who did not anticipate a spike in anxiety related to testing and conducted post-testing the day before standardized tests began may erroneously conclude that their intervention was not effective because of this confounding variable. **Intervening** or **mediating variables** explain relationships or connections between other variables. For example, attachment style (IV) influences argument beliefs (mediating variable), which influence conflict tactics used in romantic relationships (DV) (Ricco & Sierra, 2017). Finally, **moderating variables** affect the strength of relationships between other variables by increasing, decreasing, or reversing relationships. For example, loneliness (IV) and trauma symptoms (IV) predicted post-traumatic growth (DV) (Zeligman et al., 2017). Closer investigation illustrated that loneliness moderated these relationships. The researchers concluded that "feelings of loneliness may exacerbate trauma symptoms or likewise hinder individuals from being able to grow following their trauma" (p. 440).

Applications to Research and Program Evaluation

When reviewing research, pay careful attention to how authors utilize theory in their work. They should present constructs in a way that allows you to understand *what* was studied and *how* it was operationalized into variables. Finally, you should be able to determine why specific variables were included, how those variables link to the theoretical framework of the study, and how they were measured. The checklist near the end of this chapter will provide you with some questions helpful for considering how researchers integrate theory, define constructs, and utilize variables within their studies. The material in Chapter 5 will help you understand more nuances in the process of measuring variables.

When designing applied research and program evaluations, these concepts remind us of the importance of having a clear theoretical rationale or foundation for the programs we develop and the constructs we intend to influence. They also remind us of the importance of being thoughtful about how we operationalize constructs (abstract ideas) into variables (things that can be measured). At the most fundamental level, these elements influence what we are able to learn from our efforts.

POPULATION AND SAMPLES

A **population** is the universe or entire group of people one is interested in studying or understanding. A **sample** is the subset of individuals one selects to participate in a specific study. Because it is rarely feasible to access an entire population, researchers must make important decisions about how they will identify and select a smaller but representative sample of individuals to participate in a study. These decisions influence the degree to which one can trust that results **generalize** to the population as a whole (in quantitative research) or are **transferable** to similar contexts (in qualitative research).

For example, a professional counselor may be interested in promoting posttraumatic growth among adults who have experienced interpersonal violence in the last year. In this case, the population of interest is adults who have experienced interpersonal violence in the past year. Clearly, it is not feasible to access everyone in the world who had that experience. However, researchers may be able to focus on those who presented to emergency rooms, police departments, or family violence centers in the county in which they work. Similarly, an evaluator at a large agency may not be able to have in-depth interviews with every person who participated in services at the agency (population); however, they could interview a subset of people who engaged at the agency (sample).

A **sampling plan** is the process a researcher or evaluator uses to narrow from population to sample. Sampling methods are divided into **probability** and **nonprobability** methods. Probability sampling involves using some type of **random sampling** so that, statistically speaking, everyone in the population has an equal opportunity of being in the sample. In quantitative research, random sampling helps ensure that study results can be generalized to the population as a whole. Nonprobability sampling does not rely on random sampling, so not everyone in the population has an equal chance of being represented in the sample. In nonprobability sampling, researchers can describe the sample to help readers assess whether results may transfer to their settings.

Probability Sampling

There are several approaches to probability or random sampling. In **simple random sampling**, one generates a list of all those in the population and then uses a random number generator or similar device to select individuals to be included in the sample. **Stratified random sampling** allows one to conduct a random sampling approach while also ensuring adequate representation within subgroups, perhaps to allow comparison across groups. For example, a multisite agency with one central hub serving 70% of clients and several smaller satellite offices dividing the remaining 30% of clients would expect simple random sampling to yield 70% of clients at the central hub and 30% of clients at the other locations combined. That may not allow enough statistical power (see Chapter 5) to understand differences in client experience across locations and would requires some careful consideration about the purpose and uses of the data. Stratified random sampling procedures allow one to specify that the sample yields 50 clients from each site, thus facilitating comparisons between groups. **Systematic random sampling** involves selecting participants in a specific, fixed interval (e.g., surveying every tenth client who presents for services at agency sites).

Cluster random sampling involves dividing the population into known groups and then sampling individuals within a random selection of clusters. Researchers may use this option if the population is divided geographically or into easily accessible groups, such as classrooms. For example, school personnel may be reluctant to allow simple random sampling of students because it would be disruptive; however, the administration may allow researchers to sample all students within several classrooms. This would only be true probability sampling if the classrooms were selected randomly *and* students were assigned to classrooms randomly. If students were assigned to classrooms based on academic achievement or behavior, a researcher may inadvertently introduce a problematic confounding variable.

Nonprobability Sampling

Feasibility, access, and philosophy of research design all influence researchers' decisions to use nonprobability sampling. In most qualitative research designs, for example, there are very strong reasons to select individuals who can best give voice to an experience. The main types of nonprobability sampling include convenience, snowball, and purposive sampling.

Convenience sampling is just as it sounds: selection of participants based on convenience and access. For example, an evaluator may collect data from individuals who attend counseling on Monday and Wednesday mornings when they are already on site or from students in a classroom for which they already have access. It is quite likely that those who attend services on weekday mornings are somehow different from those who attend services on evenings or weekends; this may be further confounded if a certain specialist is present or groups operate only on certain days. Alternatively, researchers may distribute a call for participants and include all those who initiate a response to the call, perhaps missing the voices of those not likely to initiate contact. **Snowball sampling** is often used when a population is difficult to define or to access. In this instance, participants nominate others they believe to meet the participation criteria, thus generating a "snowball" of potential participants for the study.

Purposive sampling is also just as it sounds: selection of participants based on a very clear, predefined purpose. This may include identification or nomination of experts and intentional work to ensure the sample is as homogeneous (**typical case sampling**) or diverse (**maximum variation sampling**) as possible. For example, an evaluator might ask staff members to identify clients who are best able to speak to the impact of a specific service or decide to sample a site that is performing quite well to better understand factors contributing to its success. Researchers looking to develop competencies to provide trauma counseling may use purposive sampling to identify experts who have published on trauma services and practitioners who have been specializing in trauma work for ten years or more. Certainly, those sampled for these studies are not generalizable to the whole; however, they may yield information that advances knowledge and understanding.

Applications to Research and Program Evaluation

When reviewing research, look for details regarding the population of interest and the sampling methods utilized. This should include clear attention to criteria for inclusion in the study, criteria for exclusion in the study, description of sampling methods, and rationale for both sampling method and numbers of participants. As will be discussed in Chapter 5, the number of participants needed for research or program evaluation varies greatly depending on methodology and data analysis methods utilized. Writers should describe the sample obtained in a clear and comprehensive manner. At a minimum, this should include attention to gender, race, ethnicity, and age; writers should include additional demographic and contextual information relevant to the study. By attending to these elements, you will be better able to determine whether the sample is intended to be generalizable or whether the sample is transferable to practice in your counseling setting.

When designing program evaluations, counselors can keep concepts of population and sampling in mind. By being explicit about the population of focus and the methods of accessing the population, we can ensure that we design methods that help us understand what we need to know about our counseling interventions and programs. As with strong written research, it is important to be intentional about sampling methods used and characteristics of the resulting sample. Box 4.2 includes a checklist for creating a sampling procedure.

BOX 4.2 CHECKLIST FOR CREATING A SAMPLING PROCEDURE (FITZPATRICK ET AL., 2023)

1. Is the design a case study? (If not, proceed to step 2.)
   a. What unit is of interest (e.g., individuals, classrooms, school, district, agency)?
   b. How many units are necessary to achieve the desired depth and understanding?
   c. Should the units represent a range of characteristics, a typical unit, or unusual units on one or more dimensions?
   d. What characteristics are of interest in selection?
   e. By what means will the cases be identified?
2. Is generalizing the results beyond the sample a priority?
   a. How would you define the sampling unit (type of unit, critical characteristics)?
   b. Is there a sampling frame that might contain most, if not all, of the sampling units? How can units in the sampling frame that do not represent the sample be eliminated? How can you identify units that may have been omitted from the sampling frame?

c Are you interested in examining the responses of small subgroups? If so, consider stratifying to ensure obtaining a sufficient number of the subgroup.

DATA COLLECTION PROTOCOLS

All research and program evaluation designs require some sort of data collection tools and protocols. Researchers study a wide variety of constructs to answer a wide variety of research questions; these questions may or may not be directly focused on counseling practice. There is certainly value in understanding how constructs relate to each other or the essence of an experience for which we will design a responsive counseling intervention or program.

The measures we select must align with the purpose of the applied research or program evaluation question. For counselors, this often means not only whether our interventions work, but also how they are delivered and experienced. In Chapter 2, you learned about two primary types of objectives relevant to counseling interventions and programs: process and outcome. When it comes to striving toward our ethical imperative to offer counseling services with a reasonable probability of success and evaluating our effectiveness on an ongoing basis, two specific types of data collection measures become particularly important: process and outcome.

Process measures help us understand how or how well a program or intervention is delivered. We often use satisfaction indices as a process indicator. Although satisfaction does not tell us if a program worked, satisfaction is an important quality measure that affects overall success. Another important process measure involves fidelity. Fidelity refers to the degree to which one adheres to standardized curricula or procedures and must be assessed by those who are deeply familiar with the program. After all, it is hard to conclude whether an intervention works if service providers didn't implement the intervention with a reasonable degree of fidelity.

Outcome measures help us understand the degree to which an intervention or program reaches the intended goal. Strong outcome measures can help us understand the knowledge, behaviors, or skills with which one starts and ends a program. Not all outcome measures require formal assessment tools. When we use formal assessment measures, we may select from a wide variety of options, including self-report measures, other-report measures (e.g., an instrument completed by a caregiver on behalf of a child), or behavior observation protocols.

Program evaluators often consider the following priorities for selecting outcome measures: relevant and appropriate to the client group, easy to administer, useful and easy to interpret, appropriate evidence of reliability and validity for context, sensitive to change, and relatively inexpensive (Royse et al., 2015). See Table 4.1 for an overview of process and outcome measures related to program evaluation and intervention research.

Regardless of whether we are studying counseling process and outcomes, we most often collect data through surveys and instruments, archival records, and interviews.

TABLE 4.1 Process and Outcome Measures (Jazieh, 2020; Kilbourne et al., 2018)

	Process Measures	Outcome Measures
Definition	Metrics based on the activities, steps, or procedures taken to achieve goals	Metrics representing the effects or results of an intervention or program
Purpose	Understanding how or how well an intervention or program is delivered	Understanding the relationships between an intervention or program and an associated outcome
Examples	Satisfaction surveys, waitlist times, number of sessions, types of services received, fidelity measures	Grades, standardized test scores, retention rates, symptom reduction, diagnostic remission, sustained employment
Uses	Identifying areas for improvement or predicting the success of interventions and programs	Identifying the overall success and effectiveness of interventions and programs

The sections below provide a brief overview of these three types of measures with a special emphasis on measuring counseling processes and outcomes.

Surveys and Instruments

Researchers and program evaluators often rely on instruments for data collection. We may use instruments to directly observe participants or have participants or individuals familiar with participants (e.g., teachers, parents, partners) complete a variety of types of instruments (Sheperis et al., 2017). "Surveys are information collection methods used to describe, compare, or explain individual and societal knowledge, feelings, values, preferences, and behavior" (Fink, 2025, p. 1). Surveys can utilize a wide variety of response methods, including yes/no questions, multiple-choice questions, rating or ranking scales, or open-ended questions. Surveys have the benefit of often being quick and easy to administer, score, and analyze.

More specifically, we may directly observe using rating scales, observation forms, flowcharts, and performance checklists. Instruments completed by participants may include questionnaires, self-checklists, attitude scales, personality inventories, achievement and aptitude tests, and performance tests.

Of key concern in reviewing research and developing projects is whether surveys measure what they are believed to measure in that specific context, a concept known as **test score validity** (discussed in depth in Chapter 5). When at all possible, researchers and evaluators should use instruments that have been formally developed and assessed for the specific use. If you *needed* to know if you had a fever, you would probably prefer to take your temperature using a thermometer that had been tested over time rather than using the back of your hand to guesstimate a temperature. Similarly, if assessing the impact of an intervention on symptoms of depression, it would be far better to utilize one of the widely available, well-established instruments available than to create a single-item rating of depression or develop several homemade questions aimed at assessing that construct.

Although discussion regarding instrument development is beyond the scope of this book, it is important to consider whether and why a researcher uses established instruments, modified instruments, or tools created for the purposes of the study. If a researcher is unable to locate an appropriate instrument for the research or evaluation question, developing a customized tool may be the most appropriate step. Regardless, research reports should include transparent information regarding the nature of the instruments used and a rationale for using them. This should include the number and nature of items, connection to the construct(s) of interest, evidence of test score validity for the intended purpose, evidence of reliability, and methods for computing and interpreting scores. You will learn more about how to understand and incorporate measures in your work throughout this text. Chapter 5 includes a more detailed exploration of validity and reliability concepts in measurement. Chapter 8 includes focused attention on methods for surveying groups of people, and Chapter 15 provides practical steps for identifying assessment measures.

Existing Records

Existing records are often used within program evaluation (Fitzpatrick et al., 2023) and may also be relevant to researchers. Existing records may be particularly useful in understanding the impact of programs and services in mental health sites. Depending on your setting, you may have access to existing records that are useful as process or outcome measures. Many agencies routinely conduct assessments to determine service eligibility, gather information regarding functioning and life circumstances, and re-administer assessments to determine progress. Counselors in mental health or offender services may have access to possible outcome metrics such as recidivism rates, readmission rates, passed drug screens, sustained employment, and independent living. They will also keep track of process indicators such as wait time, type of services rendered, and frequency of services offered. In addition, school counselors have access to metrics such as school attendance, grades earned, promotion/retention rates, standardized test scores, and disciplinary action. These can all serve as outcome measures embedded in easily-accessible records or metrics in our settings.

I (Casey) once collaborated on a project aimed at using archival data from a community counseling clinic to develop a model to understand which adolescents were most likely to persist in counseling and which were most likely to terminate prematurely (Holm & Barrio Minton, 2016). Use of existing records was particularly helpful because clients who have dropped out of services are highly unlikely to respond to requests for interviews or to complete surveys regarding their reasons for discontinuing. In the end, this project helped counselors at the agency identify those who were at risk for dropout with strong accuracy, thus informing proactive steps to retain them.

There are a number of limitations to using existing records for research and program evaluation. These include missing or incomplete data; concerns with data accuracy; data available only in overly aggregated form; unknown, different, or changing definitions of data elements; data needing to be linked across programs and agencies; and confidentiality and privacy considerations (Hatry, 2015). Still, the benefits of using existing records likely outweigh the risks and is worthy of consideration.

Interviews

Researchers and evaluators may use individual or focus group interviews to generate an in-depth understanding of participant experiences in qualitative research and evaluation. Individual interviews may allow for exploration of personal experiences and insights. Focus groups tend to engage six to ten individuals in the group process to generate interactions between participants that lead to greater depth of information, including contrasting opinions. Just as individual interviews may allow intimacy for more depth of perspective, focus groups may help generate data that would not have otherwise emerged. Although they can be time-consuming, interviews allow researchers to clarify, probe, and follow up with responses, thus yielding data that would be otherwise impossible to gather using archives or surveys.

Intentionality in development of the **interview guide** is especially critical when conducting interviews. It is important to develop the guide in such a way that it allows conversation to flow while also ensuring depth of coverage regarding the topics of interest. After reviewing hundreds of semi-structured interview guides, Kallio et al. (2016) suggested that questions should be participant-oriented, not leading, clearly worded, single-faceted, and open-ended. They further suggested that interview guides include main themes and follow-up questions. Main themes should be presented in a logical order from warm-up to more in-depth or personal questions, often ending on lighter themes. Each main theme should allow for predesigned and/or spontaneous follow-up questions. Interview guides may also include nondirective probing techniques to facilitate the flow of interviews. We explore these topics in greater depth in Chapter 7.

Applications to Research and Program Evaluation

When reviewing research, consider the nature of data collection protocols as described. The methodology section should be written so that you can understand how researchers went about collecting data. This should include a clear description of and rationale for instruments, existing data, and/or interviews used in the research process. Understanding this process helps you better understand how data were collected and assess the strengths and limitations of the design.

When developing program evaluations, start with a clear understanding of the goals and purposes for the evaluation. By first understanding what you want to know, you will be better equipped to determine how you can know it. Then, each step of data collection should be carefully constructed to help inform the overall question.

INTERVENTIONS

As will be discussed in Part II, not all research designs include interventions or treatments. By definition, a program evaluation is focused on an intervention that is theoretically assumed to increase personal well-being or meet a community need of some sort. Thus, it is important that researchers and evaluators are clear and transparent about the specific interventions utilized in the program. In quantitative designs, interventions serve as independent variables intended to influence a dependent or outcome variable. Thus, research and evaluation reports should include a clear description of interventions involved in the design. This may include descriptions of numbers and duration of sessions, curricula or protocols utilized, qualification of those providing interventions, and steps taken to ensure **treatment fidelity**.

As you learned about in depth in Chapter 2, treatment fidelity involves "methodological strategies used to monitor and enhance the reliability and validity of behavioral interventions" (Bellg et al., 2004, p. 444). We may use a wide variety of strategies to make sure we implement the intervention as designed or are transparent about difficulties in implementation. Treatment fidelity strategies may be embedded in program designs (e.g., ensuring equivalent time), provider training, treatment delivery, and consumer experience.

Applications to Research and Program Evaluation

When reviewing research, we should first look to determine whether the researchers used an intervention. If an intervention is utilized, the article should provide sufficient details or links to resources to understand and learn more about the specific intervention implemented. Additionally, look for evidence of treatment fidelity in study procedures. You should leave the intervention section with a clear understanding of what was done, why it was done, and whether or how the intervention might work in your setting.

When conducting evaluations, it is important to provide a clear understanding of the specific nature of the intervention or program as it is designed. This may include specifics regarding:

- type of counseling services (e.g., individual, group, couple, family, classroom guidance),
- theory or model utilized (e.g., Relational-Cultural Theory, social-emotional learning curriculum),
- timing of services (e.g., 60 minutes once weekly for 6 weeks),
- personnel or service providers involved (e.g., school counselors employed by the school, research team members employed by a primary investigator), and
- overall target of experience (e.g., increase prosocial behaviors, decrease trauma symptoms).

By being transparent regarding the nature of programs offered, you will better position yourself to evaluate whether services were delivered as expected and whether those services had intended impacts as explored in Chapter 3.

DESIGN VALIDITY AND TRUSTWORTHINESS

Whether you are reviewing research or designing program evaluations, you will want to know the degree to which you can trust the results. There are several concepts specific to quantitative design, qualitative design, and program evaluation that relate to the validity or trustworthiness of work.

Design Validity in Quantitative Research

In quantitative research, ensuring the validity of findings requires careful attention to various factors that can influence results or limit their generalizability There are four major types of validity in quantitative research designs:

> (a) **statistical conclusion validity** (i.e., degree to which the researcher has come to the correct conclusions through statistical analyses), (b) **internal validity** (i.e., degree of certainty with which one can conclude causal relationships), (c) **construct validity** (i.e., degree a chosen variable captures the hypothetical construct), and (d) **external validity** (i.e., degree the relationship can be generalized).
>
> (Heppner et al., 2016, ch. 7)

Threats to validity can arise at multiple stages of the research process and may affect both internal validity (i.e., how confidently we can attribute changes to the intervention) and external validity (i.e., how well the results can be applied beyond the context studied). All research designs include strengths, limitations, and a balance of different threats to validity. For example, although experimental laboratory studies may be very tightly controlled in a way that leads one to know with a very high degree of certainty that an intervention produced an effect, the degree of control inherent in laboratory settings is rarely found in the messy real-world settings in which we live and work. In this case, experimental laboratory studies trade high internal validity for low external validity. Table 4.2 contains a number of common threats to validity, descriptions, and examples relevant to counseling.

TABLE 4.2 Threats to Validity in Quantitative Research

Threat	Description	Example
Selection	Bias that results from the selection of participants that do not reflect the broader population, limiting generalizability.	A study uses only clients from a university clinic that is frequented by faculty families.
History	Specific events occurring between measurements may influence participant experiences and affect findings.	A natural disaster occurs during a school counseling intervention study.
Maturation	The natural tendency of participants to grow and change over time, independent of the intervention.	Individuals in a grief counseling group exhibit reduced sadness over several months.

Threat	Description	Example
Regression to the mean	The changes in scores among participants who were selected based on very high or low scores, toward the group average over time, independent of the intervention.	Clients with severe depression show improvement without any treatment.
Testing	Exposure to a test or survey can influence responses on later administrations, affecting measured outcomes.	A student scores higher on the second administration of an IQ test due to familiarity with the items.
Instrumentation	Changes in the measurement tools, observers, or scoring procedures may result in differences mistaken as changes in outcomes.	A different researcher scores post-tests with more leniency.
Attrition	The distortion of observed effects due to the loss of participants within a sample over time, especially with extreme symptoms or responses.	Highly distressed clients drop out before completing the post-assessment.
Halo effect	An initial positive impression of a participant may unconsciously influence the appraisal of their outcomes by observers or raters.	A counselor perceives more client progress because of likability.
Population effects	The sample studied may not adequately resemble the population the findings are intended to represent.	A study on trauma is conducted with veterans but generalized to civilian clients.
Multiple intervention interference	When multiple interventions occur simultaneously, it can be difficult to determine which contributed to observed changes.	Clients attend both group therapy and receive school-based mentoring.
Context dependent effects	The effects found in one setting may not replicate in another due to the characteristics of the context.	A mindfulness program works well in schools but not in a correctional facility.
Hawthorne effect	Participants may modify behaviors or perform differently due to the experience of being observed or studied.	Youth in a group counseling intervention for conflict resolution demonstrate improved peer interactions during observation period.

Trustworthiness or Methodological Integrity in Qualitative Research

Qualitative researchers rarely refer to validity. Rather, they often refer to **trustworthiness** in the research process. Trustworthiness refers to the quality of the product. These include concepts such as credibility (i.e., extent to which findings ring true), transferability (i.e., extent to which work is described in a way that it can be applied in other contexts), dependability (i.e., evidence that findings are consistent and could be repeated), and confirmability (i.e., evidence that findings can be corroborated by others) (Lincoln & Guba, 1985). **Methodological integrity** is more practice-oriented, focusing on the quality of the research process as it relates to decisions made in alignment with the specific goals and method of a given study.

The nature of qualitative research is such that researchers are important instruments in the process; they cannot simply turn to participants for corroborations. For this reason, qualitative scholars have developed a number of critical questions, such as:

- Are the data adequate?
- Is the researcher perspective in data collection managed to enhance fidelity?
- Are data contextualized?
- Can the data lead to insights relevant to the project goals when analyzed using the method under study?
- Is the researcher perspective in data analysis managed to enhance fidelity?
- Are the findings meaningful contributions toward the project goal?
- Are the findings grounded within the data that support their understanding?
- Are the meanings of fidelity coherent with one another? (Levitt et al., 2017, p. 11)

Levitt et al. (2017) proposed several strategies researchers can use to ensure methodological integrity in qualitative research.

Validity in Program Evaluation

Although validity and trustworthiness principles transfer to program evaluation design to some extent, these principles alone are not sufficient for evaluating the quality of program evaluation designs. The Joint Committee on Standards for Educational Evaluation developed sets of standards to guide program evaluation. Their work includes sets of criteria to support the following key principles in real-life evaluation settings:

- *Utility*—the extent to which evaluation results meet the needs of intended users; emphasizes credibility, relevance, and meaningful use
- *Feasibility*—the extent to which the evaluation is effective and efficient; emphasize practical procedures and responsible use of resources that fit within the context of the program
- *Propriety*—the extent to which the evaluation is ethically and legally responsible; focus on responsiveness to users, safeguarding rights, promoting transparency, and managing conflicts of interest
- *Accuracy*—the extent to which the evaluation produces truthful and dependable findings; focus on sound methods and reasoning in context of the program

- *Evaluation Accountability* – the extent to which the evaluation is well-documented and continuously improved; focus on internal and external review

(Yarbrough et al., 2010)

Applications to Research and Program Evaluation

When reviewing research, look for ways in which the authors talk about validity (in quantitative work) and/or trustworthiness or methodological integrity (in qualitative work). When reviewing theoretical frameworks, sampling, data collection procedures, and interventions, you should be able to see steps taken to boost the integrity of the research. In addition, researchers should be transparent about limitations or shortcomings of the study, highlighting these within the discussion or limitations sections and proposing future steps to remedy weaknesses observed in the study.

When designing program evaluations, you will want to attend to the core questions raised by Yarbrough and colleagues (2010) earlier. Parts II and III of this book will help you begin to see how to build pieces for a strong counseling intervention or program evaluation design. In the meantime, you may find Box 4.3 helpful for working your way through a methods section of an article.

BOX 4.3 CHECKLIST FOR CRITIQUING METHODS SECTION OF AN ARTICLE

- What is the theoretical basis or framework for this study?
- What variables are included in this study? How are they connected to the theoretical framework for the study?
- To what degree does the author operationalize the variables?
- How was each variable measured?
- Who was the population of interest for this study?
- What were inclusion and exclusion criteria for the study?
- What sampling methods did the researchers use?
- What do I understand about characteristics of participants in this study?
- What recruitment procedures did the authors use for this study?
- What data collection procedures did the authors use for this study?
- To what degree do I understand strengths and limitations of data collection measures (i.e., instruments, observations, interviews) utilized?
- (if applicable) To what degree do I understand the intervention used for this study?
- (if applicable) To what degree do I have confidence in the steps taken to ensure treatment fidelity in this study?
- What evidence does the author provide of validity (quantitative) or trustworthiness (qualitative)?
- What validity (quantitative) or trustworthiness (qualitative) threats appear to be present but are not discussed in the article?
- To what degree are the authors transparent about study strengths and limitations?

CHAPTER SUMMARY

This chapter included an overview of common methodological concepts found across different types of research designs. We started with attention to theory, constructs, and variables; noted considerations related to populations and samples; reviewed common types of data collection protocols; discussed considerations related to interventions; and introduced concepts related to validity and trustworthiness of designs. In each section we provided considerations for reviewing research articles and sample applications to designing counseling interventions and program evaluations.

RESOURCES

- Joint Committee on Standards for Educational Evaluation, *Program Evaluation Standards.* https://evaluationstandards.org/program/
- Office of Behavioral & Social Sciences Research, *e-Source Introductory Social and Behavioral Science Training Materials.* https://obssr.od.nih.gov/training/online-training-resources/esource
- Research Methods Knowledge Base, https://conjointly.com/kb/

REFERENCES

Bellg, A. J., Borrelli, B., Resnick, B., Hecht, J., Minicucci, D. S., Ory, M.,. . .Treatment Fidelity Workgroup of the NIH Behavior Change Consortium. (2004). Enhancing treatment fidelity in health behavior change studies: Best practices and recommendations from the NIH Behavior Change Consortium. *Health Psychology: Official Journal of the Division of Health Psychology, American Psychological Association*, *23*(*5*), 443–451. https://doi.org/10.1037/0278-6133.23.5.443

Fink, A. (2025). *How to conduct surveys: A step-by-step guide* (7th ed.). Sage.

Fitzpatrick, J. L., Sanders, J. R., Worthen, B. R., & Wingate, L. A. (2023). *Program evaluation: Alternative approaches and practical guidelines* (5th ed.). Pearson.

Hatry, H. P. (2015). Using agency records. In *Handbook of practical program evaluation* (4th ed., pp. 325–343). Jossey-Bass.

Heppner, P. P., Wampold, B. E., Owen, J., Thompon, M. N., & Wang, K. T. (2016). *Research design in counseling* (4th ed.). Cengage.

Holm, J. M., & Barrio Minton, C. A. (2016). A predictive model of adolescent persistence in counseling. *Children and Youth Services Review*, *67*, 161–167. https://doi.org/10.1016/j.childyouth.2016.06.005

Jazieh A, R., (2020). Quality measures: Types, selection, and application in health care quality improvement projects. *Global Journal on Quality and Safety in Health Care*, *3*(4), 144–146. https://doi.org/10.36401/JQSH-20-X6

Joiner, T. (2009). *The interpersonal theory of suicide: Guidance for working with suicidal clients* (1st ed.). American Psychological Association.

Kallio, H., Pietilä, A. M., Johnson, M., & Kangasniemi, M. (2016). Systematic methodological review: Developing a framework for a qualitative semi-structured interview guide. *Journal of Advanced Nursing*, *72*(*12*), 2954–2965. https://doi.org/10.1111/jan.13031

Kerlinger, F. N., & Lee, H. B. (2000). Constructs, variables, and definitions. In *Foundations of behavioral research* (4th ed., pp. 39–61). Wadsworth.

Kilbourne, A. M., Beck, K., Spaeth-Rublee, B., Ramanuh, P., O'Brien, R. W., Tomoyasu, N., & Pincus, H. A. (2018). Measuring and improving the quality of mental health care: A global perspective. *World Psychiatry*, *17*, 30–38. https://doi.org/10.1002/wps.20482

Lent, R. W., Brown, S. D., & Hackett, G. (1994). Toward a unifying social cognitive theory of career and academic interest, choice, and performance. *Journal of Vocational Behavior*, *45(1)*, 79–122. https://doi.org/10.1006/jvbe.1994.1027

Levitt, H. M., Motulsky, S. L., Wertz, F. J., Morrow, S. L., & Ponterotto, J. G. (2017). Recommendations for designing and reviewing qualitative research in psychology: Promoting methodological integrity. *Qualitative Psychology*, *4(1)*, 2–22. http://dx.doi.org.proxy.lib.utk.edu:90/10.1037/qup0000082

Lincoln, Y. S., & Guba, E. G. (1985). *Naturalistic inquiry*. Sage.

Ma, J., Batterham, P. J., Calear, A. L., & Han, J. (2016). A systematic review of the predictions of the interpersonal – Psychological theory of suicidal behavior. *Clinical Psychology Review*, *46*, 34–45. https://doi.org/10.1016/j.cpr.2016.04.008

Merriam-Webster. (2025). *Definition of theory*. www.merriam-webster.com/dictionary/theory

Office of Behavioral & Social Sciences Research. (n.d.). Social and behavioral theories. *e-Source Behavioral & Social Sciences Research*. https://obssr.od.nih.gov/sites/obssr/files/Social-and-Behavioral-Theories.pdf

Ricco, R. B., & Sierra, A. (2017). Argument beliefs mediate relations between attachment style and conflict tactics. *Journal of Counseling & Development*, *95*(2), 156–167. https://doi.org/10.1002/jcad.12128

Rogers, C. R. (1961). *On becoming a person: A therapist's view of psychotherapy*. Houghton Mifflin.

Royse, D., Thyer, B. A., & Padgett, D. K. (2015). *Program evaluation: An introduction to an evidence-based approach* (6th ed.). Cengage.

Sheperis, C. J., Young, J. S., & Daniels, M. H. (2017). *Counseling research: Quantitative, qualitative, and mixed methods (2nd ed.)*. Pearson.

Shoffner, M. F., Newsome, D., Barrio Minton, C. A., & Wachter Morris, C. A. (2015). A qualitative exploration of the STEM career-related outcome expectations of young adolescents. *Journal of Career Development*, *42*(2), 102–116. https://doi.org/10.1177/0894845314544033

Yarbrough, D. B., Shula, L. M., Hopson, R. K., & Caruthers, F. A. (2010). *The program evaluation standards: A guide for evaluators and evaluation users* (3rd. ed). Corwin.

Zeligman, M., Bialo, J. A., Brack, J. L., & Kearney, M. A. (2017). Loneliness as moderator between trauma and posttraumatic growth. *Journal of Counseling & Development*, *95*(4), 435–444. https://doi.org/10.1002/jcad.12158

CHAPTER 5

Understanding Measurement and Statistical Concepts

In Chapter 4, we reviewed methodological concepts often used when designing applied research and program evaluation projects. This chapter includes an overview of concepts and terms you will often see in research articles and evaluation reports that are focused on measuring variables or conducting statistical analyses. We open by exploring the levels of variables we may work with and methods for using descriptive statistics to understand their characteristics. Next, we explore concepts related to the validity and reliability of test scores. Finally, we describe hypothesis testing and some inferential statistics you may find reported in the literature before exploring tools to understand their statistical, practical, and clinical significance. If you have not yet participated in a statistics course, we will introduce you to the language you can expect to see in quantitative research and program evaluation reports. If you have already studied statistics, this chapter will serve as a refresher. For each area, we include basic definitions and brief practical discussions regarding why these concepts matter when reading research or designing program evaluations. You will also find some summary charts to help you organize your thoughts.

BOX 5.1 CHAPTER LEARNING OUTCOMES

- Understand levels of measurement
- Describe types of descriptive statistics, including measures of central tendency and indices of variability
- Name key considerations related to reliability and validity of test scores
- Identify what different types of inferential statistics (e.g., t-tests, ANOVA, correlations, regression) are designed to do
- Understand different types of significance (e.g., statistical, practical, and clinical) you will read about in research reports
- Comprehend a results section of a research or evaluation report

DOI: 10.4324/9781003586210-6

LEVELS OF VARIABLES

As discussed in Chapter 4, a **variable** "is a property that can take on different values. It is a symbol to which values are assigned" (Kerlinger & Lee, 2000, p. 59). Variables can be **quantitative** or **qualitative** in nature and are represented across different levels of measurement—nominal, ordinal, interval, and ratio—that are broadly considered either categorical or continuous.

Qualitative, also known as **categorical variables**, are not measurable in the sense that they do not have a natural order, and there is no intrinsic meaning to the number assigned to them. In this case, the level of measurement is **nominal**. Type of counseling services is an example of a qualitative or categorical variable that is nominal in nature. For the purpose of statistical analysis, we may decide that individual services = 1, group services = 2, and family services = 3. Demographic variables such as gender, race, ethnicity, and partnership status are also categorical or nominal in nature. In each of these examples, the assignment of a number to a characteristic has no intrinsic meaning beyond saving space on a spreadsheet.

Quantitative variables are numerical in nature, and the values assigned to them have some intrinsic meaning in that they can be ordered. This meaning varies depending on whether the quantitative variable is ordinal, interval, or ratio in nature. **Ordinal** variables are ordered and can be ranked; however, there is no even spacing between the variables. For example, some systems use a continuum of services to meet different levels of need. We may conceptualize that outpatient services = 1, intensive outpatient services = 2, partial hospitalization services = 3, and inpatient services = 4. Alternatively, one might conceptualize level of impairment as mild = 1, moderate = 2, and severe = 3. Or we might ask people to rate their satisfaction with services as very dissatisfied = 1, dissatisfied = 2, satisfied = 3, and very satisfied = 4. Although we can place these variables in order, we cannot infer that those who are "very satisfied = 4" are twice as satisfied as those who are "dissatisfied = 2."

The **interval** and **ratio** levels of measurement are ordered *and* have even spacing between points on the scale. These are also known as **continuous variables**. The primary difference between them is that the interval level of measurement does not have a true zero (e.g., a score indicating complete absence of something), whereas the ratio level of measurement does have a true zero. Level of impairment as assessed via a formal assessment instrument will yield data we generally treat as interval in nature. Technically, however, many assessment scores derived are ordinal because they reflect rankings based on underlying constructs rather than equal units with a true zero. On the other hand, number of counseling sessions completed is assessed at the ratio level. There is a true zero, and we can reasonably conclude that someone who completed ten sessions engaged in twice as much counseling as someone who completed five sessions. Because we generally treat interval and ratio data the same in statistical analysis, we refer to this level of measurement as interval–ratio.

Level of measurement is important because it influences how we handle the related data and make meaning from our observations. As we will explore in the following section, some descriptive statistics can only be applied to certain levels of measurement. In addition, inferential statistics commonly used in research and program evaluation use assumptions that require variables to be at certain levels of measurement.

DESCRIPTIVE STATISTICS

When looking at any given dataset, researchers and evaluators tend to start with descriptive statistics. Descriptive statistics include metrics designed to help us know what our variables look like. This section includes attention to measures of central tendency and indices of variability. Because these are designed to help us visualize data, we start by attending to the shapes of distributions. In this section, we use a running example of number of counseling sessions attended with a counselor over the last year. This counselor has seen a total of 30 individual clients this year, and the number of sessions attended were as follows: 1, 1, 1, 1, 1, 1, 1, 1, 1, 1, 2, 2, 2, 2, 3, 3, 3, 4, 5, 6, 6, 8, 8, 10, 12, 15, 18, 20, 40, 56.

Using Distributions to Visualize Data

Distributions are ways of visualizing data. How we visualize data will depend on the type of data we are working with. At the simplest level is the **frequency distribution,** and this is most often used when working with nominal or ordinal data. Consider the simple bar chart in which we see types of services clients at our hypothetical agency attended.

In some instances, it may be helpful to portray group frequency data in a **histogram**. For example, it would be unwieldy to visualize the age of every client at the agency, but a grouped visualization may be meaningful. Alternatively, we might want

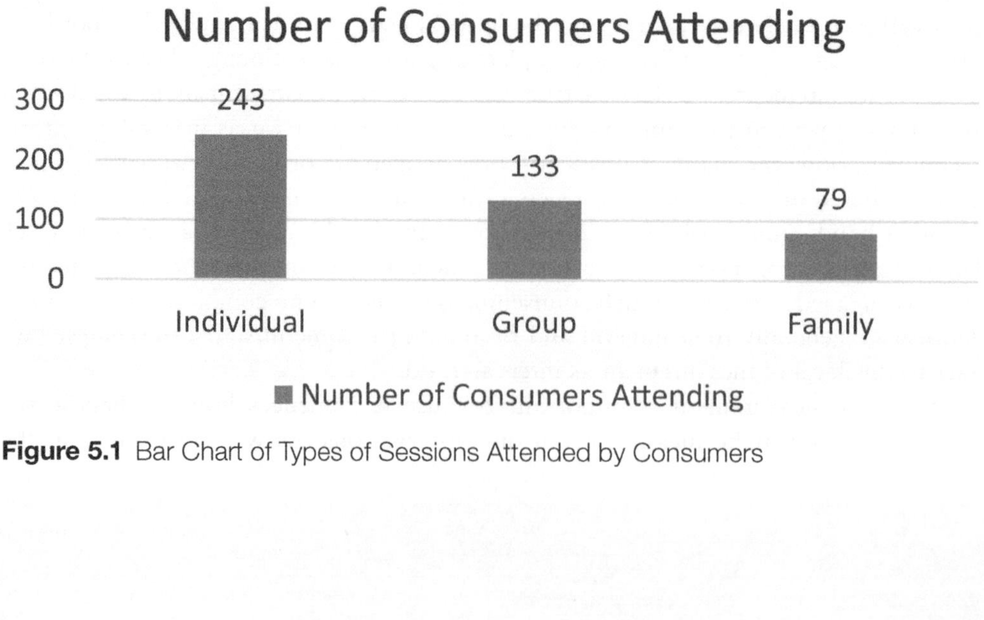

Figure 5.1 Bar Chart of Types of Sessions Attended by Consumers

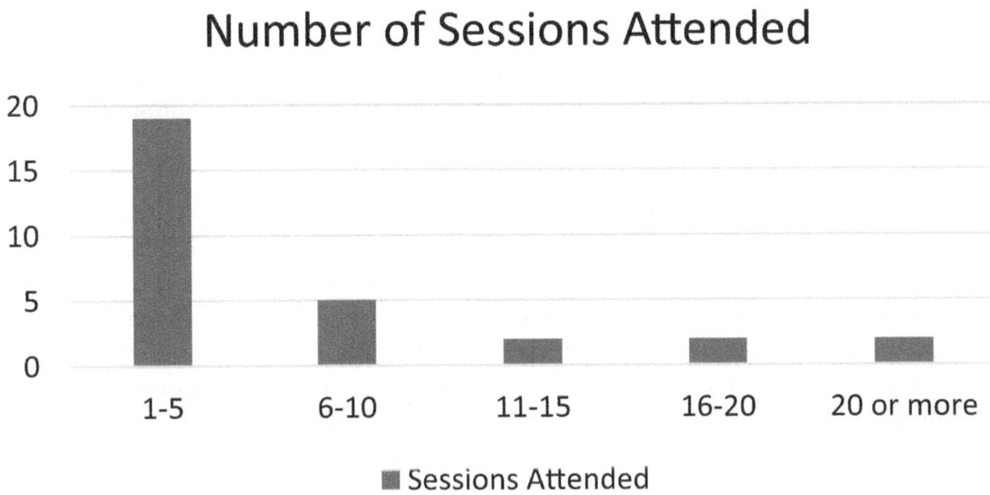

Figure 5.2 Histogram of Number of Sessions Attended by Consumers

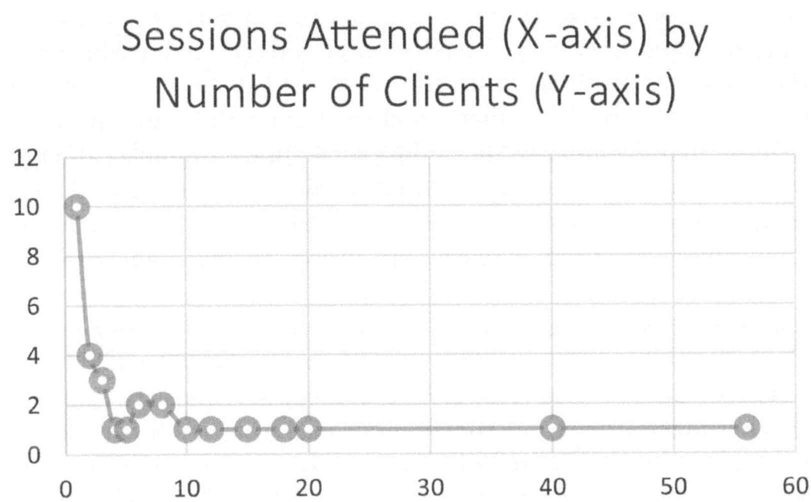

Figure 5.3 Scatterplot of Number of Sessions Attended by Consumers

a quick look at the number of sessions attended by the clients in our running example. Shall we?

When working with continuous, interval–ratio-level data, we are also able to chart each data point onto a continuous **probability distribution** or a **scatterplot**. This helps us understand something more about the shape of our data. We will return to the concept of distributions later in this section. A full exploration of distributions is beyond the scope of this text. If this concept is new to you, you may wish to check out the free text and video tutorials available via http://onlinestatbook.com.

Measures of Central Tendency

Measures of central tendency are used to describe a collection of data or a dataset. These are concise ways of representing what we might see in a distribution. Measures of central tendency include mode, median, and mean.

The **mode** is the most common or frequently occurring value in a dataset. A mode can be computed using any level of data; however, mode is the *only* measure of central tendency that can be used when working with nominal or categorical data. For example, if we find that 243 clients engaged in individual services, 133 clients engaged in group services, and 79 client systems engaged in family services, individual is the modal, or most common, category of services. We can also apply mode to interval–ratio data. For example, when examining number of counseling sessions attended, we find that ten clients attended one session, four clients attended two sessions, three clients attended three sessions, and so forth. The mode number of sessions completed was one. The mode of interval–ratio variables, such as assessment scale results, may not have much intrinsic meaning because the variables may take on so many different values.

The **median** is the middle value or score in a dataset. Because values must be placed in order to determine the median, a median can only be computed for **ordinal** and **interval–ratio**-level data. A median tells us the value for which exactly one half of the cases are below the observation and one half of the cases are above the observation. To compute the median number of counseling sessions attended, we sort the dataset in order and find the middle value. In the example earlier, the counselor saw 30 clients. The median would fall between the fifteenth (three sessions) and sixteenth (three sessions) case. Thus, the median number of sessions was three. If these two values were different, we would average the two middle values to identify the median.

The **mean**, or average, is the sum of all values divided by the number of observations and can be used for quantitative data. Although some will apply the concept of mean to ordinal data, we need to be careful in doing so. This may make good sense when reporting on the average satisfaction rating on a scale of 0–10; however, it would not be meaningful to report the mean level of care. In this case, mode or median would be more appropriate. To compute the mean in our running example, we add up the number of sessions offered (235) and divide by the number of clients seen (30). This yields a mean of 7.83.

There are two take-home messages for this section. First, levels of measurement influence which measures of central tendency we can use. Second, when working with ordinal or interval–ratio data, we must consider context when determining which measures of central tendency are most meaningful for interpretation. The counselor noted earlier saw 30 clients for which the mode number of sessions was 1, median number of sessions was 3, and mean number of sessions was 7.83. The mean was highly influenced by outliers, with clients who attended 40 and 56 sessions greatly outweighing values for the majority, who attended just 1 or 2 sessions. In reality, one-third of this counselor's clients did not return after the first session, and one half of this counselor's clients completed three sessions or fewer. Reporting only the mean of 7.83 would distort the picture for this counselor.

Indices of Variability

This example leads us to the importance of measures of variability. At the most basic level, variability refers to the pattern of spread within a group of scores. We are generally concerned with four measures of variability: range, interquartile range, variance, and standard deviation. These measures are used with quantitative data, generally at the interval–ratio level of measure.

The **range** is the most straightforward measure of central tendency. We compute a range by subtracting the lowest value from the highest value. In the example provided earlier, the minimum number of sessions was 1 and the maximum number of sessions was 56. Thus, the number of sessions ranged from 1 to 56, and the range was 55.

The **interquartile range** (IQR), also known as the **H-spread**, is concerned with the spread between the first quartile (25th percentile) and third quartile (75th percentile). In the section earlier, we described the median as the data point for which one half of values are above and one half of values are below (i.e., the 50th percentile). IQR helps us understand the spread between the middle 50% of values. A **quartile** simply divides the rank-ordered list into four even parts. To divide our example into quartiles, we divide the number of observations (30) by 4 and determine that we need to take the value of every 7.5th data point. Although you could do this by hand, we prefer to use an online interquartile range calculator (e.g., www.mathportal.org) to do the work for us. In this case, the first quartile is 1 and third quartile is 8. Thus, the IQR or spread between the first and third quartiles is 8–1 = 7. The following chart includes a visual representation of interquartile range in what is known as a boxplot, with the rectangular box indicating the middle 50% of values and the whiskers extending to the outer values. In this case, the boxplot helps us see that we have two extreme outliers.

Variance shows how close scores are to the middle of the distribution and "is defined as the average squared difference of the scores from the mean" (Lane et al., n.d.). We could create a table in which we list each score, subtract the mean to yield a difference, square each difference, and then average the squared differences to compute a mean. It is important to note that there is a slightly different formula when computing variance for samples compared to populations. Although it may be useful to hand-compute for the joy of learning, we prefer to use an online calculator or built-in Excel function. Doing that, we see that the variance for our running example is 151.11.

If you are wondering how to interpret the variance here, you aren't alone. You will likely prefer to think about variance in terms of **standard deviation** (SD). SD is the square root of the variance; in this case, SD = 12.29. By taking the square root of this value, we are able to interpret variability of scores based on the original scale (i.e., number of sessions). When scores are normally distributed, we expect to see 68% of scores within one standard deviation, 95% of scores within two standard deviations, and 99.7% of scores within three standard deviations of the mean. In this case, we have a standard deviation that is larger than our mean. This tells us that there is something unique about the way that our data fall. In particular, our data are asymmetrical, or have **skewness** (i.e., most observations are concentrated on one side of the distribution), *and* our data have **kurtosis** (i.e., a pattern that indicates more or less values in the tails of our distribution than would be expected). Again, http://onlinestatbook.com has some excellent tutorials designed to help you understand these concepts.

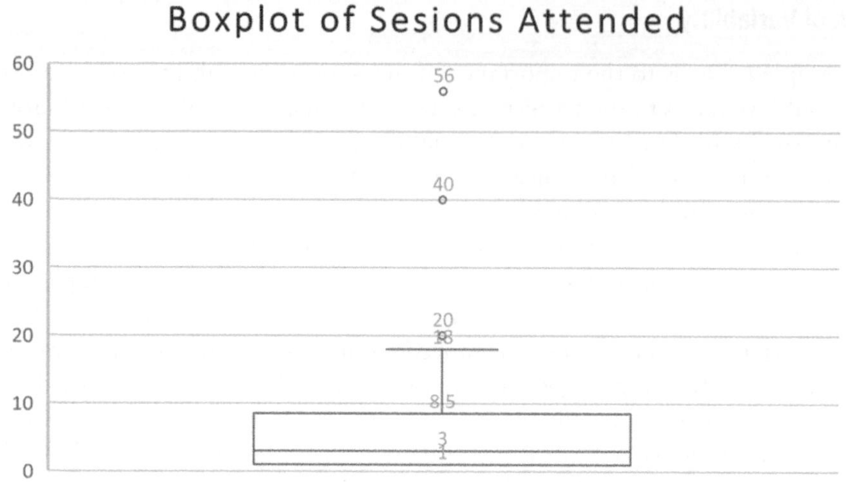

Figure 5.4 Boxplot of Number of Sessions Attended by Consumers

TABLE 5.1 Measures of Central Tendency and Indices of Variability

Measure or Index	Take-home Meaning	Value
Mode	Most frequent number of sessions	1
Median	Middle number of sessions (50th percentile)	3
Mean	Average of all sessions	7.83
Range	Difference between highest and lowest sessions	55
Interquartile range (IQR)	Range of middle 50% of cases; difference between 75th percentile and 25th percentile	7
Variance	Spreadness of scores; average squared difference of scores from the mean	151.11
Standard deviation (SD)	Spreadness of scores; square root of the variance	12.29

Before we move on to the next section, take a minute to check out how we can use descriptive statistics to describe what we have learned about the service picture for this counselor in a way that goes far beyond what the mean might tell us.

FROM VARIABLES TO MEASURES TO INFERENCES

In the last chapter, you learned about the differences between constructs (ideas that can be measured) and variables (things that take on and can be assigned values). You also learned about different types of variables (e.g., independent, dependent) you will encounter as you embark on an inquiry. Before we get into the technicalities of statistical concepts, it is important to slow down and consider just what we are measuring with the numbers we generate.

Even the most advanced statistical analysis means nothing if the scores generated for the analysis are not strong representations of the constructs they are intended to assess in that specific context. Interpreting test or assessment scores also involves recognizing the uncertainty that arises from sampling and measurement error. This is where an understanding of **confidence intervals** becomes essential. A confidence interval provides a range of values, based on a sample, in which we can reasonably expect the true value of a population score to fall. For example, an observed score of 85 might be reported alongside a 95% confidence interval of 80 to 90, indicating that we can be reasonably confident (i.e., 95%) that the true score for the population is somewhere between 80 and 90. This concept is very important for supporting accurate interpretations of scores on assessments we may use.

Validity Evidence for Test Scores

Although you may have heard someone describe a specific assessment or test as valid, this can be misleading. **Validity** is "a transitory property that is unique across instances of test use . . . there are not valid tests, just valid uses of their scores" (Lenz, 2025, p. 1). Researchers are responsible for integrating different sources of evidence to reach a conclusion regarding the degree to which test scores are valid for use in a specific context. This includes a clear focus on the intended use and interpretation of any instrument along with information regarding samples and settings used in validation. For example, if focusing on depression, it would be important to differentiate between a test intended to *screen* for depression and one intended to support a *diagnostic* decision regarding depression. Likewise, an instrument designed for adults in clinical settings would likely hold up very differently if administered to youth in school settings.

Lenz (2025) outlined five specific forms of validity evidence to consider when making a determination about test score validity in a specific context.

- Evidence based on **test content** involves considering connections between the underlying theory that informs a measure with the test format, instructions, items, and response options (e.g., a measure regarding depression includes affective, behavioral, and cognitive symptoms as operationalized by the DSM-5-TR).
- Evidence based on **response processes** involves considering how test takers engage with the test itself (e.g., a measure of youth depression involved cognitive interviews with youth to ensure that the youth understood the instructions and items).
- Evidence based on **internal structure** involves the statistical relationships between items scores and any theoretical factors or subscales (e.g., statistical tests indicate that items do indeed load onto subscales designed to assess affective, behavioral, and cognitive symptoms *and* show measurement invariance by holding steady across gender and race/ethnicity).
- Evidence based on **relations to other variables** involves considering **convergence** and **divergence** as one would expect theoretically (e.g., a measure regarding depression correlates with several other measures regarding depression and well-being in general; however, it does not correlate with age or reading ability).
- Evidence based on **consequential validity** involves considering both intended and unintended consequences of administering the instrument and the subsequent use

of scores (e.g., a measure designed to screen for depression in youth is successful in identifying those who are in need of additional supports without unduly burdening the system or alarming test takers not in need of further services).

Reliability Evidence for Test Scores

In addition to providing evidence for the validity of test scores in particular contexts, instruments should include evidence of **reliability**. In general, reliability refers to the degree to which scores are consistent. Four types of reliability estimates are relevant to formal instruments (Trochim, n.d.). **Interrater reliability** refers to the degree to which different trained raters produce similar results. This concept applies mostly when using observation protocols. **Test–retest reliability** refers to the degree to which results are stable over time. Some constructs, like personality or intelligence, are believed to be static over time. Thus, a user who takes the same instrument a few weeks or months apart should receive very similar results. Other constructs, like state anxiety, may vary from day to day or week to week; because we would like our instruments to be sensitive to change, we would expect to see lower test–retest reliability estimates. **Parallel-forms reliability** is most often used in academic testing wherein we would expect that several different versions of an instrument produce highly similar results. Finally, **internal consistency reliability** refers to the degree to which items within a particular instrument or scale are correlated to the group of items as a whole.

Counseling researchers are most often interested in internal consistency reliability (Kalkbrenner, 2024). Just as validity refers to the uses of test scores, reliability estimates are specific to the sample that represent. We might use information about reliability observed in past studies to determine whether we think an instrument will work similarly with our sample; however, we will really only know reliability after we've collected data and examined what happened with that specific sample. We most often see attention to Cronbach's coefficient alpha (α); however, that is not the only estimate of internal consistency reliability you will encounter in the literature. Table 5.2 provides a quick overview of reliability estimates and interpretation guidelines adapted from Kalkbrenner; the interpretation guidelines are just guidelines. As noted in the table, we tend to be more stringent when making **higher-stakes** decisions and more relaxed when making **lower-stakes** decisions based on test scores. In addition, internal consistency reliability estimates are just that, estimates. Confidence intervals allow us to provide more context and precision to those estimates by indicating the range where the true reliability likely falls. For example, if you see a source reference α = .84 95% CI [.80, .88], that means there is a 95% likelihood that the true Cronbach's coefficient alpha was between .80 and .88.

Understanding of test score validity and reliability will be important to you as you understand what measures researchers used to investigate their constructs and consider which instruments might be ideal for your own process and outcome evaluations. Chapter 4 included attention to different types of measures we might use in our work, and Chapter 15 includes nuts and bolts guidance on how you can go about selecting assessment measures to use in your own projects. Now that you have a foundation for understanding descriptive statistics as well as characteristics of measures used in research and program evaluation, we turn to understanding how we can use inferential statistics to answer quantitative research questions.

TABLE 5.2 Internal Consistency Reliability Estimates

Measure	Description	Tentative Guidelines for Acceptable Estimates
		lower stakes and higher stakes
Cronbach's coefficient alpha (α)	Most classic estimate based on split-half methods; focus on unidimensional scales and vulnerable to many statistical assumptions	≥ .70 (lenient for lower) ≥ .70 to .79 (acceptable for lower) ≥ .80 (conservative for lower) ≥ .90 or ≥ .95 (acceptable for higher)
McDonald's coefficient omega (ω)	Composite reliability estimate based on factor analysis; more resilient in smaller samples, with skewed items, and when items contribute different stability to scores	≥ .65 or ≥ .70 (acceptable for lower) ≥ .90 or ≥ .95 (acceptable for higher)
Omega Hierarchical (ω_H)	A derivative ω; used with multidimensional scales	≥ .80 (acceptable for lower)
Coefficient H	Composite reliability estimate based on factor analysis; based on optimal scale weighting where items that contribute more to the scale are weighted differently	≥ .70 (acceptable for lower) ≥ .80 (more stringent)

INFERENTIAL STATISTICS

Until this point, we have been exploring **descriptive** ways of using numbers and words to depict characteristics of the specific data we are examining. When we wish to infer something about relationships between two samples, a sample and a population, and/or two or more variables, we turn to **inferential statistics**. Because inferential statistics are designed to support hypothesis testing, we start with a review of that concept. Then we provide an overview of the most common types of inferential statistics you will encounter when reviewing research. We include attention to types of questions answered by the test and types of data needed to run the test. Throughout this section, we utilize the example of a school-wide eight-week group intervention for anger management.

Hypothesis Testing

A hypothesis is an assertion or statement designed to be tested through the scientific process. When using inferential statistics, we often state a **null hypothesis** indicating that there is *no relationship or difference* between variables, samples, or populations. Then, we create an **alternative hypothesis** in which we *specify a relationship or* *difference* we would expect to see if the null hypothesis was false. For example, my null hypothesis would be *an eight-week group intervention for anger management will not result in a reduction of disciplinary referrals*. My alternative hypothesis would be *an eight-week group intervention for anger management will result in a reduction of disciplinary referrals*.

Inferential statistics use probability theory to assess the degree to which a finding is likely if the null hypothesis is true. Researchers must always balance the possibility of different types of error. An **alpha** (α) or **significance level** represents the degree of chance a researcher is willing to take by mistakenly rejecting the null hypothesis and accepting the alternative hypothesis. We call this a **Type I error**. Most researchers set alpha levels at $\alpha = 0.05$ (5% chance of a Type I error); however, some researchers will restrict their alpha levels to $\alpha = 0.01$ (1% chance) or even $\alpha = .001$ (0.1% chance). When researchers conduct statistical analyses, they look for a *p*-value, an estimate regarding the likelihood of the result if the null hypothesis is false. When the *p*-value is less than or equal to the **alpha level** we set prior to analysis, we reject the null hypothesis. Type I error is a false positive. An example of a Type I error in counseling practice would be assessing someone to be at high risk of suicide when they are not at high risk. In the evaluation example we presented earlier, we would make a Type I error if we concluded the intervention was effective, even if it did not result in a change.

Type II error occurs when statistics generated lead one to fail to reject the null hypothesis (i.e., not accept an alternative hypothesis) when, in fact, there is a difference to be detected. The likelihood of making a Type II error is depicted by beta (β). Researchers are often more willing to make a Type II error, thus setting $\beta = 0.20$ (20% chance) or $\beta = 0.10$ (10% chance). **Power**, calculated as 1—β, is the probability of detecting a difference if one is present. Power is related to sample size, alpha level, standard deviation, degree of differences to be observed, and types of tests conducted. Researchers often use a computer program, like G*power, to calculate the necessary sample size. Type II error is a false negative. An example of a Type II error in counseling practice would be assessing someone as not at high risk of suicide when they are indeed at high risk of suicide. In the evaluation example we presented earlier, we would make a Type II error if we concluded the intervention was not effective, even if it did result in change.

Some researchers also refer to a concept of **Type III error**. For some, a Type III error means making the correct decision to fail to reject or reject the null hypothesis for the wrong reason. We prefer to look at Type III error as answering a question that was not the one asked. An example of a Type III error in counseling practice would be focusing on history of depression and treatment progress when the aim was to conduct a suicide risk assessment. Although depression and suicide risk are related and relevant to each other, we did not ask the questions we intended to ask. In the evaluation example we presented earlier, we would make a Type III error if we measured participants' self-reported anger management skills rather than changes in the number of disciplinary referrals.

Confidence intervals also play a key role in interpreting the results of hypothesis tests. Hypothesis testing tells us whether a result is statistically significant based on the level of precision we specified (remember, $\alpha = 0.05$ means we are willing to accept a 5% chance of a Type I error). A confidence interval rounds out this information by showing us the true range of values expected with 95% confidence. If the confidence interval does not include 0, the result is statistically significant at that corresponding confidence level. If the interval is narrow, we can believe that our estimate is more precise. If the interval is wide, there is more uncertainty around the estimates. In sum, *p*-values tell us whether an effect is likely real, and confidence intervals tell us how big that effect might be and how confident we are in the estimate.

Although it is beyond the scope of this practical text, an understanding of hypothesis testing is important for interpreting inferential statistics. If these concepts are new to you, you may wish to refer to the continuing education tutorials and resources listed at the end of this chapter.

Types of Inferential Statistics

Researchers utilize countless types of inferential statistics. The most appropriate statistical test to use depends on a variety of factors, including the specific research question or hypothesis, level of measurement of variables involved, design of relationship between data points (e.g., within participants or between participants), characteristics of descriptive data (e.g., variability, normality), and sample size. We can boil most statistical tests down to being concerned about mean differences, relationships, and predictions. The statistical tests covered in the remainder of the chapter are presented in a simplified manner. There are situations in which it may be more appropriate to use alternative statistical tests or analysis procedures. Although the types of tests covered here are not exhaustive or appropriate in every situation, they are the most often used metrics in research, and they will be the most accessible to you for evaluation purposes.

Tests Regarding Mean Differences

Analysis of variance (ANOVAs) and *t*-tests are the most common tests regarding differences between mean scores for two or more groups or points in time. Both tests are based on the same assumptions; however, *t*-tests can only compare two means, whereas ANOVAs can compare two or more means. Table 5.3 includes an overview of different types of *t*-tests and ANOVAs.

If a statistical test returns a *p*-value of $<.05$, the researcher is responsible for determining the degree of mean difference and the potential meaning for this change. When using *t*-tests, we can go directly to descriptive statistics to interpret differences between the two groups tested, and we can use what we know of practical and clinical significance to guide this interpretation. For example, if the independent samples *t*-test regarding mean differences in disciplinary referrals on the basis of gender resulted in $p = .02$, we could then consider the effect size (generally Cohen's *d*) and the mean number of referrals for boys (4.30) compared to girls (4.00) to determine whether we think a mean difference of 0.30 referrals over the course of a year is meaningful. If using ANOVAs with three or more groups, we will first have to use follow-up statistics (often based on *t*-tests) to determine *where* the difference is occurring. Then, we can repeat the process of deciding the degree to which the difference is meaningful.

TABLE 5.3 Tests Regarding Mean Differences

Test	Purpose	IV Level of Measurement	DV Level of Measurement	Sample Question
One-sample t-test	Compare mean of a sample with known mean of a population	Nominal (population vs. sample)	Interval–ratio	Is there a mean difference in the number of disciplinary referrals for students in the anger management group compared to students in the school as a whole?
Independent samples t-test	Compare means of two different samples	Nominal (sample 1 vs. sample 2)	Interval–ratio	Is there a mean difference in the number of disciplinary referrals for girls and boys?
Dependent samples (pairwise) t-test	Compare means of one group at two points in time	Nominal (time 1 vs. time 2)	Interval–ratio	Is there a mean difference in the number of disciplinary referrals one year after completing the group compared to the year leading up to the group?
One-way ANOVA	Compare means of two or more groups	Nominal (two or more categories)	Interval–ratio	Is there a mean difference in the number of disciplinary referrals by student race and ethnicity?
Within-groups, repeated measures ANOVA	Compare means of a group over two or more points in time	Nominal (two or more times)	Interval–ratio	Is there a mean difference in the number of disciplinary referrals pre-group, post-group, and six months post?
Factorial ANOVA	Compare means and interactions across two or more points in time	Two nominal variables with two or more levels each	Interval–ratio	Is there a mean difference in the number of disciplinary referrals pre-group, post-group, and six months post? Is there a mean difference in the number of disciplinary referrals by gender? Is there an interaction between change in referrals over time and gender?

Test	Purpose	IV Level of Measurement	DV Level of Measurement	Sample Question
Multivariate analysis of variances (MANOVA)	Compare means of two or more groups on two or more related dependent variables	Nominal (two or more levels)	Interval–ratio	Is there a mean difference in the number of disciplinary referrals, days suspended, and externalizing symptoms for participants in the group intervention compared to those receiving treatment as usual?
Analysis of covariance (ANCOVA)	Compare means of two or more groups on dependent variable while accounting for influence of one or more other variables	Nominal (two or more levels)	Interval–ratio	Is there a mean difference in the number of disciplinary referrals for students in the intervention compared to peers when controlling for age?
Multivariate analysis of covariance (MANCOVA)	Compare means of two or more groups on two or more related dependent variables while accounting for influence of one or more other variables	Nominal (two or more levels)	Interval–ratio	Is there a mean difference in the number of disciplinary referrals, days suspended, and externalizing symptoms for participants in the group intervention compared to those receiving treatment as usual when controlling for age?

Tests Regarding Relationships

The most common tests regarding the presence and strength of relationships between variables involve chi-square (χ^2) independence tests and correlations. The differences between tests tend to be focused on levels of data for which the tests can be used. Table 5.4 includes an overview of different ways to test for relationships among variables.

If any of the statistical tests return a *p*-value of <.05, the researcher is responsible for determining the degree of relationship detected. For example, when interpreting chi-square tests of independence, researchers look to effect size (often presented as phi or Cramer's *V*) and compare observed and expected frequency counts to understand the strength of the relationship. For Spearman and Pearson correlations, the test statistic (*r* or *rs*) serves as the effect size. These numbers will range from 0 (indicating no relationship) to +/–1.0 (indicating very strong positive or negative relationship). Again, researchers must use what they know of specific variables of question to decipher meaning in the results.

Tests Regarding Prediction

When we would like to use one or more independent variables to *predict* a dependent variable, we utilize statistical tests within the regression family. These tests vary depending on the specific number and nature of the IVs and DVs involved. Table 5.5 includes an overview of different types of regression.

As you read research articles, you will likely notice a variety of types of multiple linear regressions. For example, researchers can determine whether they would like to

TABLE 5.4 Tests Regarding Relationships

Test	Purpose	Level of Measurement	Sample Question
Chi-square (χ^2) test of independence	Determine whether two categorical variables are related	At least two nominal variables with two or more categories each	Is referral to anger management group (yes/no) independent of race/ethnicity?
Spearman rank-order correlation	Determine degree to which two ordinal-level (or higher) variables are related	Two ordinal variables OR one ordinal and one interval–ratio variable	Is there a relationship between student satisfaction with anger management group (measured on 4-point scale) and number of disciplinary referrals following group?
Pearson product-moment correlation	Determine degree to which two interval-ratio variables are related	Two interval–ratio variables	Is there a relationship between student GPA and number of disciplinary referrals?

TABLE 5.5 Tests Regarding Prediction

Test	Purpose	IV Level of Measurement	DV Level of Measurement	Sample Question
Simple linear regression	Use one interval–ratio variable to predict scores on another	Interval–ratio	Interval–ratio	Does GPA predict number of disciplinary referrals?
Multiple linear regression	Use two or more interval–ratio variables to predict scores on an interval–ratio variable	Two or more interval–ratio variables (note: can do special coding of nominal variables)	Interval–ratio	Do gender, GPA, standardized test scores, and perceived family support predict number of disciplinary referrals?
Logistic regression	Use two or more interval–ratio variables to predict a categorical outcome	Two or more interval–ratio variables (note: can do special coding of nominal variables)	Nominal with two levels	Do gender, GPA, standardized test scores, and perceived family support predict referral to anger management group?

enter all variables into a regression equation at one time (simultaneous regression) *or* intentionally place them in blocks so that the models first account for some variables and then determine the degree to which adding other variables enhances how well the model predicts the dependent variable (hierarchical regression). In each case, the statistical tests produce data to help researchers determine whether and how much the variables combine to predict the dependent variable. The resulting statistical data allow researchers to determine which specific variables contribute to the models and the degree to which they do so.

Types of Significance

There are three primary types of significance we must consider when using inferential statistics: statistical, practical, and clinical (Thompson, 2002). We have already introduced the concept of **statistical significance**. Each statistical test will produce several metrics to determine the probability that there is a relationship among the situations specified. This probability is reported as a p-value. If the *p-value* is less than the pre-selected α-level, one rejects the null hypothesis and concludes there is indeed a "statistically significant" result.

That sounds important, right? We often assume that there must be something very special about a "significant" finding or else it wouldn't be, well, *significant*. And perhaps the smaller the *p*-value, the more significant my results? Right? Not quite. The likelihood of obtaining a statistically significant result (i.e., rejecting the null hypothesis) is directly related to a number of measurement and sample characteristics, most importantly, sample size. The bigger our sample, the more we are able to detect teeny-tiny differences. Statistical significance also assumes generalizability of the study sample to the population *and* stability of the constructs investigated. However, humans are beautifully complex, and the constructs we tend to study are unstable even when participants interact with measures in similar ways (Balkin & Lenz, 2021).

Thus, all findings must be considered in light of two additional types of significance: practical and clinical. **Practical significance**, often assessed via effect sizes, provides an estimate of the *strength* of relationships or impacts among variables. "Effect size is a universal term that refers to any of the metrics that counselors use to represent and interpret the practical, real-world impacts of their observed outcomes" (Balkin & Lenz, 2021, p. 229). For example, if a statistical test indicates that students who completed the anger management group had fewer disciplinary referrals than those who did not, we should want to know (a) how much difference was found and (b) how much of that difference could be attributed to the intervention compared to how much could be attributed to error. Statisticians will use a variety of indices to account for effect size. In addition, we must interpret effect size in context of what we know about the specific field of study. For example, a 10% reduction in disciplinary referrals may not matter as much as a 10% reduction in cancer risk.

A number of scholars have proposed general guidelines for computing and interpreting effect sizes. The specific effect size measures used are directly related to the statistical test and nature of the variables. If you are working with dichotomous variables, you will also find references to odds ratios that compare the likelihood of an outcome happening in one group to the likelihood of it happening in another group. If the odds ratio is 1, there is no difference in likelihood of the outcome between the groups, whereas an odds ratio of 2 means the outcome is two times more likely to occur in one group compared to the other. For example, imagine implementing a program to support high school graduation. An odds ratio of 2 would indicate that students who were in the intervention were twice as likely to graduate than those who did not receive the intervention.

Effect sizes are a bit different when working with continuous variables as they focus on the strength of effect than the odds of an outcome. In this case, look for effect size estimates such as Cohen's d, Glass's Δ, Hedge's g, eta[2] (η^2), Phi φ, and Cramer's V. Also remember that correlations (r) and regressions (R^2) return test statistics that also serve as estimates of effect size. You will see confidence intervals appear in literature regarding effect size as well. In parallel with the other examples in this chapter, a 95% confidence interval would provide us with a reasonable estimate of the true range of the effect size, further supporting interpretation of effects as small, medium, or large. See Balkin and Lenz (2021) and Watson et al. (2016) for additional guidance on effect size. Additionally, we included a link to an online effect size calculator in the resources section at the end of this chapter. Table 5.5 includes some guidance on interpreting effect sizes adapted from Balkin and Lenz (2021).

TABLE 5.5 Interpreting Effect Sizes

Inferential Statistic	Effect Size	Interpretation		
		Small	Medium	Large
Chi-square (χ^2)	Odds ratio	1.68–3.46	3.47–6.70	≥ 6.71
t test, ANOVA	Cohen's *d*, Hedges's *g*	0.20–0.49	0.50–0.79	≥ 0.80
	Cohen's *f*	0.10–0.24	0.25–0.39	≥ 0.40
Bivariate correlation	Pearson's *r*	.10–.29	.30–.49	≥ .50
Chi-square (χ^2)	Cramer's *V*	.10–.29	.30–.49	≥ .50
Spearman rank correlation	ρ	.10–.29	.30–.49	≥ .50
ANOVA, Repeated measures ANOVA	η^2	.01–.05	.06–.13	≥ .14
Multiple regression	R^2	.02–.12	.13–.25	≥ .26

Finally, **clinical significance** refers to the degree to which findings matter to real people in their real-life settings. Some argue that there are no statistical indices or magical tests to determine clinical significance. Rather, we must use what we understand of our clients and students to make these decisions. Let's imagine that the average participant in our running example had four disciplinary referrals, including two suspensions, in the academic quarter leading up to the anger management program. During the academic quarter following the conclusion of the group, the average participant had two disciplinary referrals with no suspensions. Statistical tests indicated that the changes were statistically significant, and effect size estimates indicated a "large" effect. From a real-life standpoint, we see a 50% reduction in referrals *and* we have reason to believe those referrals may have been less severe, as evidenced by a shift to zero suspensions. In all, we might use our clinical expertise to conclude that the program had a very strong impact on participants.

Some researchers believe that it is possible to use statistical strategies to approximate clinical significance (Balkin & Lenz, 2021). These might include estimations based on **percent improvement** from pre-test to post-test. Others look to a **reliable change index,** which is calculated by dividing the difference between pretest and posttest by the standard error of difference. Still others estimate clinical significance through **normative group comparisons**. See Lenz (2020) for more details regarding how to estimate and report clinical significance based on percent improvement.

BOX 5.2 CASE STUDY

Carlson et al. (2018) examined the impact of individual-oriented relationship education on conflict-related relationship behaviors and overall perceptions of relationship equality among a sample of 230 participants from a low-income community. The researchers used the *Intimate Justice Scale* (IJS) as a measure of relationship equality (interval–ratio data) and used cutoff scores for the IJS to place participants into intimate partner violence (IPV) risk categories (ordinal data). They used the *Continuum of Conflict and Control Relationship Scale* (CCC-RS) as a measure of conflict-related relationship behaviors (interval–ratio data). Participants completed both assessments and a demographic form prior to participating in a 12-hour workshop series over the course of one month. The researchers supervised facilitators to ensure fidelity to the intervention. Immediately following the conclusion of the workshop, participants completed the assessments again. Thus, the article represents a single-group design.

The method section of the article indicates that the researchers explored the nature of their descriptive data and preliminary inferential statistics, such as correlations among variables, to ensure they were able to run the most appropriate statistical analyses. Then they used repeated measures mixed between multivariate analysis of variance (MANOVA) with the following variables:

- Within-subjects independent variable: time of assessment (i.e., pre-vs. post-)
- Between-subjects independent variable: violence severity group determined by IJS scores
- Dependent variables: relationship equality (IJS scores), controlling violence, and conflict repair (all CCC-RS subscales)

In the results section, the authors reported "[a] significant interaction existed between time and violence severity group, Wilks's Λ =.88, $F(8, 450) = 3.29$, p =.001, η^2 =.06" (p. 149). In short, this result tells us that participants who had different levels of IPV risk had statistically significant, different responses to the intervention, requiring researchers to examine these results separately. Next, the researchers provided evidence regarding how they concluded that the intervention resulted in changes for those with some or severe violence risk; however, it did not affect those with no violence risk. Carlson et al. provided readers with tables of pre- and post-test means and standard deviation scores and evidence of effect size (η^2) to help readers interpret practical significance.

In the discussion section, the authors attended to statistically significant changes as well as areas that did not change or appeared to worsen. They concluded that the workshop had the greatest impact on those who started the intervention with the greatest severity levels. In the discussion, the researchers addressed clinical significance as they discussed real-life implications of this finding for those who are experiencing IPV and are not advised to participate in couples counseling.

CHAPTER SUMMARY

This chapter included an overview of measurement and statistical concepts you will find when reading research and program evaluation studies. We included attention to levels of variables; descriptive statistics, including measures of central tendency and indices of variability; and inferential statistics focused on differences between groups, relationships between variables, and prediction of variables. We closed the chapter with attention to three types of significance: statistical, practical, and clinical, including a case study intended to help you work through the results section of a published research study focused on a single-group counseling intervention.

RESOURCES

- G*Power. www.gpower.hhu.de/
- Introduction to Hypothesis Testing. www.youtube.com/watch?v=VK-rnA3-41c
- Mathportal.org. www.mathportal.org/calculators/statistics-calculator/
- Online Statistics Education: An Interactive Multimedia Course of Study. http://onlinestatbook.com
- Scales of Measurement: Nominal, Ordinal, Interval and Ratio Scale. www.youtube.com/watch?v=hZxnzfnt5v8
- Social Science Statistics. www.socscistatistics.com/
- Types of Data: Nominal, Ordinal, Interval/Ratio. www.youtube.com/watch?v=hZxnzfnt5v8
- Research Methods Knowledge Database. https://conjointly.com/kb/

REFERENCES

Balkin, R. S., & Lenz, A. S. (2021). Contemporary issues in reporting statistical, practical, and clinical significance in counseling research. *Journal of Counseling & Development*, *99*(2), 227–237. https://doi.org/10.1002/jcad.12370

Carlson, R. G., Wheeler, N. J., & Adams, J. J. (2018). The influence of individual-oriented relationship education on equality and conflict-related behaviors. *Journal of Counseling & Development*, *96*(2), 144–154. https://doi.org/10.1002/jcad.12188

Kalkbrenner, M. T. (2024). Choosing between Cronbach's coefficient alpha, McDonald's coefficient omega, and coefficient *H*: Confidence intervals and the advantages and drawbacks of interpretative guidelines. *Measurement and Evaluation in Counseling and Development*, *57*(2), 93–105. https://doi.org/10.1080/07481756.2023.2283637

Kerlinger, F. N., & Lee, H. B. (2000). Constructs, variables, and definitions. In *Foundations of behavioral research* (4th ed., pp. 39–61). Wadsworth.

Lane, D. M., Scott, D., Hebl, M., Guerra, R., Osherson, D., & Zimmer, H. (n.d.). *Online statistics education: An interactive multimedia course of study*. http://onlinestatbook.com/2/index.html

Lenz, A. S. (2020). Estimating and reporting clinical significance in counseling research: Inferences based on percent improvement. *Measurement and Evaluation in Counseling and Development*, *53*(4), 289–296. https://doi.org/10.1080/07481756.2020.1784758

Lenz, A. S. (2025). Making sense of test score validity in counseling assessment. *Measurement and Evaluation in Counseling and Development*, *58*(1), 1–6. https://doi.org/10.1080/07481756.2025.2445995

Thompson, B. (2002). "Statistical," "Practical," and "Clinical,": How many kinds of significance do counselors need to consider? *Journal of Counseling & Development*, *80*(1), 64–71.

Trochim, W. M. (n.d.). *Research methods knowledge base*. https://conjointly.com/kb/

Watson, J. C., Lenz, A. S., Schmit, M. K., & Schmit, E. L. (2016). Calculating and reporting estimates of effect size in counseling outcome research. *Counseling Outcome Research and Evaluation*, *7*(2), 111–123. https://doi.org/10.1177/2150137816660584

CHAPTER 6

Addressing Ethical, Legal, and Cultural Considerations

Just as counselors are responsible for attending ethical, legal, and cultural considerations throughout our clinical work, we must take special care to ensure our applied research and program evaluation activities are conducted in ways that honor our ethical principles while meeting the unique contextual needs of the communities we serve. In this chapter, we provide a brief overview of ethical and legal standards related to evaluation alongside some practical strategies for managing them. The second half of this chapter includes a summary of cultural considerations in applied research and program evaluation, complete with some steps you may take to ensure your efforts are culturally responsive and relevant to those you serve. The chapter ends with resources for further study.

BOX 6.1 CHAPTER LEARNING OUTCOMES

- Identify ethical standards related to applied research and program evaluation
- Implement strategies to ensure adherence to ethical and legal standards during applied research and program evaluation activities
- Ensure research and program evaluation are culturally responsive and sustaining

BOX 6.2 CASE VIGNETTES

- Maria is a school counseling intern conducting a project on peer mentoring. She plans to use a short survey during group to assess students' sense of belonging before and after six weeks in the program. Maria plans to share her findings in her capstone paper for her graduate program and hopes to be able to present them during a local conference later in the year.

DOI: 10.4324/9781003586210-7

- Rural Mental Health Services evaluates services using anonymous feedback forms. One client provides particularly critical feedback within the context of their experience being the only openly nonbinary individual in the program.
- Jay leads a counseling group for teens in juvenile detention. He wants to assess program effectiveness through a self-report questionnaire, but he worries the clients might feel obligated to participate, especially if they believe it is tied to their case outcomes.
- A counselor educator designs what they believe to be a revolutionary approach to teaching essential counseling skills. They decide to evaluate the effectiveness of their approach by analyzing skills demonstrated in a series of video-recorded role plays students completed as part of a course assignment.

ETHICAL PRINCIPLES AND STANDARDS

The counseling profession is grounded in foundational ethical principles such as autonomy, nonmaleficence, beneficence, justice, fidelity, and veracity (ACA, 2014; Van Hoose, 1986). Just as professional counselors have an ethical imperative to plan interventions and programs with "reasonable promise of success" and to evaluate the effectiveness of their programs and services (ACA, 2014, p. 4), we are responsible for conducting research and evaluation activities in a manner that upholds our ethical principles. Although research tends to be regulated more stringently than program evaluation (more on that in the next section), we are responsible for attending to ethical best practices, regardless of more legalistic status.

A number of organizations have developed ethical standards relevant to conducting research and program evaluation. In this section, we provide a brief overview of standards published by the Office of Research Integrity (ORI; Steneck, 2007), American Counseling Association (2014), and American Evaluation Association (2018). We recommend you take a moment to review these documents in full: all resources are linked at the end of this chapter.

The U.S. Department of Health and Human Services published an *Introduction to the Responsible Conduct of Research* (Steneck, 2007) to "provide a practical overview of the rules, regulation, and professional practices that define the responsible conduct of research" (p. xii). The ORI noted that research should be guided by shared values, including honesty, accuracy, efficiency, and objectivity. In addition, there are minimal standards that *must* be followed (e.g., legal requirements) and standards that *should* be followed (e.g., best practices). Table 6.1 includes a summary of ORI's key concepts; the original source includes elaboration on each point and references to additional resources for understanding requirements and recommendations.

As noted in *Introduction to the Responsible Conduct of Research* (Steneck, 2007), professional organizations also set standards for engagement in research. Section G of

TABLE 6.1 Key Concepts in Responsible Conduct of Research

Concept	Summary
Rules of the road	There are four sources of rules for responsible conduct of research: professional codes, government regulations, institutional policies, and personal convictions.
Research misconduct	Research misconduct can take many forms; there are procedures for reporting and investigating misconduct, as well as protections for whistleblowers and those accused of misconduct.
Protection of human subjects	Research that involves human subjects must comply with federal, state, and local laws and regulations; these include specifications regarding which research is subject to regulation, processes for project approval, training, and ongoing compliance.
The welfare of laboratory animals	Research that involves laboratory animals must comply with rules, policies, and guidelines; these include specifications regarding activities subject to regulation, processes for project approval, training, and ongoing compliance.
Conflicts of interest	Key motivations for research include advancing knowledge, making discoveries that benefit individuals and society, furthering professional advancement, and securing personal gain and satisfaction; conflicts of interests are not inherently wrong, but special steps are taken when identifying conflicts of interest related to financial gain, work commitments, and intellectual and personal matters.
Data management practices	Data management practices must include attention to ownership, collection, storage, and sharing.
Mentor and trainee responsibilities	Mentorship should include clear understanding of basic responsibilities, commitment to appropriate work environment, supervision and review, and a focus on preparing trainees to become successful researchers.
Collaborative research	Collaborative research should include attention to complex roles and relationships, common interests, management requirements, and cultural differences; this requires clear attention to roles and relationships, management plans, and attention to interdisciplinary differences.
Authorship and publication	Research publications should include full and fair description of work, accurate reports of results, and open assessment of findings; this includes attention to authorship, complete attention to publication elements, and avoidance of unethical publication practices (e.g., honorary authorship, salami publication, duplicate publication, and premature public statements).
Peer review	Peer review is used to make decisions regarding funding, publication, personnel, and reliable research; peer review should include careful attention to meeting deadlines, assessing quality, judging importance, preserving confidentiality.

(Adapted from Steneck, 2007)

the *Code of Ethics* (ACA, 2014) offers a number of standards specific to engagement in research and publication. Although these standards are expressly related to research, they provide strong guidance for ensuring ethical practice when conducting program evaluations. Table 6.2 includes a reprint of these standards.

Finally, the American Evaluation Association developed *Guiding Principles for Evaluators* (2018), noting that they reflect the organization's core values and "are intended as a guide to the professional ethical conduct of evaluators" (p. 1). These standards were designed to guide professional evaluators; however, they will also apply to program evaluation work you may do within your agencies and schools. Table 6.3 includes a summary of each of the five major sections of the principles; you can view the principles in their entirety on the organization's webpage.

Taken together, these standards illustrate the importance of attending to ethics throughout the applied research and program evaluation process. The documents highlight responsibility for minimal compliance with legal considerations alongside the use of ethical best practices. Ethical best practices focus on steps taken for ensuring protection of human participants (e.g., informed consent, confidentiality and privacy controls), accurate analysis and reporting, and that our efforts "do good" for the individuals and communities we serve.

TABLE 6.2 American Counseling Association *Code of Ethics* (2014) Section G Research and Program Evaluation

Code	Statement
Introduction	Counselors who conduct research are encouraged to contribute to the knowledge base of the profession and promote a clearer understanding of the conditions that lead to a healthy and more just society. Counselors support the efforts of researchers by participating fully and willingly whenever possible. Counselors minimize bias and respect diversity in designing and implementing research.
G.1 Research Responsibilities	
G.1.a Conducting Research	Counselors plan, design, conduct, and report research in a manner that is consistent with pertinent ethical principles, federal and state laws, host institutional regulations, and scientific standards governing research.
G.1.b Confidentiality in Research	Counselors are responsible for understanding and adhering to state, federal, agency, or institutional policies or applicable guidelines regarding confidentiality in their research practices.
G.1.c Independent Researchers	When counselors conduct independent research and do not have access to an institutional review board, they are bound to the same ethical principles and federal and state laws pertaining to the review of their plan, design, conduct, and reporting of research.

Code	Statement
G.1.d Deviation from Standard Practice	Counselors seek consultation and observe stringent safeguards to protect the rights of research participants when research indicates that a deviation from standard or acceptable practices may be necessary.
G.1.e Precautions to Avoid Injury	Counselors who conduct research are responsible for their participants' welfare throughout the research process and should take reasonable precautions to avoid causing emotional, physical, or social harm to participants.
G.1.f Principal Researcher Responsibility	The ultimate responsibility for ethical research practice lies with the principal researcher. All others involved in the research activities share ethical obligations and responsibility for their own actions.
G.2. Rights of Research Participants	
G.2.a Informed Consent in Research	Individuals have the right to decline requests to become research participants. In seeking consent, counselors use language that 1. accurately explains the purpose and procedures to be followed; 2. identifies any procedures that are experimental or relatively untried; 3. describes any attendant discomforts, risks, and potential power differentials between researchers and participants; 4. describes any benefits or changes in individuals or organizations that might reasonably be expected; 5. discloses appropriate alternative procedures that would be advantageous for participants; 6. offers to answer any inquiries concerning the procedures; 7. describes any limitations on confidentiality; 8. describes the format and potential target audiences for the dissemination of research findings; and 9. instructs participants that they are free to withdraw their consent and discontinue participation in the project at any time, without penalty.
G.2.b Student/ Supervisee Participation	Researchers who involve students or supervisees in research make clear to them that the decision regarding participation in research activities does not affect their academic standing or supervisory relationship. Students or supervisees who choose not to participate in research are provided with an appropriate alternative to fulfill their academic or clinical requirements.
G.2.c Client Participation	Counselors conducting research involving clients make clear in the informed consent process that clients are free to choose whether to participate in research activities. Counselors take necessary precautions to protect clients from adverse consequences of declining or withdrawing from participation.

(Continued)

TABLE 6.2 (Continued)

Code	Statement
G.2.d Confidentiality of Information	Information obtained about research participants during the course of research is confidential. Procedures are implemented to protect confidentiality.
G.2.e Persons Not Capable of Giving Informed Consent	When a research participant is not capable of giving informed consent, counselors provide an appropriate explanation to, obtain agreement for participation from, and obtain the appropriate consent of a legally authorized person.
G.2.f Commitments to Participants	Counselors take reasonable measures to honor all commitments to research participants.
G.2.g Explanations after Data Collection	After data are collected, counselors provide participants with full clarification of the nature of the study to remove any misconceptions participants might have regarding the research. Where scientific or human values justify delaying or withholding information, counselors take reasonable measures to avoid causing harm.
G.2.h Informing Sponsors	Counselors inform sponsors, institutions, and publication channels regarding research procedures and outcomes. Counselors ensure that appropriate bodies and authorities are given pertinent information and acknowledgment.
G.2.i Research Records Custodian	As appropriate, researchers prepare and disseminate to an identified colleague or records custodian a plan for the transfer of research data in the case of their incapacitation, retirement, or death.
G.3 Managing and Maintaining Boundaries	
G.3.a Extending Researcher–Participant Boundaries	Researchers consider the risks and benefits of extending current research relationships beyond conventional parameters. When a nonresearch interaction between the researcher and the research participant may be potentially beneficial, the researcher must document, prior to the interaction (when feasible), the rationale for such an interaction, the potential benefit, and anticipated consequences for the research participant. Such interactions should be initiated with appropriate consent of the research participant. Where unintentional harm occurs to the research participant, the researcher must show evidence of an attempt to remedy such harm.
G.3.b Relationships with Research Participants	Sexual or romantic counselor–research participant interactions or relationships with current research participants are prohibited. This prohibition applies to both in-person and electronic interactions or relationships.
G.3.c Sexual Harassment and Research Participants	Researchers do not condone or subject research participants to sexual harassment.

Code	Statement
G.4 Reporting Results	
G.4.a Accurate Results	Counselors plan, conduct, and report research accurately. Counselors do not engage in misleading or fraudulent research, distort data, misrepresent data, or deliberately bias their results. They describe the extent to which results are applicable for diverse populations.
G.4.b Obligation to Report Unfavorable Results	Counselors report the results of any research of professional value. Results that reflect unfavorably on institutions, programs, services, prevailing opinions, or vested interests are not withheld.
G.4.c Reporting Errors	If counselors discover significant errors in their published research, they take reasonable steps to correct such errors in a correction erratum or through other appropriate publication means.
G.4.d Identity of Participants	Counselors who supply data, aid in the research of another person, report research results, or make original data available take due care to disguise the identity of respective participants in the absence of specific authorization from the participants to do otherwise. In situations where participants self-identify their involvement in research studies, researchers take active steps to ensure that data are adapted/changed to protect the identity and welfare of all parties and that discussion of results does not cause harm to participants.
G.4.e Replication Studies	Counselors are obligated to make available sufficient original research information to qualified professionals who may wish to replicate or extend the study.
G.5 Publications and Presentations	
G.5.a Use of Case Examples	The use of participants', clients', students', or supervisees' information for the purpose of case examples in a presentation or publication is permissible only when (a) participants, clients, students, or supervisees have reviewed the material and agreed to its presentation or publication or (b) the information has been sufficiently modified to obscure identity.
G.5.b Plagiarism	Counselors do not plagiarize; that is, they do not present another person's work as their own.
G.5.c Acknowledging Previous Work	In publications and presentations, counselors acknowledge and give recognition to previous work on the topic by others or self.
G.5.d Contributors	Counselors give credit through joint authorship, acknowledgment, footnote statements, or other appropriate means to those who have contributed significantly to research or concept development in accordance with such contributions. The principal contributor is listed first, and minor technical or professional contributions are acknowledged in notes or introductory statements.

(Continued)

TABLE 6.2 (Continued)

Code	Statement
G.5.e Agreement of Contributors	Counselors who conduct joint research with colleagues or students/supervisors establish agreements in advance regarding allocation of tasks, publication credit, and types of acknowledgment that will be received.
G.5.f Student Research	Manuscripts or professional presentations in any medium that are substantially based on a student's course papers, projects, dissertations, or theses are used only with the student's permission and list the student as lead author.
G.5.g Duplicate Submissions	Counselors submit manuscripts for consideration to only one journal at a time. Manuscripts that are published in whole or in substantial part in one journal or published work are not submitted for publication to another publisher without acknowledgment and permission from the original publisher.
G.5.h Professional Review	Counselors who review material submitted for publication, research, or other scholarly purposes respect the confidentiality and proprietary rights of those who submitted it. Counselors make publication decisions based on valid and defensible standards. Counselors review article submissions in a timely manner and based on their scope and competency in research methodologies. Counselors who serve as reviewers at the request of editors or publishers make every effort to only review materials that are within their scope of competency and avoid personal biases.

Reprinted with permission from American Counseling Association (2014). *Code of ethics*. Author.

TABLE 6.3 American Evaluation Association *Guiding Principles for Evaluators* (2018)

AEA Principle	Summary
Systematic Inquiry: Evaluators conduct data-based inquiries that are thorough, methodical, and contextually relevant.	Guiding principles highlight the importance of adhering to technical standards, exploring limitations and strengths of questions and methods, communicating accurately, owning limitations, giving context to findings, and considering ethical implications of emerging technologies.
Competence: Evaluators provide skilled professional services to stakeholders.	Guiding principles highlight the importance of having appropriate skills to conduct evaluations, recognizing bounds of competencies, building competencies needed within cultural context, and engaging in ongoing professional development.

AEA Principle	Summary
Integrity: Evaluators behave with honesty and transparency in order to ensure the integrity of the evaluation.	Guiding principles highlight the importance of open and truthful communication; disclosures of conflict of interest; communication regarding changes to evaluation plans; clear attention to "stakeholders', clients', and educators' values, perspectives, and interests" regarding the evaluation; transparency in reporting method and results; careful communication around potentially misleading methods or conclusions; and disclosure regarding financial support.
Respect for People: Evaluators honor the dignity, well-being, and self-worth of individuals and acknowledge the influence of culture within and across groups.	Guiding principles highlight the importance of fair attention to stakeholders' perspectives and interests, adherence to ethical considerations, actions to maximize benefits and mitigate risks, and informed consent regarding contributions to the evaluation.
Common Good and Equity: Evaluators strive to contribute to the common good and advancement of an equitable and just society.	Guiding principles highlight the importance of balancing stakeholder interests while promoting integrity of evaluation, identifying the "evaluation's potential threats to the common good," mitigating potential impacts related to inequality, balancing transparency with confidentiality protections, and mitigating bias and power within the evaluation.

Note: Abstracted from American Evaluation Association (2018). *Guiding principles for evaluators*. American Evaluation Association. For complete document, see www.eval.org/About/Guiding-Principles

LEGAL CONSIDERATIONS

When we engage in applied research and program evaluation, we are responsible for adhering to federal, state, and local laws related to our practices. You have likely heard of how the German government conducted torturous medical experiments during World War II, ultimately resulting in international trials and the development of the Nuremberg Code, a set of ethics to guide medical experimentation. In the United States, the Tuskegee syphilis study involved studying long-term impacts of untreated disease among 399 Black men who believed they were receiving treatment; the study went on for 40 years, 26 of which took place after penicillin was determined to be an effective treatment (Centers for Disease Control, 2024). Over time, legal regulations have developed in the face of well-publicized international and domestic human rights violations in the name of research.

Common Rule

In response to the gross injustices of the Tuskegee syphilis study, the National Research Act (Public Law 93–348) was signed into law in 1974, leading to the creation of a commission to consider

> (i) the boundaries between biomedical and behavioral research and the accepted and routine practice of medicine, (ii) the role of assessment of risk-benefit criteria in the determination of the appropriateness of research involving human subjects, (iii) appropriate guidelines for the section of human subjects for participation in such research and (iv) the nature and definition of informed consent in various research settings.
>
> (Office for Human Research Protections, 2018)

This led to what is now known as the *Belmont Report*, a document that serves as the foundation of legal requirements related to research. Currently, the "Common Rule" refers to the Federal Policy for the Protection of Human Subjects (45 Code of Federal Regulations part 46) and includes requirements related to institutional review boards (IRBs), informed consent, and assurances of compliance as they apply to research conducted by federal departments or agencies, including those that receive federal support (i.e., colleges and universities). The Common Rule discussed in this chapter was last updated in 2018.

Although research activities are bound by legal regulations highlighted in this section, program evaluation activities are not regulated as closely. Most notably, quality improvement (QI) and quality assurance (QA) efforts are not considered research and thus are not subject to the Common Rule. The Office for Human Research Protections offers a flow chart for determining whether an activity is research involving human subjects (Figure 6.1).

The Common Rule also exempts some research projects from IRB review. However, the Office for Human Research Protections warns against allowing researchers to make their own determinations of exempt status due to an inherent conflict of interest. Instead, university IRBs will review proposed studies to determine whether an exemption applies. Figure 6.2 includes a flowchart illustrating research projects that may be eligible for exemption. This is particularly relevant because counselors often produce applied research using these methods.

At the most fundamental level, it is important to consider whether the activities in which you are about to engage may comprise "research" and thus be subject to regulation. Figure 6.1 may help you make this determination. If an activity is indeed research, it will need IRB approval. IRB approval will involve submission of study materials and procedures to an objective committee that will conduct a risk–benefit assessment to ensure project methods adhere to fundamental ethical practice and legal requirements.

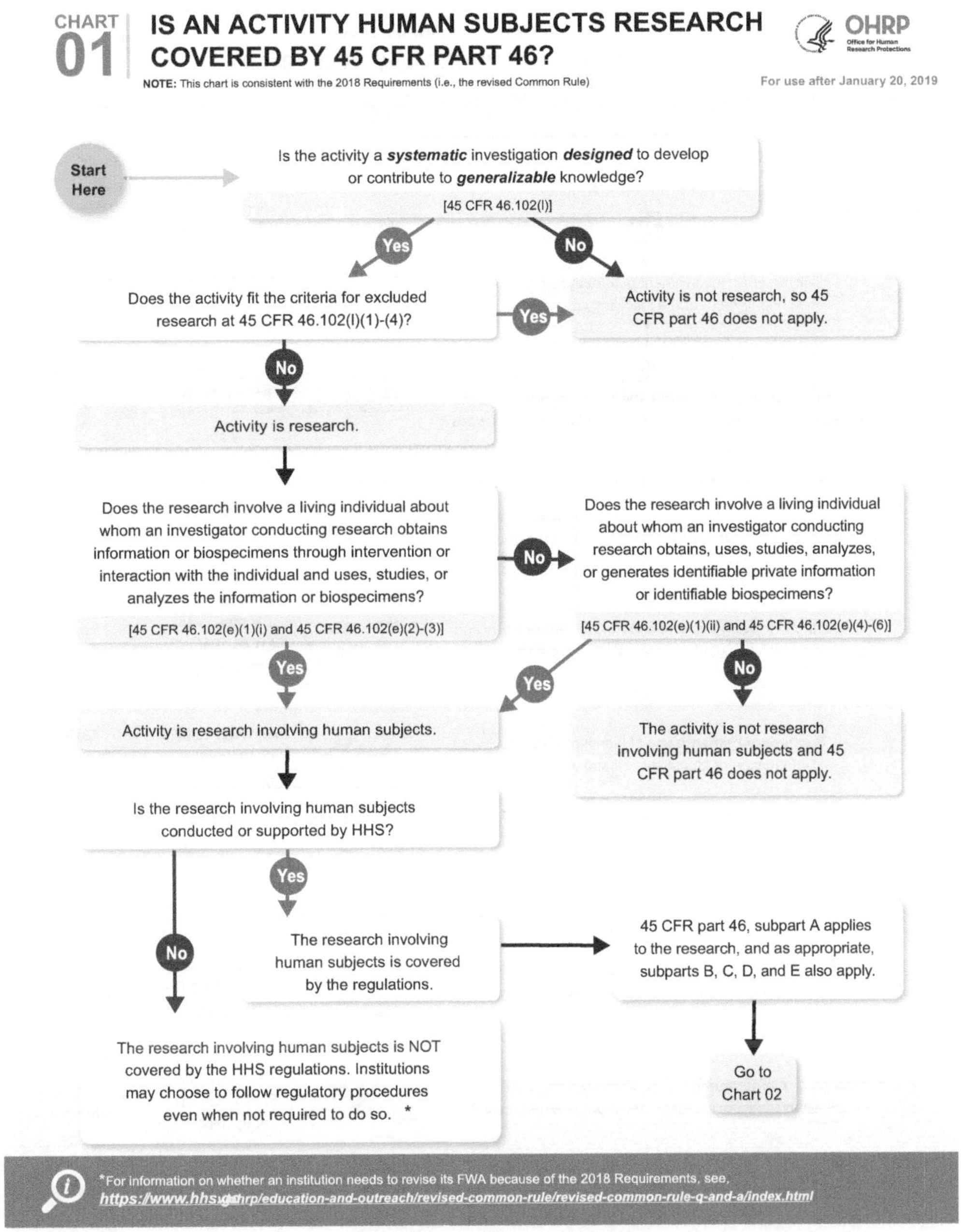

Figure 6.1 Is an activity human subjects research covered by 45 CFR Part 46?

Reprinted from U.S. Department of Health and Human Services, Office for Human Research Protections (2018). *Chart 1: Is an activity human subjects research covered by 45 CFR Part 46?* www.hhs.gov/ohrp/regulations-and-policy/decision-charts-2018/index.html#c1

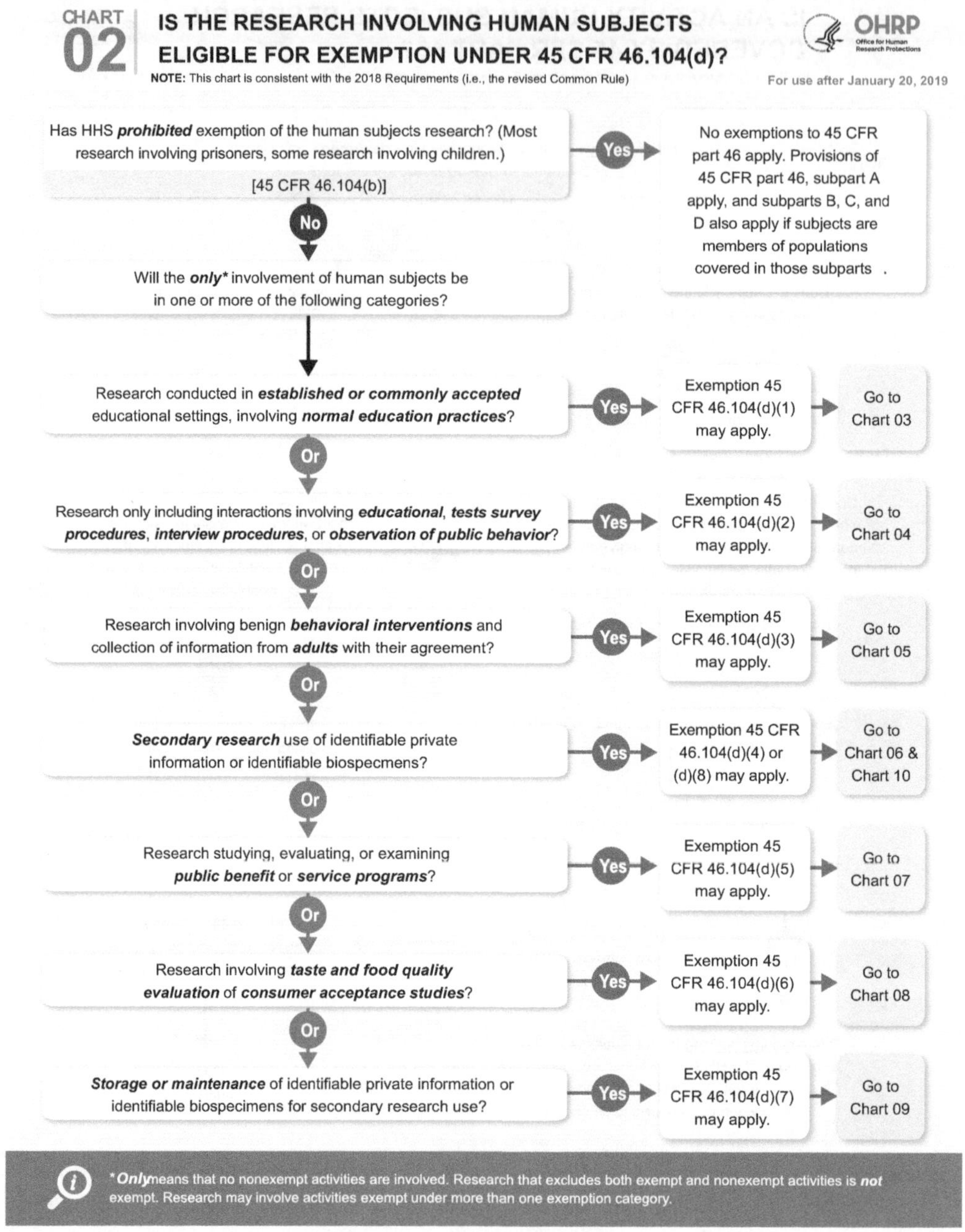

Figure 6.2 Is the research involving human subjects eligible for exemption under 45 CFR 46.104(d)?

Reprinted from U.S. Department of Health and Human Services, Office for Human Research Protections (2018). *Chart 2: Is the research involving human subjects eligible for exemption under 45 CFR 46.104(d)?* www.hhs.gov/ohrp/regulations-and-policy/decision-charts-2018/index.html#c1

A full exploration of legal considerations related to securing IRB approval for research is beyond the scope of this chapter. You may find it helpful to consult the resources listed at the end of this chapter. If you are uncertain regarding whether your activities comprise research, you may consult an IRB within your affiliated college, university, or institutional setting. If your unit does not have an IRB, you may contact an IRB at a public institution near you for consultation. Alternatively, you may seek out services of an independent review board.

BOX 6.3 CHECKLIST: PRACTICAL STRATEGIES FOR MANAGING ETHICAL AND LEGAL CONSIDERATIONS

- Have I confirmed whether my project qualifies as human subjects research covered by 45 CFR Part 46?
- Have I secured IRB approval or consulted an IRB if unsure?
- What protections are needed to ensure informed consent (and assent if applicable) is clear, voluntary, and appropriate to participants' context?
- What steps are needed to ensure participants do not experience coercion when making decisions about participating?
- What protections are needed to ensure participants are not unduly influenced by evaluation or study procedures?
- What protections are needed to ensure participant anonymity, confidentiality, and/or privacy?
- Are confidentiality and data security measures clearly established?
- What protections are needed to protect participants against possible risks or negative experiences?
- Does the project team have the relevant expertise to conduct the activity as planned?
- Does the project team have the relevant expertise to analyze data generated as planned?
- Do all involved parties understand how findings will be used?
- Have I planned how to share results in ways that are accessible to the communities I serve?

Other Legal Regulations

In most cases, your evaluation activities will fit under the quality assurance/improvement (QA/QI) umbrella and not be subject to the Common Rule and related IRB requirements. Still, you have ethical and legal obligations to ensure your activities protect the rights of participants. For example, if you are examining program outcome data, you must ensure that individual level data are handled in a manner that protects privacy as required by the Health Insurance Portability and Accountability Act (HIPAA) and/or Family Educational Rights and Privacy Act (FERPA), as applicable to your setting. In addition, you must take special steps to ensure individuals engage freely in program evaluation activities. This is especially important for vulnerable populations such as children, people with disabilities, and those who are engaged with the correctional system. This means all parties need to understand how their information is used, are not coerced or otherwise pressured to engage in QA/QI activities, and are protected from potential retaliation should they share negative information about a program or process.

BOX 6.4 CASE VIGNETTES REVISITED

Now that you've had a chance to consider ethical and legal considerations related to applied research and program evaluation, let's reconsider the cases from the beginning of the chapter.

- How can Maria determine whether her project qualifies as research, program evaluation, or quality improvement? What steps should she take to ensure informed consent and/or assent from students and/or their guardians? What additional considerations arise if she wants to publish or present findings publicly? How might her dual role as intern and evaluator influence students' responses?
- Even though the Rural Mental Health Services form was anonymous, what confidentiality risks might still exist? What ethical responsibilities does the agency have when presenting or responding to the feedback? How could the evaluator handle identity-specific quotes that could indirectly identify the client?
- What strategies can Jay use to ensure that participation is truly voluntary in this setting? What ethical concerns arise around power and coercion in correctional environments? How should Jay explain the purposes of the questionnaire and address misconceptions? Should Jay pursue IRB consultation or approval for this activity?
- What are the ethical implications of evaluating teaching strategies using course-required assignments? Do students need to give separate consent for their course videos to be used in a study? How can confidentiality and FERPA protections be handled when using student work in research? How might the power differential between faculty and students affect participation or consent?

CULTURAL CONSIDERATIONS

Just as we are responsible for attending to ethical and legal considerations in applied research and program evaluation activities, we are responsible for attending to cultural considerations in these activities. In fact, attending to culture *is* an ethical obligation. We have highlighted cultural considerations throughout this book. Certainly, we must attend to culture when we are considering the relevance of interventions for any given client or client group and developing programs for the unique communities and schools we serve. We must consider cultural responsiveness when entering spaces and selecting measures to capture program outcomes. Culture will be present when we conduct focus groups and interviews to understand the experiences of consumers. And, finally, culture will be at play as we analyze data and make recommendations regarding programs and practices.

BOX 6.5 CASE VIGNETTE

Dr. Nguyen is partnering with a local nonprofit that provides trauma-informed counseling for refugee youth ages 11–17. The program leaders want to evaluate the effectiveness of the intervention in reducing trauma symptoms and enhancing overall well-being. Dr. Nguyen selects several commonly used standardized scales that have evidence of validity primarily with English-speaking adolescents in U.S. public schools.

The staff express concern that some items on the measures don't reflect the lived experiences of the youth they serve—many of whom have experienced displacement, grief, financial hardship, and shifts in family roles. In early pilot testing, younger participants struggle to understand the vocabulary, and several teens systematically skip the same few questions. A few caregivers ask whether the questions are appropriate, particularly ones that inquire about independence and emotional openness.

Unsure of how to proceed, Dr. Nguyen considers whether to revise the instruments or include alternative measures. She wonders how to balance the need for valid outcomes with the developmental, cultural, and linguistic differences of the youth and families served within the program.

It is impossible to separate culture and context in the evaluation process, and active engagement from a variety of parties is essential for a successful, relevant evaluation. Recommendations for culturally responsive evaluation (Tomis, 2025) include strong parallels to the Multicultural and Social Justice Counseling Competencies (Ratts et al., 2016). Counselors need to begin with **self-awareness** and understanding, especially as it relates to their own cultural identities and experiences with the communities served. Just as counselors must work to understand client worldview and experiences, those conducting evaluations should first center **context** of the community and intervention or program in focus through a strength-based lens. Culturally responsive evaluation also requires operating with **humility and respect** in relationships, which includes taking the time to slow down, build relationships, and **understand community and culture** before jumping into the business of an evaluation. It may take quite a bit of time to develop engaged and trusting relationships, especially given historical abuses of power and a drive-by approach where academics may enter spaces to swoop up data and never return (Barrio Minton et al., 2021). Just as with selecting counseling and advocacy interventions, counselors are responsible for working alongside community partners to determine specific evaluation procedures that work within the unique cultural context of those we serve. Any strong evaluation will end with **disseminating findings** in accessible and transparent ways that further benefit the community—you'll learn more about this process in Chapter 17.

Although designed for medical settings, the CDC offers an extensive document in which they propose *Practical Strategies for Culturally Competent Evaluation* (Centers for Disease Control and Prevention, 2014). This publicly available guide includes in-depth discussion regarding the importance of cultural competency in evaluation, as well as practical steps to take in each of six stages of program evaluation. Although we note key points in Box 6.6, please reference the entire document for further exploration and specific self-reflection prompts to guide you through this important process. By drawing upon your multicultural and social justice counseling competencies and using the guiding reflection questions offered by the CDC, you will build capacity to attend to culture throughout your applied research and program evaluation process.

BOX 6.6 PRACTICAL STRATEGIES FOR CULTURALLY COMPETENT EVALUATION (ADAPTED FROM CENTERS FOR DISEASE CONTROL AND PREVENTION, 2014)

1 Engage partners.
   a Assess cultural self-awareness.
   b Engage partners that reflect the diversity of the community.
   c Lay clear ground rules for participation to establish equality.
   d Teach basic evaluation skills along the way.
   e Create a diverse advisory team to help with planning, implementing, and interpreting findings from the evaluation.
   f Build trust.
2 Describe the program.
   a Clarify the partners' perceptions of the program.
   b Affirm what is known about the social and historical context of the program.
   c Highlight community strengths and assets, including the talents and expertise of the members.
   d Use models that resonate with the community.
3 Focus the evaluation design.
   a Ensure that the evaluation questions reflect the partners' values.
   b Consider how aspects of culture might influence an evaluation's design and implementation.
4 Gather credible evidence.
   a Ensure that multiple perspectives are represented when determining "what counts as credible evidence."

   b Select data collection instruments that are culturally responsive for the population of focus.
   c Factor in cultural and linguistic distinctions when planning data collection.
   d Adapt data collection processes to the partner context.
5 Justify conclusions.
   a Recognize potential cultural implications during data analysis.
   b Involve multiple partners in interpreting data.
   c Ensure that many partners' voices are heard when making judgments.
6 Ensure the use of evaluation findings and share lessons learned.
   a Ensure that recommendations are generated through an inclusive process.
   b Tailor the dissemination of evaluation results to partner and community needs.
   c Encourage the use of evaluation information to enhance practice.

Culturally Responsive Research in Action

Professional counselors have a number of resources available to support our engagement in culturally responsive research. Phipps et al. (2025) provided a Culturally Sensitive Research Conceptual framework to help counselors address longstanding biases in research and ways of knowing while working toward equity and justice. This framework includes four steps with corresponding prompts and discussion questions to guide counselors through the process of considering their own orientation and purpose in research, explicating design and methodological decisions as they relate to the unique populations served, integrating analysis and skills within community, and reporting on findings in ways that are relevant, respectful, and impactful.

Specific approaches to counseling research are also well-suited to culturally responsive research. Decolonizing methods and relational-cultural theory (RCT) are also well-aligned for building respectful, engaged, collaborative relationships with marginalized communities (Hipolito-Delgado et al., 2025). Specifically, decolonizing perspectives include questioning Western assumptions, deficit-frameworks, and power dynamics through critical reflexivity. These can pair with RCT frameworks that center mutuality and connection in the context of power and oppression. In addition, community-based participatory research (CBPR) aligns with the MSJCCs and is ideal for bridging research-practice gaps in ethical and culturally relevant ways (Trott et al., 2024). Likewise, research approaches that center dialogue, storytelling, art, or movement may be well-aligned to the cultural beliefs and values of diverse communities. By pulling from these traditions, counselors can help ensure that their research questions and processes are aligned with our commitments to celebrating human dignity and diversity.

BOX 6.7 CHECKLIST FOR DESIGNING CULTURALLY RESPONSIVE RESEARCH

- Have I reflected on my own cultural identities, biases, and positionality before designing the project?
- Have I consulted with or partnered with individuals or groups from the community being studied?
- Does the research question reflect issues or needs identified by the community?
- To what degree are the constructs and measures culturally relevant and appropriate for the population of focus?
- To what degree have I planned to use methods (e.g., interviews, surveys, focus groups) that are congruent with cultural values and practices?
- Have I ensured participation is voluntary and inclusive?
- Have I established protocols to build trust and meaningful relationships before and during the research?
- Have I considered power dynamics and created ways for community voices to shape the process and interpretation?
- Are dissemination plans accessible, useful, and empowering to the communities involved?
- Have I committed to sharing credit and benefits with the community (e.g., co-authorship, training, local presentations)?

BOX 6.8 CASE VIGNETTE REVISITED

Now that you've had an opportunity to learn a bit about how cultural considerations are present in counseling research, let's revisit the Dr. Nguyen's situation. By reflecting on the following questions, you will position yourself to both critique research with attention to cultural considerations and to design more responsive interventions.

1. How might the cultural backgrounds and life experiences of youth in the program shape how they interpret and respond to the standardized measures?
2. What might the observed patterns of skipped questions indicate?
3. How could Dr. Nguyen ensure the measures are developmentally appropriate for youth across the entire 11–17-year-old age range?
4. What are the potential consequences of using standardized instruments that may not reflect participants' cultural or developmental realities?
5. How could Dr. Nguyen respectfully involve caregivers and staff in identifying the constructs most relevant for the community served?

6. How could Dr. Nguyen collaborate with staff and family members to design data collection methods that are responsive to communication norms and community values?
7. How can Dr. Nguyen ensure that the research is framed in empowerment rather than deficit?

CHAPTER SUMMARY

This chapter focused on practical resources for attending to ethical, legal, and cultural considerations throughout applied research and program evaluation practices. This includes attending to both minimal and best practices related to responsible conduct of research and program evaluation. In addition, we reviewed strategies for determining whether your work represents research that falls under the Common Rule or falls within the QI/QA umbrella. Even when our activities do not fall under the Common Rule, it is important to protect participants and ensure appropriate privacy protections within your specific setting. Finally, we reviewed the importance of cultural responsiveness throughout the research and program evaluation process. Resources from the CDC (2014), UConn Extension (Tomis, 2025), and within the counseling profession provide practical guides for attending to cultural considerations in your applied research and evaluation activities.

RESOURCES

- American Counseling Association Code of Ethics. www.counseling.org/docs/default-source/default-document-library/ethics/2014-aca-code-of-ethics.pdf
- American Evaluation Association *Guiding Principles for Evaluators*. www.eval.org/About/Guiding-Principles
- CITI Program. https://about.citiprogram.org/en/homepage/
- Office for Human Rights Protections (www.hhs.gov/ohrp) and The Belmont Report. www.hhs.gov/ohrp/regulations-and-policy/belmont-report/index.html
- Office of Research Integrity https://ori.hhs.gov/ and *Introduction to the Responsible Conduct of Research*. Retrieved from https://ori.hhs.gov/ori-introduction-responsible-conduct-research
- Phipps, G. S., Anandavalli, S., Moh, Y. S., & Jenkins, K. (2025). Inquiry with intention: Fostering cultural sensitivity in counseling research. *Counselor Education and Supervision*, Online first. https://doi.org/10.1002/ceas.12340
- Tomis, S. (2025). Culturally responsive extension program evaluation. UConn Extension Publication EXT 115. https://doi.org/10.61899.ucext.v2.115.2025
- Wester, K. L. (2011). Publishing ethical research: A step-by-step overview. *Journal of Counseling & Development*, *89*(3), 301–307.

REFERENCES

American Counseling Association. (2014). Code of ethics. Author.

American Evaluation Association. (2018). Guiding principles for evaluators. https://www.eval.org/About/Guiding-Principles

Barrio Minton, C. A., Gibbons, M. M., & Hightower, J. M. (2021). Community-engaged research and evaluation in counseling: Building partnerships and applying program evaluation. *Journal of Counseling & Development*, *99*(2), 210–220. https://doi.org/10.1002/jcad.12368

Centers for Disease Control. (2024). *About the untreated syphilis study at Tuskegee*. https://www.cdc.gov/tuskegee/about/index.html

Centers for Disease Control and Prevention. (2014). *Practical strategies for culturally competent evaluation*. Atlanta, GA: U.S. Department of Health and Human Services.

Hipolito-Delgado, C. P., Kwag, D., & Sharma, J. (2025). Relationships and collaboration: engaging in research with marginalized communities. *Counselor Education and Supervision*, *64*(2), 278–286. https://doi.org/10.1002/ceas.12338

Office for Human Research Protections. (2018). The Belmont report. www.hhs.gov/ohrp/regulations-and-policy/belmont-report/read-the-belmont-report/index.html

Phipps, G. S., Anandavalli, S., Moh, Y. S., & Jenkins, K. (2025). Inquiry with intention: Fostering cultural sensitivity in counseling research. *Counselor Education and Supervision*, Online first. https://doi.org/10.1002/ceas.12340

Ratts, M. J., Singh, A. A., Nassar-McMillan, S., Butler, S. K., & McCullough, J. R. (2016). Multicultural and Social Justice Counseling Competencies: Guidelines for the counseling profession. *Journal of Multicultural Counseling and Development*, *44*(1), 28–48. https://doi.org/10.1002/jmcd.12035

Steneck, N. H. (2007). *Introduction to the responsible conduct of research*. American Psychological Association. https://doi.org/10.1037/e638422011-001

Tomis, S. (2025). *Culturally responsive extension program evaluation*. UConn Extension Publication EXT 115. https://doi.org/10.61899.ucext.v2.115.2025

Trott, A., Suri, T., & Chávez, T. A. (2024). A CBPR approach to multicultural and socially just counseling research. *Counselor Education and Supervision*, *63*(4), 379–391. https://doi.org/10.1002/ceas.12305

Van Hoose, W. H. (1986). Ethical principles in counseling. *Journal of Counseling & Development*, *65*(3), 168.

CHAPTER 7

Using Literature to Support Counseling Research and Practice

By now, you have likely heard multiple instructors and authors comment about the importance of using evidence to support counseling practice. Terms like *evidence-informed*, *evidence-supported*, and *evidence-based practices* appear throughout accreditation standards and in the literature, and the need to bridge research and practice inspired this text. This chapter opens with a recap of evidence-based practice before building upon the foundational understanding that you've developed regarding the purposes of research and program evaluation, how interventions and programs work, and methodological and statistical concepts that cut across all types of literature. Now, it's time to put the wheels into motion. In the first part of this chapter, we will try to demystify what you will find in peer-reviewed journal articles and evaluation reports. In the second part of this chapter, we focus your attention to some practical tools for searching the literature and locating resources beyond the university library. We outline some go-to places to search for resources before providing guidance for how you might evaluate these resources within your unique context. We conclude with a case study and a few resources for assessing the quality and relevance of research for practice.

BOX 7.1 CHAPTER LEARNING OUTCOMES

- Understand the relevance of literature for informing counseling practice
- Describe standard components of journal articles
- Identify evidence-based practices using a variety of methods, including those that do not require access to a university library
- Critique literature regarding evidence-based practices with special attention to your client population and setting

EVIDENCE-BASED PRACTICE

We opened Chapter 1 with a discussion regarding the importance of blending art and science in counseling. Although less tangible relational qualities are clearly vital for counseling outcomes, we also have a compelling charge to ensure we offer interventions

DOI: 10.4324/9781003586210-8

and programs that have a reasonable promise of success. We live in an era of accountability, and counselors across a variety of settings are responsible for justifying their choice of approaches and producing evidence that our services make a difference in the lives of those we serve.

To recap Chapter 1, evidence-based practice features the "integration of the best available research within clinical expertise in the context of patient characteristics, culture, and preferences" (APA Presidential Task Force on Evidence-based Practice, 2006, p. 273). Identifying specific practices supported by research is one very important leg of a three-legged stool with responsiveness to client characteristics and reference to clinical expertise comprising the other two legs (Melchert et al., 2024; Tolin et al., 2015). Although all resources may be useful in some way, not all sources of evidence are equal. For example, a meta-analysis of 30 different outcome studies likely offers more compelling evidence than any single study included in the analysis. However, specific articles included in the analysis may tell us something valuable about the nuances of implementation with our specific population or context.

When designing counseling interventions and programs (see Chapter 2), we must integrate what we know about evidence-supported practices and what we know of our unique client population with high-quality accessible resources. Although we hope that all counselors will be lifelong learners, our learning shifts as we enter the world of practice. In most settings, our time is filled with client contact and administrative responsibilities. Much of what we learn will come from conferences, continuing education, and what we can access through our Internet browsers. With limited exceptions for those who write grants to fund programs, we will rarely conduct extensive literature reviews or write papers to support our counseling decisions. Thus, we need a practical strategy for identifying best practice resources that is both accessible and realistic for life as a professional counselor.

DEMYSTIFYING JOURNAL ARTICLES

Now that you have a working understanding of types of research, methodological considerations, and measurement and statistical concepts, it's time to see how these elements work together. In Part II of this text, you will learn about hallmarks and quality indicators of specific of types of research questions and methods you will encounter in peer-reviewed research. Understanding of the specific design choices in any given study will be important for assessing the quality of the article and the degree to which you can have confidence in the findings as relevant to your practice. For now, let's dive into the sections you can expect to find in a journal article. We recommend that you read this section alongside a recently published article from your favorite professional counseling journal so you can see reporting standards in action.

The American Psychological Association (APA) publishes a set of *Journal Article Reporting Standards* (JARS; https://apastyle.apa.org/jars) that are commonly used across journals in our discipline. These provide guidelines to authors that are specific to quantitative (JARS-Quant), qualitative (JARS-Qual), and mixed methods (JARS-Mixed) research. The APA also offers a guide for discussing race, ethnicity, and culture in journal articles (JARS-REC), as well as a number of supplemental JARS guidelines for specific research design types. As a result, many counseling and psychology journals now require that authors submit manuscripts in accordance with JARS. When authors use JARS to present their work, they do so in a systematic, predictable manner that should make your job as a reader easier. You can access JARS through the link above, so this section includes just a synopsis to guide your journey through an article.

Journal articles should open with a descriptive **title** and information about the **authors**, including funding, possible conflicts of interest, and contact information. They should also include an **abstract** that provides a very concise overview of the purpose of the study, participants, method, and findings.

The **introduction and literature review** will typically span several pages and articulate the focus of the issue or concern in a compelling way. Within the first page, you should have a clear understanding of why the problem is important to study, particularly in the context of counseling practice or policy. In the pages to follow, the authors should provide a concise yet thorough review of relevant literature to help readers understand what is already known and what remains unknown about the topic. For example, if the article focuses on a counseling intervention for anxiety among elementary-aged youth, the literature review might begin with data on the increasing prevalence of anxiety disorders in children post-COVID. Then, the authors might provide an overview of evidence-based practices for treating childhood anxiety with a larger focus on a specific intervention that is promising for addressing childhood anxiety. The review should end with a summary of findings from previous research, limitations, and unanswered questions. For example, if existing interventions are promising but have all been conducted with youth in grades 3–5 while children are having earlier-onset anxiety, there would be a good reason to investigate developmental adaptations for youth in grades K–2. In all, this section should end with a clear statement of the problem or need and plainly stated research questions or hypotheses that were addressed in the study.

The **method** section should open with a clear statement of the specific design utilized in the study. Remember, Chapters 8–14 of this text include details that will help you understand the purposes and characteristics of most methods you will encounter. Next, the article should clearly provide the inclusion and exclusion criteria and characteristics of the resulting participant sample. At a minimum, authors should disclose age, sex or gender identity, race, and ethnicity. Authors may also include additional details relevant to the unique sample or context. Qualitative articles should also include a description of the researchers, including their positionality and experiences or assumptions related to the topic of focus (i.e., reflexivity). Next, authors should provide details regarding procedures for recruiting and selecting participants or other data sources. Read these sections carefully so you can assess the degree to which the participant sample may or may not generalize or transfer to your setting.

Qualitative and quantitative articles will diverge a bit at this point. However, you can expect to see clear and transparent reporting of any instruments or assessment tools used in the research as well as specific steps taken for data collection. The method section should conclude with a detailed accounting of the strategies researchers used to analyze their data. Qualitative studies should have an additional section on methodological integrity. In short, by the end of the method section, you should be able to answer the question "what happened here?" In other words, who was in the study, what they did, and how researchers worked with data to construct results or findings.

The **results** (quantitative) or **findings** (qualitative) section will appear next. This section will vary considerably depending on the specific nature of the inquiry. In quantitative research, you can expect to see research questions covered systematically. This will include results of inferential statistics inclusive of statistical, practical, and clinical significance (see Chapter 5). In qualitative research, authors will present findings such as themes, categories, theories, or models that emerged from their analysis. You can expect them to use participants' words to illustrate the findings and deepen meaning and understanding.

The final section of any article is the **discussion**. In the discussion section, authors will work to interpret their findings in light of existing literature. They should compare and contrast their results with those from other sources, offering possible interpretations for surprising or new findings. After a brief discussion, authors should offer a transparent assessment of the limitations of their study prior to transitioning to implications for future research and practice. Implications are "next steps" or marching orders. The recommendations authors make here should have a transparent link to their unique findings.

It may be tempting to read just the introduction and skip to the discussion and counseling implications. We encourage you to slow down and take time with the article as a whole. The method and results/findings sections have important information you will need to be able to digest in order to assess the nature and strength of evidence presented and the relevance of the article for informing your own practice or inquiry. A resource at the end of this chapter includes some reflection questions you might find helpful for guiding your assessment of any article or piece of evidence.

NAVIGATING LIBRARY RESOURCES

If you have the luxury of access to an academic library, it is important to understand the many resources available to you. Most libraries offer a number of **databases** for searching. These digital collections of articles, books, and industry reports are often specific to subject matter. Some resources, like Academic Search Complete or ProQuest Central are appropriate for broad searches. Other sources, like PsychINFO (psychology), ERIC (education), and CINAHL (nursing and allied health) are discipline-specific. Some resources (e.g., Scopus, Web of Science) include only citations and abstracts, while others include full-text articles. Don't shy away from citation-only resources; many universities integrate them with other tools that allow you to easily access PDF downloads from their collection. In all, it will be up to you to select databases that are appropriate to your study. Most universities have extensive help documents, subject matter guides, and tutorials to help you understand the resources at your disposal. Professional counseling has roots in both psychology and education. If your institution does not have a specific counseling or counselor education subject guide, check out the guides for psychology and education.

Once you've identified the database(s) most appropriate for your search, it is important to formulate quality searches. Effective literature searches rely on carefully selected keywords. Because researchers and practitioners often use different terms to describe similar concepts, limiting your search to a single word or phrase may yield incomplete results. For example, a researcher interested in the counseling relationship might miss key studies that use related terms such as therapeutic alliance, working alliance, helping relationship, or rapport. This is why we recommend searching for the terms you *think* you will need. Pay careful attention to subject terms and keywords that pop up in your initial findings, using those findings to adjust your search approach. This initial step may help you to identify additional terms to use in your search.

Once you've identified your keywords or subject terms, you are ready to form search strings to identify literature related to your questions. To do this, we recommend careful use of Boolean operators to refine your search results. Check out Box 7.2 for some search tips and examples.

BOX 7.2 TIPS AND TRICKS FOR SEARCHING DATABASES

Boolean Operators

Boolean operators help us combine keywords to narrow or broaden our searches. There are three main types of operators:

- AND narrows your search, telling the database you want results that include all of your terms (e.g., trauma AND counseling)
- OR broadens your search, telling the database you want results that include any of the terms (e.g., counseling OR therapy OR intervention)
- NOT excludes results, telling the database you want to filter out results with a certain term (e.g., trauma NOT loss; addiction NOT alcohol)

There are several other tools to use when creating search strings:

- Quotation marks tell the engine to look for exact phrases (e.g., "post-traumatic growth" or "counseling relationship")
- An asterisk tells the engine to look for all variations of a word up to that point (e.g., counsel* will return counselling, counseling, counselor, and counsellor; therap* will return therapy, therapist, and therapeutic)
- Parenthesis allow us to create complex searches. For example
  - (counsel* OR therapy OR intervention) AND (trauma* OR PTSD OR post-traumatic stress)
  - ("cultural humility" OR "multicultural competence") AND ("therapeutic alliance" OR "counseling relationship" OR "working alliance" OR "therapeutic relationship")
  - ("mental health" OR wellness or well-being or wellbeing) AND ("college students" OR "emerging adult*")

Clear as mud? Practice a bit, and you'll get the hang of it in no time. We find it much more fulfilling to sift through 50 hits on our topic area than 50,000. There's one more highly under-utilized resource at your disposal. At the risk of a gross overgeneralization that warrants some hypothesis testing, we can think of only one group of professionals who enjoy being helpful even more than counselors do: **librarians!** We strongly recommend making use of your library's tutorials and resources. If you find yourself lost or wanting to fine-tune your process, reach out to your librarian. They have a wealth of resources at their fingertips. In our experience, most won't stop until you have access to the resources you desire and have the skills to implement on your own in the future.

LOCATING RESOURCES BEYOND THE UNIVERSITY LIBRARY

Whether you are a student now or you were in the past, you are likely well aware of the riches of resources available to you through a university library. The university library is a go-to place for locating peer-reviewed research to support coursework or counseling practices. Of course, academic and public libraries also offer books. We've skipped over that part because we are fairly sure you understand that piece. But what happens when you don't have access to the same search engines? Or what happens when you find a promising article and you click through only to find that it will cost you $49 to view, a steep price to pay out of pocket and the reality that you might realize on page two that the article is not useful for your needs?

The resources presented in the next part of this chapter may be important workarounds if you don't have access to a university library. However, you likely have more access to traditional resources than you think. In addition to offering physical and digital books for loan, public libraries offer access to databases that feature peer-reviewed journal articles. Many university libraries—especially those at public universities—are open to the public, even if they require a visitor pass or a library card. Some may charge a nominal fee for semester-long access. You may not be able to surf these resources from the convenience of your office or while cuddled under a blanket with your favorite pet, but a field trip to a brick and mortar library will likely yield a computer terminal with access to the resources we hope you engaged throughout your graduate study. Additionally, if you are working in a school or have a child in school, you likely have access to their academic library databases, some of which will allow remote access. Finally, a number of journals are moving to open-access or hybrid formats where researchers pay a fee to make articles available to the public. Public universities and grant funders will often pay these fees, especially for meta-analyses, systematic reviews, or rigorous clinical trials that offer the most promising evidence for practice. In all, check out your access options before you assume that you do not have access to current research.

Although accessing public or university libraries is an important step for locating research regarding evidence-based practices, there are a few other resources you should consider in your work. In the following sections, we address best practice guidelines, clearinghouses and registries, federal resources, and university partnerships as resources to consider.

Best Practice Guidelines

Best practice guidelines or statements are most often developed and endorsed by a cadre of experts using their interpretation of the research literature and clinical expertise. Often, professional organizations will commission the development of these guidelines and then endorse or adopt them, formatting them in a way that is readily accessible to practitioners. Scholars who are operating independently may also develop best practice guidelines. In some cases, these guidelines will be published on organization websites; however, they may also appear in peer-reviewed journals. As with any resource, it is important to consider the quality and context of the source, perhaps giving more weight to guidelines developed and adopted by a professional community compared to those developed independently.

The Substance Abuse and Mental Health Services Administration (SAMHSA) Evidence-Based Practices Resource Center (www.samhsa.gov/libraries/evidence-based-practices-resource-center) provides a list of organization websites on which you can find best practice guidelines that were vetted by the organization. To be included in the guide, the websites must include specific information, pay attention to multiple evidence-based practices, and be free to access. The web guide includes a listing of resources specific to substance abuse prevention, substance abuse treatment, prevention of mental health disorders, mental health treatment, and adult evidence-based practices.

Additionally, you may find the following tips helpful for locating best practice guidelines:

- Identify general professional organizations (e.g., American Counseling Association, American Psychological Association) or specialty-focused organizations (e.g., International Society for Traumatic Stress Studies, Anxiety and Depression Association of America, National Child Traumatic Stress Network) relevant to the topic. Look for a link that indicates resources or tools for practitioners.
- Search for variations of your topic using terms such as "best practice," "best practice guidelines," and "practice statement."
- Using a library database, search using variations of your topic and terms such as "best practice," "best practice guidelines," and "practice statement."

Although this list is not comprehensive, you may find the following websites helpful for identifying best practice guidelines:

- American Counseling Association Competencies & Exemplary Practices: www.counseling.org/resources/competencies
- American Counseling Association Practice Briefs: www.counseling.org/resources/practice-briefs
- American Mental Health Counselors Association Practice Guidelines: www.amhca.org/events/publications/practiceguidelines
- American Psychiatric Association Clinical Practice Guidelines: www.psychiatry.org/psychiatrists/practice/clinical-practice-guidelines

- American Psychological Association Approved Standards and Guidelines: www.apa.org/research-practice/standards-guidelines
- American Psychological Association Professional Practice Guidelines: www.apa.org/practice/guidelines/index.aspx
- Anxiety and Depression Association of America Clinical Practice Tools: https://adaa.org/resources-professionals/practice-guidelines-tools
- International Society for Traumatic Stress Studies Clinical Resources: https://istss.org/clinical-resources/
- National Association of Social Workers Practice Standards and Guidelines: www.socialworkers.org/Practice/Practice-Standards-Guidelines
- SAMHSA Evidence-Based Practices Resource Center: www.samhsa.gov/libraries/evidence-based-practices-resource-center

Clearinghouses and Registries

Some organizations offer clearinghouses or registries related to evidence-based programs. Most generally, a clearinghouse operates as an intermediary between two groups. A clearinghouse may provide an online space for scholars who developed interventions and programs to share information and evidence in support of them. Then, potential consumers of the programs or practices (i.e., counselors) can come to one convenient place to locate resources.

Sometimes clearinghouses offer registries or searchable lists of resources on a particular topic. Registries may include opportunities for those who have developed programs or practices to share information about the method as well as evidence to support use. As with any resource, clearinghouses and registries vary in quality, with some approving all programs submitted and others using a rigorous peer review process to determine what to include.

The SAMHSA, a federal agency, offers the Evidence-Based Practices Resource Center (previously known as the National Registry of Evidence-Based Programs and Practices). The center

> aims to provide communities, clinicians, policy-makers and others in the field with the information and tools they need to incorporate evidence-based practices into their communities or clinical settings. The Resource Center contains a collection of scientifically-based resources for a broad range of audiences, including Treatment Improvement Protocols, toolkits, resource guides, clinical practice guidelines, and other science-based resources.
>
> (SAMHSA, 2024)

You may locate additional registries and clearinghouses by searching for your topic or population of focus and adding terms such as "clearinghouse" or "registry."

Federal Resources

We have already previewed SAMHSA as an important federal resource for locating evidence-based practices. You may also find a number of other federal resources helpful for locating evidence-based practices and even engaging in (often free) continuing education related to these practices. Generally, domain names for federal resources end in.gov, letting you know that this is a government-funded or sponsored resource.

Although this list is not comprehensive, you may find the following federal resources helpful starting points for identifying best practices and related training:

- Administration for Children and Families: www.acf.hhs.gov
- Centers for Disease Control and Prevention: www.cdc.gov
- Child Welfare Information Gateway: www.childwelfare.gov
- Department of Education: https://ed.gov
- National Center for PTSD: www.ptsd.va.gov/
- National Institute on Drug Abuse: www.nida.nih.gov/
- National Institute of Mental Health: www.nimh.nih.gov
- Substance Abuse and Mental Health Services Administration (SAMHSA): www.samhsa.gov

University Partnerships

Although not a formal search tool, we would like to remind you that you need not set out on your quest for evidence-based interventions and programs alone. As you complete work within your agency or school, remember that universities and faculty members are often more than happy to develop and sustain community partnerships, especially when those partnerships support the mission of the university. Graduate students routinely participate in field placements that are part of university partnership: the agency or school provides clinical experience and supervision, and the university provides well-prepared personnel to offer services and run programs. CACREP accreditation standards even require that programs provide ongoing technical assistance and consultation to agencies and schools where students are placed.

We close this section by reminding you to seek out university partnerships beyond graduation. You may well find yourself connected with a faculty member who has content expertise related to your area of focus or possesses evaluation expertise that can help you get funded and justify your programs. Like many counselor educators, we routinely engage with community partners and nonprofits as they plan and evaluate their services. University partners may be quite familiar with the best practice literature, have access to traditional library resources (on more than one occasion, the first author has happily sent relevant articles along to a community collaborator), and long for a connection to the type of place that inspired their academic journey in the first place.

Additionally, authors across disciplines tend to be delighted to know that someone beyond the ivory tower is using their work. If you come across an article that's behind a paywall but you think might be helpful to your practice, you can typically find the author's contact information at the very beginning or end of the article. Reach out and let the author know you are a practicing counselor who thinks their article "From Scales to Fur: Comparing the Therapeutic Impact of Goldfish, Ferrets, and Dogs" would be helpful for your practice. Many authors are permitted to share copies of their articles for individual use. You won't know unless you ask, and we hope you ask.

BOX 7.3 CASE STUDY

In Chapter 8, you'll meet a school counselor who surveyed community members at Prairieview Middle School as part of a broader needs assessment related to bullying in the school. The needs assessment indicated strong evidence of bullying in the school environment, with over three quarters of students indicating that students are teased about clothing or physical appearance and over one half agreeing that bullying is a problem at the school. About two thirds of students reported being bullied at school during this school year, including 30% who were bullied once a week or more. In response to the needs assessment, the school board allocated additional funding for a staff in-service training and a bullying program for students.

The school counselor searched Google for "evidence-based bullying programs" and immediately found several promising hits related to the topic. In addition to a number of state-sponsored websites, she identified www.stopbullying.gov. The webpage included a section specific to what schools can do, and the counselor was able to find some concrete resources to guide school policy and the staff in-service training. She also found a section titled "research resources" that included well-cited fact sheets, resource summaries, and infographics.

Further examination of search results brought the school counselor to School-Based Bullying Prevention at www.ojjdp.gov. Through this resource, she was able to link to a practice profile that highlighted common practice components, outlined meta-analysis outcomes, and linked her to related programs. For each program, she was able to review a synopsis including a description of the program, evaluation outcomes, evaluation methodology, cost, details for implementation, and original sources. Together, these resources provided the team a strong starting point for considering the usefulness of these policies and programs for their unique school.

EVALUATING RESOURCES IN CONTEXT

Once you have identified best practice resources and other literature to support your counseling practice, it is important to evaluate the quality and relevance of the source for your population and focus. Sure, a 20-session intervention may be lovely and well supported by the literature, but if structural constraints are such that you have, at most, 6 sessions, that 20-session intervention isn't going to be of much use to you (unless, of course, you use data to advocate for a change in policy—but that's another chapter). You may also find a program that promises the moon; however, closer inspection indicates a domain that ends in.com, a steep price point, and no mention in any scholarly literature despite website claims. How can you know whether this program would be a good investment? Or what should you do with that program that was piloted on a

White, upper-middle-class population and assumes heavy parental involvement when you are in an agency working primarily with ethnically diverse clients in foster care?

The examples here highlight the importance of reviewing the technical quality of resources *and* relevance for your unique context. The information provided throughout this book will establish a foundation for your critique. For example, if you are reviewing an article focused on a randomized control trial, you may find it helpful to check out Chapter 12 to see how closely the authors adhered to guidelines for that methodology. The checklist in this chapter provides some core questions you can use to determine the usefulness of any resource for your specific practice needs.

BOX 7.4 CHECKLIST FOR EVALUATING RESOURCES FOR PRACTICE

- What is the **nature** of the piece I am reviewing? Is it a peer-reviewed article, consensus or best practice statement, or general access website?
- Who is the **author** of the piece I am reviewing? Is it an individual, a group of individuals, or an organization? What are their credentials and motivations?
- What do I know about the **source** of the piece I am reviewing? How well respected and well vetted does the source appear to be?
- Where does the piece I am reviewing **fall on the hierarchies** of evidence? Does it report meta-analyses or systematic reviews, introduce new data in the form of experimental studies, report descriptive data, or focus on expert opinion or experience?
- To what degree does the source provide necessary details regarding the **intervention or program** of focus? Do I understand what exactly was studied? How well would the intervention or program translate to my work setting?
- To what degree does the source provide necessary details regarding the **population** of focus? Do I understand who was studied and why they were included? How well does the population compare to the population I serve in my work setting?
- To what degree does the source provide necessary details regarding **measures** used to evaluate change? Do I understand what was measured and why? How well do the measures included resonate with my understanding of the population I serve in my setting?
- To what degree does the source provide necessary details regarding **statistical procedures** used to evaluate the intervention or program? Do I understand the numbers presented?
- Does the author provide a clear explanation of the practical and clinical significance of findings?
- To what degree does the source discuss **limitations** to the study? Does an understanding of limitations change my interpretation of the critique?

CHAPTER SUMMARY

This chapter included practical strategies for using literature to inform practice. After briefly revising the concept of evidence-based practice, we introduced APA's JARS and stepped through different sections you can expect to find in a peer-reviewed journal article. We also provided tips and tricks for searching academic databases and navigating the university library. Next, we explored how you can access research articles and other forms of evidence to inform the selection of programs and practices relevant to your work. In particular, we highlighted public library and university resources that may still provide free or inexpensive access to articles, methods for identifying best practice guidelines, potential clearinghouses or registries for review, federal resources, and university partnerships. Finally, we introduced the importance of reviewing resources with careful attention to practicalities in your unique setting and with your unique population. The checklist provided will help you further evaluate these resources.

RESOURCES

- American Psychological Association *Journal Article Reporting Standards* https://apastyle.apa.org/jars
- How to Search for Relevant Literature FAST using Boolean Operators, www.youtube.com/watch?v=u0KVJ0lj8rw&t=47s
- Tutorial: How to Read and Comprehend Scientific Research, www.youtube.com/watch?v=t-2K6mJkSWoA

REFERENCES

APA Presidential Task Force on Evidence-based Practice. (2006). Evidence based practice in psychology. *American Psychologist*, *61*(4), 271–285. https://doi.org/10.1037/0003-066X.61.4.271

Melchert, T. P., Halfond, R. W., Hamdi, N. R., Bufka, L. F., Hollon, S. D., & Cuttler, M. J. (2024). Evidence-based practice in psychology: Context, guidelines, and action. *American Psychologist*, *79*(6), 824–837. https://doi.org/10.1037/amp0001253

Substance Abuse and Mental Health Services Administration. (2024). *Evidence-based practices resource center*. www.samhsa.gov/libraries/evidence-based-practices-resource-center/about

Tolin, D. F., McKay, D., Forman, E. M., Klonsky, E. D., & Thombs, B. D. (2015). Empirically supported treatment: Recommendations for a new model. *Clinical Psychology: Science and Practice*, *22*(4), 317–338. https://doi.org/10.1111/cpsp.12122

PART II
Using Research and Program Evaluation in Practice

CHAPTER 8

Surveying Groups of People

Counselors and researchers alike use surveys as a relatively easy way to gather information regarding attitudes, knowledge, or experiences. We may report these findings in terms of descriptive statistics such as averages and frequencies, or we may use inferential statistics to examine whether attitudes, knowledge, or experiences are related to other variables (more on this in Chapter 9) or change over the course of counseling services or programs (more on this in Chapters 10 to 12). Professional counselors have some very good reasons to survey groups of people. For example, we may wish to understand the needs of community members, experiences seeking services in a program, or satisfaction with services in a program. Well-designed survey methodology allows us to get at this information in a simple, straightforward manner.

This chapter introduces you to essential activities for surveying groups of people. Because we expect this is the design you will use most frequently, we also include an overview of the survey research process in general. We pay special attention to three types of survey designs mental health professionals are most likely to use in agency or school practice: (a) needs assessments, (b) process evaluations, and (c) satisfaction estimation. We apply elements of each method to a case study of a school-based bullying concern.

BOX 8.1 CHAPTER LEARNING OUTCOMES

- Develop rese arch questions consistent with the use of survey methodology
- Articulate key features of needs assessments, process assessments, and satisfaction estimation
- Design, plan, carry out, record, and analyze results of surveys for needs assessments, process evaluations, and satisfaction estimations
- Communicate findings from surveys using a variety of methods
- Identify and critique data associated with surveys

DOI: 10.4324/9781003586210-10

BOX 8.2 CASE STUDY

Over the last year, faculty and staff within a Title I middle school in a rural, midwestern area noted increases in detentions and suspensions related to bullying. They also logged an increased number of phone calls from parents concerned about bullying that occurred on district buses and on school grounds after dismissal. Demand for attention to the bullying problem shifted to the public arena following a well-publicized student death by suicide in a neighboring county and subsequent release of social media posts highlighting the cyberbullying the student endured. After a particularly charged town hall meeting, school officials tasked the school counselor with leading a multidisciplinary group focused on understanding the bullying problem and proposing a strategy for school-wide attention to the problem.

OVERVIEW OF SURVEY RESEARCH METHODS

What Are Survey Methods?

Survey methods involve the use of written or oral questionnaires to gather information from a group of people about their attitudes, knowledge, behaviors, or experiences. Most surveys involve responding to a written questionnaire on paper or online; however, we can also administer surveys orally, with interviewers asking questions and marking down responses in person or by phone. When implementing survey designs, researchers and program evaluators are most concerned with reaching a representative sample and designing items to answer questions about that group's attitudes, knowledge, behaviors, or experiences.

When Are Survey Methods Indicated?

There are three primary reasons for conducting surveys: meeting policy or program needs, evaluating programs, and generating research (Fink, 2025). All survey designs are intended to answer questions regarding participants' attitudes, knowledge, behaviors, or experiences. Although surveys may stand on their own, they are often used in conjunction with other sources of information or evaluation designs described in this book. With this in mind, let's take a deeper look into how survey methods may be helpful in your work as a counselor. In each example, we think back to the opening case study to illustrate questions we may answer using surveys.

Meeting Policy or Program Needs

We should design interventions and programs based on data from a number of involved parties. Program staff may use surveys in attempts to determine the prevalence or impact of specific experiences on their constituents. This activity is often known as a needs assessment, and we cover it in greater detail later in this chapter. For example, a school counselor may survey students or staff regarding experiences related to bullying. These surveys could be attitudinal in nature to inform understanding of how much these groups of stakeholders see bullying as a problem in their school. The surveys could be behavioral in nature with a focus on the frequency with which one experienced, witnessed, or perpetrated specific bullying behaviors. Finally, surveys could assess interest holders' interest in different types of interventions and programs related to bullying. Together, we could use this information to understand the problem of bullying among the student body and design interventions, programs, or policies responsive to the unique needs in this group. We might ask questions such as:

- How do students at Prairieview Middle School rate the school culture and climate related to bullying?
- How do teachers at Prairieview Middle School rate the school culture and climate related to bullying?
- How do parents or guardians of students at Prairieview Middle School rate the school culture and climate related to bullying?

Evaluating Programs

Surveys are often a hallmark of program evaluation designs. As we will explore in future chapters, many program evaluation designs use validated self-report instruments to assess the degree to which attitudes, beliefs, or behaviors change as a result of participating in programs. For example, self-report surveys may be the method through which an evaluator determines that students who participated in a school-wide bystander intervention program were more likely to perceive themselves as willing and able to intervene when witnessing bullying compared to those who did not participate in the program. We may also use supplemental surveys to understand important parts of stakeholders' experiences within interventions and programs.

As will be discussed in depth later, we often use surveys to determine the degree to which a program was implemented as designed. For example, we could use surveys to assess participants' knowledge or understanding following specific intervention curricula or as a check to determine whether practice role-plays were implemented as planned during a certain lesson. Finally, program evaluators use satisfaction surveys to understand individuals' overall experiences with an intervention or program. Because satisfaction estimation is often standard practice in agencies and schools, we also cover this activity later in this chapter. For example, we might ask:

- To what degree is Prairieview Middle School's bystander intervention program being implemented as planned?
- To what degree do faculty and staff of Prairieview Middle School report satisfaction with the bystander intervention program?
- To what degree do students of Prairieview Middle School report changes in school culture and climate related to bullying as a result of the implementation of the bystander intervention program?

Generating Research

Researchers may utilize survey methodology in attempts to understand attitudes, knowledge, behaviors, or experiences among a sample of individuals with the intent of generalizing this understanding to a larger population. Survey research is often correlational or predictive in nature, allowing researchers to test hypotheses regarding connections between phenomena (see Chapter 9). For example, to better guide understanding about bullying and inform effective intervention methods, we may survey a representative sample of students to determine whether experiences of bullying vary by demographics such as age, gender, race, ethnicity, or academic performance. In so doing, we may find that middle school girls report higher instances of relational bullying compared to boys who report higher instances of physical bullying. We may also learn that students identifying as transgender or non-binary report substantially higher instances of all types of bullying. This knowledge may help us better reach all students by developing a relational bullying module within a curriculum highly focused on physical bullying. The findings could also help school staff tailor prevention strategies or adjust school policies to address the unique needs of students at high risk of bullying.

Similarly, researchers may wish to determine relationships between bullying and other social attitudes or earlier experiences, perhaps identifying indicators that might be used in prevention or early intervention. Although this book is primarily focused on helping you apply research principles to your practice, you will likely find yourself using survey research reports to understand your client population. For example, we might ask: Are there statistically significant differences in experiences of bullying based on racial and ethnic identity, gender identity, and grade?

SURVEY RESEARCH PROCESS

The process of designing and implementing surveys tends to be quite similar, regardless of our specific research questions. Although some scholars will present more complicated models (Fink, 2025; Rea & Parker, 2014), we believe most survey design breaks into four main steps: (a) determining the purpose and focus of the survey, (b) selecting or designing a survey instrument, (c) specifying sampling procedures, (d) and administering the survey.

Determining the Purpose and Focus of the Survey

The first step in any applied research or program evaluation is to determine the specific purpose and focus of the survey. You should be able to answer the questions what, where, when, who, and why. The what should include clear attention to attitudes, knowledge, behaviors, and/or experiences you would like to understand. We must also determine who is in the best position to provide responses, and when they are best able to do so. Most often, we would like to go directly to the source to understand perspectives. However, there may be times when mental health professionals, teachers, parents, or caregivers are situated to provide additional context or more objective accounts. We should have a clear rationale for each decision we make about the purpose and focus of the survey.

Selecting or Designing a Survey

Next, we must select or design a survey for implementation. Specific design decisions will depend on the purpose and focus of the survey, the availability of existing measures, and the nature of the population of focus. Our decision whether to use paper, online, phone, or in-person data collection strategies will influence the types of questions we can ask, the time and resources required to implement, and overall project design. Table 8.1 includes a summary of different types of survey administration formats, including their advantages and disadvantages (Fink, 2025; Rea & Parker, 2014).

Before going through the work of designing a survey, it is important to determine whether you are able to locate an existing, already-validated survey that meets your needs and is relevant to your population. For example, a number of inexpensive, well-established satisfaction indices will likely provide you with a more accurate understanding of satisfaction than a survey you create. If you want to understand something

TABLE 8.1 Types of Survey Administration Formats

Type	Advantages	Disadvantages
Paper surveys	Time and cost savings over interview methods; convenient; no time constraints; anonymity; reduced interviewer-induced bias; complexity; can include visual aids	Requires more time; lower response rates due to self-selection; lack of interviewer involvement; incomplete open-ended questions
Online surveys	Convenient; rapid data collection; cost-effective; no time constraints; ease of follow-up; confidentiality and security; may reach specialized populations more easily; can include complexity and visual aids	May not be accessible or appropriate for all populations; lower response rates due to self-selection; lack of interviewer involvement
Phone surveys	Rapid data collection; possible cost savings; some degree of anonymity; interviewers can ensure questions are understood and instructions are followed	Less control over interview situation; difficulty establishing credibility and trust; lack of visual materials; less complexity of design; requires training of interviewers
In-person interviews	Flexibility; greater complexity; ability to contact hard-to-reach populations; interviewers can ensure questions are understood and instructions are followed	High cost; interviewer-introduced bias; reluctance to cooperate; greater stress; less anonymity; requires training of interviewers

of behaviors, symptoms, or experiences, you will likely be better off using established instruments than creating your own, especially when it comes to using outcome measures. Chapters 4 and 5 include foundations that should help you understand characteristics of assessment instruments; Chapter 15 includes practical guidance on identifying instruments for use in a broad range of applied research and program evaluation designs.

If you must create a survey, the success of your survey will depend on the quality of your questions. This process generally starts with determining the information that is of interest to you, including details or subcomponents that are important to understand. In essence, this step requires that you define your constructs (i.e., the abstract ideas you wish to operationalize). When it comes time to write items, you will need to make several decisions. You must decide whether you would like to use open-ended questions or closed-ended questions. Open-ended questions may allow you to understand greater detail or nuance; however, they take more time for participants to answer, participants are more likely to skip them, and they are more difficult to analyze. If using open-ended questions, you might choose to prompt participants to provide one, two, or three things they liked best and liked least about a program (Fink, 2025), thus giving some direction and focus to responses. Closed-ended questions are easier to answer, easier to analyze, and may help you access more sensitive information. However, closed-ended questions are more sensitive to random responding and may not help you understand your questions in depth. Sometimes program evaluators will use "other, please specify" or open-ended follow-up questions to help capture these distinctions.

Fink (2025, pp. 44–49) offered the following rules for writing closed-ended questions:

- Each question should be meaningful to respondents.
- Use standard language rules.
- Make questions concrete.
- Avoid biased words and phrases.
- Check your own biases.
- Use caution when asking for personal information.
- Each question should have only one thought.

If using closed-ended items, you will need to decide which response format to use. Response formats vary widely and depend on the nature of your questions. In some cases, a simple yes or no response will suffice. In others, you may want participants to select one or more nominal items from a multiple-choice list. In yet other cases, you may use ordinal scales or ask participants to rank-order responses. For example, a Likert-type scale usually uses 5 points: 1 = strongly disagree, 2 = disagree, 3 = neither agree nor disagree, 4 = agree, and 5 = strongly agree. Some researchers prefer to eliminate the middle point, thus "forcing" a choice (e.g., 1 = strongly disagree, 2 = disagree, 3 = agree, 4 = strongly agree). Of course, you may choose to use other rating scales depending on the nature of your questions or participants. Many online resources provide guidance regarding possible response formats.

Once you have constructed items and response formats, it is time to construct the overall survey. This includes developing introductory information, writing instructions, and deciding the order of questions. Typically, you should start with more general, less sensitive information and build toward more specific and sensitive information. The survey should be built in a logical manner, with order of questions easing participants through the exercise without introducing bias. You may also want to include notes or images to help participants understand when you are changing topics, response formats, or instructions. Box 8.3 includes a checklist for deciding question order.

BOX 8.3 CHECKLIST FOR GUIDING QUESTION ORDER (FINK, 2025, P. 72)

- For any given topic, ask relatively objective questions before the subjective ones.
- Move from the most familiar to the least.
- Follow the natural sequence of time.
- See to it that all questions are independent.
- Relatively easy-to-answer questions (including demographic questions such as age or occupation) should be asked at the end.
- Avoid many questions that look alike.
- Sensitive questions should be placed well after the start of the survey but also well before its conclusion.
- Questions should be in logical order.

The survey should be formatted in a way that eases administration and conveys a professional appearance. If the survey is to be administered orally, it is important to train interviewers to ensure consistency in administration. Finally, pilot-test the survey with a few members of your target population to ensure that the items and instructions make sense to them. This is particularly important when considering developmental, cultural, and linguistic characteristics of the population you are serving. When working with a general population of adults, we will strive to write at a sixth to eighth grade reading level. However, we will need to adjust based on unique context. By seeking feedback early in the process and revising the survey instrument accordingly, you increase the chances that your survey will yield useful data.

In addition to selecting or creating the survey, you will want to attend to key demographic information so you can describe and understand who has responded (and not responded) to your survey. Depending on your sample size and nature of your questions, collecting this information may allow you to assess interactions between demographic variables and your survey items. For example, we may find that single parents in the sample see childcare as essential to engaging in services at an agency; we might have missed this distinction if we only reported the percentage of total participants needing childcare. At the very least, plan to collect information about age, gender identity, and racial and ethnic identity. Depending on your population of focus, you might also want to report things like grade level, partnership status, and current or past participation in services.

Specifying Sampling Procedures

As discussed in Chapter 4, **population** refers to the entire group we are interested in understanding. The population may be all clients seeking services at an agency, all students in a school, or all adolescents in the United States. In some cases, a population is small and well-defined enough that it is feasible to survey all members. For example, we could feasibly survey all students in a middle school or all consumers who completed a specific program at a school or agency. However, when the population is large or not clearly defined, it is not feasible or cost-effective to survey all members of the population. The **sample** refers to the specific group we select in efforts to represent the population as a whole. If you need to refresh, please review Chapter 4 for an overview of probability and nonprobability sampling methods and considerations.

Prior to determining a sampling plan, it is important to be clear regarding inclusion and exclusion criteria for the survey. Inclusion criteria include things that all people in the sample must have in common. For example, I might decide that one must be at least 18 years of age and have completed at least five sessions of a program. Exclusion criteria are not the opposite of inclusion criteria. Rather, exclusion criteria are other reasons someone should not participate in a survey. I might decide to exclude individuals who are enrolled in other services at the agency out of concern that their responses might not be specific to my program of interest. The sample size you need will depend on the specific nature of the survey and planned analyses, especially if you plan to use inferential statistics to compare groups (see Chapter 5). In addition, the sampling plan will vary depending on the anticipated response rate, especially because some types of surveys and survey scenarios yield very low response rates.

Administering the Survey

Once we have determined the scope of the survey, selected or designed the survey protocol, and specified sampling procedures, it is time to administer the survey. Although not always necessary for program evaluation, some work settings will require that surveys go through an institutional review board process to ensure adequate human subjects protections (see Chapter 6). Even if formal approval is not necessary, it is important to review the survey plan with administrators in your agency or school to ensure their understanding and support of the process. In addition, you should develop an administration plan which includes a timeline and steps to be taken to secure the sample, administer the survey, gather responses, troubleshoot difficulties that arise during the process, and begin analysis. Part III of this book includes practical guidance for navigating many of these steps.

BOX 8.4 CHECKLIST OF INDICATORS OF A QUALITY SURVEY DESIGN

- Purpose and focus of the survey are well defined and logically connected.
- There is a logical connection between the purpose of study/evaluation, related research/evaluation questions, and analytic strategy.

- Survey has clear evidence of validity and appropriateness for purpose; if evaluator is not able to use existing survey, questions are well constructed and presented in logical order.
- Sampling procedures are appropriate to purpose and focus of the survey.
- Survey administration procedures are appropriate to design.
- If used, data meet statistical model assumptions required for analyses.
- If used, estimates of statistical significance are computed and reported.
- If used, estimates of practical significance are computed and reported.
- Tables and visual depictions support reporting of findings.

TYPES OF SURVEY DESIGNS

The survey steps outlined earlier apply to a wide variety of surveys used in applied research and program evaluation. However, there are three primary areas in which master's-level counselors will likely find themselves using simple survey designs. These designs often involve survey methodology, but they may involve the use of other types of data to corroborate findings. In this section, we include an overview and practical considerations for conducting needs assessments, process evaluations, and satisfaction estimations.

Needs Assessment

Core Features

"Needs assessment is a process for figuring out how to close a learning or performance gap. It involves determining what the important needs are and how to address them" (Sleezer et al., 2014, p. 17). Needs assessments generally include input from a variety of individuals such as consumers, community members, administrators, and organization staff. Although needs assessments tend to include surveys at some level, they also include other forms of data such as results from focus groups, review of records, and expert interviews (see Chapter 7).

Intended Uses and Design Considerations

Needs assessments have four primary uses: securing resources, modifying policy, improving services, and enhancing partnerships (Royse et al., 2009). First, needs assessments are used to secure or advocate for resources. Agencies and schools may rely on grant or contract funding to support services. Funders often require that groups present a clear, data-based rationale regarding the particular need the funding will address. Even within systems, we may use needs assessment data to advocate for resources, develop services, or expand programs. Although other forms of data are included when advocating for resources, needs assessments often include survey results regarding needs expressed by stakeholders.

Second, we may use needs assessments to modify policy or present a rationale regarding a need for a change in policy. In addition to considering interviews and records, policy modifications may be based on surveys regarding stakeholders' opinions of current policies or prospective policy changes.

Similarly, we may use needs assessments to improve services. For example, surveys could help us understand which services are desired by the community, how the community would like to access services, and when community members are able to access services. They may also inform understanding regarding the perception of the agency in the community. Finally, needs assessments can be used to establish or strengthen partnerships. This may include results of survey data regarding gaps or inconsistencies in services.

As with all designs, it is critical to consider the purpose, intended use, and audience when designing the specific needs assessment. Royse et al. (2009) noted that assessments can include attention to four different types of needs:

- Normative need as determined by experts.
- Expressed need as noted in consumer requests for services and engagement in services.
- Felt need as expressed by consumers.
- Comparative need as seen when comparing population information with service within an agency.

Thus, we will shift the focus of our needs assessment to match our intended purpose. For example, we might want to know about client awareness of services, availability of services, accessibility of services, or acceptability of services (Royse et al., 2009) in order to advocate for resources or design responsive programs.

When designing needs assessments, we must consider sources of data that correspond to the intended use and audience of the needs assessment. This will often include surveys of stakeholders with special attention to design considerations summarized earlier in this chapter. Data sources can include documentation of need as noted in agency or school referral records, focus groups and interviews with key stakeholders (see Chapter 13), or results of larger community needs assessments or expert studies regarding needs in one's population. The resources featured at the end of this chapter include some practical attention to conducting needs assessments for mental health settings.

Data Analysis and Interpretation

Analysis of needs assessment surveys is often quite simple, as we most often rely on descriptive statistics. For example, we might include frequency counts for nominal and ordinal data and descriptive statistics (e.g., means, standard deviations, ranges) for interval–ratio-level data. At times, it may be appropriate to present tables of data illustrating differences in response patterns on the basis of demographic variables such as gender identity, age, or race or ethnicity.

Because surveys are usually just one component of needs assessment, analysis and interpretation must also include consideration of other data sources collected. You may wish to triangulate data from surveys with focus groups of other stakeholders and past reports. Chapter 13 includes more detailed attention to methods for analyzing qualitative data such as interviews and focus groups. Together, you can use these sets of data to paint a picture of the current situation and potential future directions.

Process or Implementation Evaluation

Core Features

Process or implementation evaluations help us determine whether an intervention or program is being implemented as planned. Process evaluation is a formative evaluation in which we consider program activities and timeline to date, individuals reached, and fidelity of implementation. Because process evaluation occurs as we roll out an intervention or program, it allows us to troubleshoot and make adjustments that can affect long-term success. A good process evaluation will also give context to outcome data, as discussed in Chapters 10 to 12. For example, if we design an exceptional program but implement it poorly, we might erroneously decide that the program design was no good. Alternatively, if we design an exceptional program and implement it well but it had very low enrollment because we offered it in a way that was not accessible to those we wished to serve, the program has limited potential impact.

Intended Uses and Design Considerations

As with all evaluations, it is important to start the design by considering the overall purpose and focus of the process evaluation. The Centers for Disease Control *Program Evaluation Framework* proposed the following process evaluation questions (Kidder et al., 2024, Table 5):

- To what extent are the program resources sufficient for successful implementation?
- How do program staff qualifications align with those needed for program implementation? What gaps exist?
- To what extent is the program being implemented as planned? What are the facilitators and barriers to implementation?
- Is the program reaching its intended audience? Why or why not?
- What are the overall program costs? How much does the program cost per unit of service?
- In what ways are or aren't program activities designed to address the drivers of health inequities?
- In what ways are the program activities tailored to the community served? Where are there opportunities for improvement?
- What is the quality of materials provided as part of the program? To what extent are they understood across a variety of intended audiences?

We may easily obtain some of these indicators (e.g., numbers of those receiving services, and demographics of those receiving services, staff characteristics, specific program activities) from program records. Other indicators may require the use of surveys or other data collection measures. For example, we may assess the quality of services by developing surveys to make sure important parts of curricula were developed as planned. Alternatively, we may use satisfaction surveys to determine participants' perceptions of the quality of services.

Data Analysis and Interpretation

As with needs assessment data, process evaluation data are often multifaceted, with survey results comprising just one component of wraparound data that may also include program records, focus groups, and interviews with key informants. Data analysis most often includes examination of frequency and descriptive statistics with triangulation of information from multiple sources.

Satisfaction Estimation

Core Features

The last few decades have seen enhanced attention to the importance of consumer experiences, culminating in federal mandates for use and sometimes publication of patient assessments of quality (Pauselli et al., 2018; Russell et al., 2015). Estimates of satisfaction are simple, straightforward, and almost always used in program evaluation. Although satisfaction data are not sufficient in the absence of outcome data, they are an important component of understanding the overall experience (Royse et al., 2015). Certainly, individuals who are satisfied with care are more likely to persist in services and engage with their treatment plans (Pauselli et al., 2018; Russell et al., 2015). By understanding consumer experiences, we can adjust programs and policies to boost overall success and experience.

Intended Uses and Design Considerations

When designing satisfaction estimations, it is important to consider which factor(s) we would like to include in the evaluation. Russell et al. (2015) identified three components of service quality:

- Interpersonal—satisfaction with relational quality between caregiver and consumer.
- Administrative—satisfaction with things like scheduling, wait times, and registration.
- Technical/clinical—perception of caregiver expertise and progress toward outcome.

Quite often, mental health professionals overestimate the importance of technical/ clinical considerations and underestimate the importance of administrative and relational considerations. A good satisfaction estimation takes multiple aspects of consumer experience into consideration. Box 8.5 includes a checklist of considerations for the use of satisfaction surveys in mental health organizations.

Because well-established satisfaction indices are available, we recommend using an established instrument to assess client satisfaction. The instrument you choose should be appropriate to the setting, language, and development of the populations served. For example, the *Client Satisfaction Inventory* (McMurtry & Hudson, 2000)

BOX 8.5 CHECKLIST FOR USE OF SATISFACTION SURVEYS IN MENTAL HEALTH ORGANIZATIONS (ROYSE ET AL., 2006, PP. 216–221)

- Use a scale that has good reliability and that has been used successfully in other studies.
- Use the same instrument on repeated occasions, and develop a local baseline of data so that departures from the norm can be observed.
- Employ at least one and possibly two open-ended questions so that the consumers of your services can alert you to any problems that you did not suspect and could not anticipate.
- In order to avoid the problem of surveying only the clients who remain in a program (and therefore would be more likely to have positive experiences than those who drop out), use a "ballot box" approach where one week is set aside when every client entering the agency is given a brief questionnaire while waiting for their appointment.
- Do not focus only on solving the problems of dissatisfied consumers, assuming that you will be able to convert them into satisfied consumers.
- If you conduct a mailed survey, do what you can to get a response rate over 50%.
- Target specific dimensions.
- Keep your expectations realistic.
- Look for behavioral indicators (i.e., attendance) to supplement the client satisfaction data.

contains either 25 items (original form) or 10 items (short form) rated on a 7-point scale. The resources at the end of this chapter and in Chapter 15 include several links you may find helpful for identifying satisfaction surveys for use in counseling settings.

As noted by Royse et al. (2015), key considerations in designing satisfaction estimations are around ensuring adequate responses. Because many clients discontinue after just a couple sessions, it would be inadequate to only survey those who complete services or reach a particular benchmark. Rather, you may wish to consider whether it would be appropriate for an administrative staff member or volunteer (not the service provider!) to conduct telephone surveys with a sample of those who attended services in the past few months, including those who did not return.

We also recommend you add two specific, open-ended questions to help you understand ratings in context. For example, you might cue clients to indicate the one or two best things about their experience and one or two changes they would recommend. This is especially important because there is evidence that qualitative satisfaction prompts tend to generate more critical (and actionable) feedback than quantitative satisfaction prompts (Royse et al., 2015). By asking for specific feedback, you open the possibility of understanding client experiences more deeply and positioning yourself to do something with information you collect.

Data Analysis and Interpretation

Like other types of surveys in this chapter, satisfaction surveys are usually best understood using simple descriptive statistics such as frequency counts, medians, and means. Keep in mind that satisfaction surveys often show high positive ratings, so any results showing less than 75% satisfaction may be a sign of concern (Royse et al., 2015). You might want to consider satisfaction scores for specific subgroups of people, programs, or service providers. No matter what the numbers say, it is important to also review open-ended qualitative comments people provide (see Chapter 13) to better understand the story behind satisfaction ratings.

PUTTING FINDINGS IN CONTEXT

When we opened this chapter, we established three primary purposes of survey design: meeting policy or program needs, evaluating programs, and generating research (Fink, 2025). It is important to present results of surveys in context by describing the purpose of the survey, specific data collection methods, participants (e.g., number and description) and response rate, and overall findings. You should also situate these findings in the greater context of the program, school, or organization, perhaps describing the programs or services examined and including additional information to triangulate findings and help readers make sense of your reports. Box 8.6 depicts a six-step guide to reporting needs assessment findings featuring, but not limited to, survey design.

BOX 8.6 BASIC FRAMEWORK FOR REPORTING NEEDS ASSESSMENT FINDINGS IN CONTEXT

Step 1: Describe purpose and focus of needs assessment

Clearly note the context in which you conducted the needs assessment, including motivation driving the assessment, time period conducted, and overall focus.

Step 2: Provide overview of data sources utilized for the needs assessment

List data sources and stakeholders (e.g., role, number) involved in each component of the needs assessment. Describe methods for gathering data, and provide evidence of validity for the data.

Step 3: Report descriptive and (if appropriate) inferential statistics related to findings

For each data source, provide a brief summary of descriptive statistics and any inferential statistics utilized to understand the data. If appropriate, include tables or graphs to help stakeholders visualize data.

Step 4: Provide plainly spoken interpretation of findings

Weave together data sources to give life to findings as a whole. Point to areas of convergence and overall themes.

Step 5: Report limitations or unanswered questions

Note limitations or unanswered questions addressed in the needs assessment. This may include conflicting results or gaps you noted.

Step 6: Develop a summative statement about findings and recommendations

Constructively integrate all the earlier steps to summarize findings and make recommendations for next steps.

Developing Impact Statements

Impact statements you develop from survey studies should be clear and direct, with careful attention not to overestimate or underestimate findings. Although it may be tempting to focus only on strengths or on limitations, present the data in a way that allows readers to draw their own informed conclusions. Try to avoid overgeneralizing findings, reaching beyond what you know, or drawing causal conclusions. For example, avoid confounding having satisfied clients or students with having an effective program.

Using Descriptive Statistics

In most instances, you will be using frequencies, means, and standard deviations to report results. For items rated on an interval scale, you may indicate proportion of participants marking each item along with an overall mean and standard deviation for the item. For items that involve interval–ratio data, provide minimum, maximum, mean, and standard deviation. Be sure to note the number of responses received and rating scales utilized so that readers can decipher what any given rating means.

Shaping Summative Findings

In the end, aim to integrate survey findings with the context of your agency or school, program, and community to help readers understand how you derived findings for needs assessment, process evaluation, or satisfaction estimation. Develop your summative statement of findings to include strengths and limitations of the current situation, using specific data to support claims.

DISPLAYING RESULTS

As with other designs, descriptive tables and graphics are helpful for depicting results. It is generally best to present these in a clearly defined table format. If you have sufficient sample size and detect important differences and trends in your data, you may wish to provide a breakdown of ratings in a table or chart. Chapter 17 will provide more in-depth guidance regarding strategies for presenting results.

BOX 8.7 CASE STUDY REVISITED

The school counselor worked with a multidisciplinary team to conduct a needs assessment related to bullying at Prairieview Middle School. This section will provide a brief application of chapter content to illustrate the use of surveys and data to support the needs assessment. Although we note data sources utilized for a broader needs assessment, we only present detailed findings for the student survey component used in this process.

Purpose of Needs Assessment

- Develop greater understanding regarding the nature and scope of bullying at Prairieview Middle School as noted by students, parents or guardians, teachers, and administrators.
- Utilize findings of needs assessment to support selection of an evidence-based bullying intervention program.

Related Questions Guiding the Evaluation

- What is the prevalence and nature of disciplinary action related to bullying at Prairieview Middle School?
- How do students at Prairieview Middle School rate school culture and climate related to bullying?
- How do teachers and staff at Prairieview Middle School rate school culture and climate related to bullying?

Overview of Data Sources

- Examination of school records related to disciplinary action and referrals related to bullying or suspected bullying over the last three academic years.
- Teachers in grades 6 to 8 were invited to complete the Secondary School Teacher/Staff Version of the *Authoritative School Climate Survey* (Cornell, 2019) during in-service development.
- Focus group of students who self-reported witnessing bullying among peers.
- Students in grades 6 to 8 were invited to complete the Secondary School Student Version of the *Authoritative School Climate Survey* (Cornell, 2019) during a homeroom period in November 2024. A total of 88.12% (n = 245) students completed the survey. The ASCS is a nationally normed survey instrument that yields a number of subscales. For this assessment, we utilized subscales related to student engagement; school disciplinary structure; prevalence of teasing and bullying; bullying by teachers; aggressive attitudes;

victim experiences; bullying experiences; and demographic items, including grades, suspension status, and personal demographics. Attitudes scales were rated on scales ranging from 1 = Strongly disagree to 4 = Strongly agree; experiences were rated as follows: 1 = Never, 2 = Once or twice, 3 = About once per week, and 4 = More than once per week. Cronbach's alphas observed for this administration ranged from .72 to .88.

Putting Findings into Context

Students largely felt engaged at their school ($M = 3.10$, $SD = 0.79$), although 16.7% of students had mean scores indicating they disagreed or strongly disagreed with these statements. Students had divergent perspectives on disciplinary structure ($M = 2.62$, $SD = 0.77$), with just 55.9% of students agreeing or strongly agreeing with items related to fair rules and punishments. As is indicated in the table that follows, students reported witnessing teasing and bullying at the school, most often related to appearance. Although students reported lower instances of teasing related to race/ethnicity or sexual orientation, these results should be viewed in context of this school's demographic composition of 85% White.

TABLE 8.2 Results of Praireview Climate Survey

	Strongly Disagree	Disagree	Agree	Strongly Agree	M	SD
Students in this school are teased about clothing or physical appearance	1%	23%	27%	49%	3.24	0.84
Students in this school are teased or put down because of their race or ethnicity	30%	35%	25%	10%	2.15	0.96
There is a lot of teasing about sexual topics at this school	8%	33%	30%	29%	2.80	0.95
Bullying is a problem at this school	3%	44%	28%	25%	2.75	0.87
Students in this school are teased or put down about their sexual orientation	6%	40%	28%	26%	2.74	0.91

Students at this school reported direct experiences related to bullying that are concerning, with 65% of students being bullied at school this year and 12% of students reporting bullying more often than once a week. Verbal and social bullying appeared to be most prevalent, with cyberbullying and physical bullying least prevalent. Results are illustrated in the following stacked bar graph.

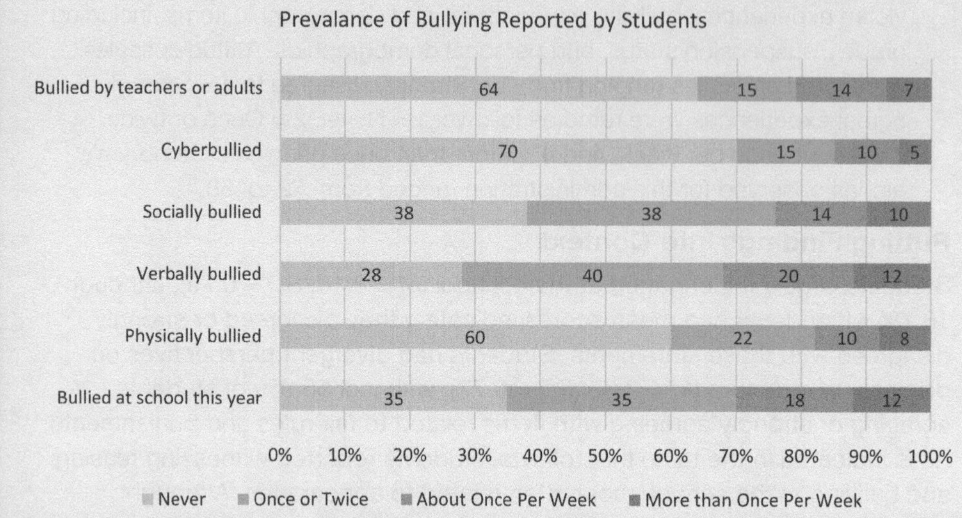

Figure 8.1 Stacked Bar Graph of Prairieview Climate Survey Results

CHAPTER SUMMARY

This chapter presented initial concepts and tools to design, develop, and implement survey designs. With this information in hand, you are ready to begin using survey tools to perform the three most fundamental program evaluation tasks master's-level counselors will use: needs assessments, process evaluations, and satisfaction estimations. We illustrated these concepts and tools with a case example of a middle school counselor conducting a needs assessment related to a problem of bullying in their school. By referencing the checklists presented in this chapter and the supplemental tools noted throughout, you are ready to begin understanding needs and experiences of your students, clients, and communities more fully.

RESOURCES

- Agency for Healthcare Research and Quality, CAHPS mental health surveys, www.ahrq.gov/cahps/surveys-guidance/mental-health/index.html
- Center for Mental Health, What makes a good mental health needs assessment? www.centreformentalhealth.org.uk/publications/what-makes-a-good-mental-health-needs-assessment/
- Centers for Disease Control and Prevention, *CDC Approach to Program Evaluation*. www.cdc.gov/evaluation/php/about/index.html
- Centers for Disease Control and Prevention, *CDC Program Evaluation Framework*. www.cdc.gov/evaluation/php/evaluation-framework/index.html
- Community Tool Box, *Assessing Community Needs and Resources*. https://ctb.ku.edu/en/table-of-contents/assessment/assessing-community-needs-and-resources/

- CSQ Scales, *Client Satisfaction Questionnaires*. www.csqscales.com
- Fink, A. (2025). *How to conduct surveys: A step-by-step guide* (7th ed.). Sage.
- Rea, L. M., & Parker, R. A. (2014). *Designing and conducting survey research* (4th ed.). Wiley.
- National Center for School Mental Health (2023). School mental health quality guide: Needs assessment and resource mapping. University of Maryland School of Medicine. www.schoolmentalhealth.org/media/som/microsites/ncsmh/documents/quality-guides/Needs-Assessment-&-Resource-Mapping.pdf
- National Training and Technical Assistance Center for Child, Youth, and Family Mental Health (2025). Children's Mental Health Initiative (CMHI): Needs assessment template and guidelines. https://nttacmentalhealth.org/resource/child-mental-health-initiative-cmhi-needs-assessment-template-and-guidelines-2025/

REFERENCES

Cornell, D. (2019). *The authoritative school climate survey and the school climate bullying survey: Research summary*. https://virginia.app.box.com/s/2v4fubb4mri8elq1w7rn16shd-vnlf2mk/file/1086708979372

Fink, A. (2025). *How to conduct surveys: A step-by-step guide* (7th ed.). Sage.

Kidder, D. P. Fierro, L. A., Luna E., et al. CDC program evaluation framework. (2024). *Morbidity and Mortality Weekly Report*, *73*(6), 1–37. http://dx.doi.org/10.15585/mmwr.rr7306a1

McMurtry, S. L., & Hudson, W. W. (2000). The client satisfaction inventory: Results of an initial validation study. *Research on Social Work Practice*, *10*(5), 644–663. https://doi.org/10.1177/104973150001000506

Pauselli, L., Galletti, C., Verdolini, N., Paolini, E., Gallucci, D., Balducci, P. M.,. . .Compton, M. T. (2018). Predictors of client satisfaction with outpatient mental health clinic services in Italy and New York. *Community Mental Health Journal*, *54*(5), 562–570. https://doi.org/10.1007/s10597-017-0196-6

Rea, L. M., & Parker, R. A. (2014). *Designing and conducting survey research* (4th ed.). Wiley.

Royse, D., Staton-Tindall, M., Badger, K., & Webster, J. M. (2009). *Needs assessment*. Oxford University Press.

Royse, D., Thyer, B. A., & Padgett, D. K. (2015). *Program evaluation: An introduction to an evidence-based approach* (6th ed.). Cengage.

Royse, D., Thyer, B. A., Padgett, D. K., & Logan, T. K. (2006). *Program evaluation: An introduction* (4th ed.). Thompson.

Russell, R. S., Johnson, D. M., & White, S. W. (2015). Patient perceptions of quality: Analyzing patient satisfaction surveys. *International Journal of Operations & Production Management*, *35*(8), 1158–1181. https://doi.org/10.1108/IJOPM-02-2014-0074

Sleezer, C. M., Russ-Eft, D. F., & Gupta, K. (2014). *Practical guide to needs assessment* (3rd ed.). Wiley.

CHAPTER 9

Predicting Relationships between Variables

An ecological perspective of development and well-being supports the notion that all people, places, and psychological spaces are connected in meaningful ways, and these elements have varied degrees of relationships and influence to one another (Cook, 2015; McLaren & Hawe, 2005). Without too much consideration, you can likely enumerate many events and personal characteristics that are related to one another either directly or through indirect ripple effects. Freud (1905) believed that the degree of psychosexual conflict resolution would be reflected in the amounts of fixations and neurosis later in life. Adler (1927/2014) proposed that birth order predicted interaction with others over the lifespan. Lenz and Oliver (2017) suggested that certain family characteristics forecast the emergence of self-protective strategies in adulthood. Flückiger et al. (2018) proposed that the working alliance between counselor and client predicted about 30% of therapeutic outcomes. Although focused on different variables, each of these cases is similar because there is a proposition that if we know enough about one phenomenon, we can fairly confidently predict another. What distinguishes Freud's and Adler's propositions from those of more contemporary colleagues is the preponderance of evidence to support conclusions and guide evidence-based practices.

This chapter introduces designs you can use to evaluate relationships between two or more variables in an effort to describe associations, predict a clinically relevant criterion, or forecast an event occurring. Specific methods covered in this chapter include bivariate correlations, linear regression, and logistic regression. Elements of each method will be applied to a case study of experiences in a substance use treatment facility.

BOX 9.1 CHAPTER LEARNING OUTCOMES

- Develop research questions consistent with use of predictive methods
- Design, plan, carry out, record, and analyze the results of predictive studies
- Communicate findings from predictive studies using a variety of methods
- Identify and critique data associated with predictive studies

DOI: 10.4324/9781003586210-11

BOX 9.2 CASE STUDY

A partial hospitalization program in a metropolitan area of the Midwest region of the United States is providing a six-week dialectical behavior therapy for adolescents (DBT-A; Rathus & Miller, 2015) intervention. During the intake process, clients and their guardians provide information related to demographics, biopsychosocial variables, current psychiatric symptoms, and treatment history. Additionally, clients complete surveys throughout the treatment process to monitor treatment aspects believed to promote therapeutic progress with DBT-A such as mindfulness, distress tolerance, emotion regulation, interpersonal effectiveness, and parent–child communication. Because there is little evidence for use of DBT-A with adolescents, especially within partial hospitalization settings, the clinical director is interested in identifying which client and intervention characteristics predict positive treatment outcomes. The program administrator is particularly interested in these findings as a means to promote admissions and coverage decisions by third-party payors.

OVERVIEW OF PREDICTIVE DESIGNS

What Are Predictive Designs?

Predictive research and evaluation designs rely on inspecting the statistical relationships among theoretically linked variables to understand their direction and magnitude. Unlike experimental designs, there is no manipulation of any variables or any true outcome associated with the program. Rather, predictive designs depict relationships between variables expressed through correlation statistics. Instead of stimulating change among dependent variables through manipulation (e.g., exposure to an intervention), these designs rely on *predictor variables* such as age or number of previous psychiatric hospitalizations to estimate amounts of *criterion variables* such as symptom reduction or likelihood for readmission that can be predicted. Therefore, predictive designs depend on the prudent use of measures intended for the sample. Although it is possible to use categorical data, most predictive studies will attempt to represent associations among continuous data associated with participant characteristics, intervention/program features, or the presence of a specific construct. Relatedly, these designs are convenient and accessible given that data of interest can be obtained by researchers in a single effort or are usually already collected by a program.

Core Features of Predictive Designs

Regardless of their complexity, all predictive designs share some common features that ground our ability to test hypotheses evaluate programs. First, all predictive designs rely on estimations of **covariance** between scores that depict the direction of the relationship between scores representing variables as they move together in a *positive relationship* or away from one another in a *negative relationship*. Second, **correlation coefficients** such as Pearson's *r* or Spearman's rho (*rs*) are often used to add information about the magnitude of covariance between scores that can be interpreted similarly regardless of which scales or scores are used. Third, despite the value of evaluating correlation coefficients, due to their non-experimental nature it is imperative to recall that **correlation does not equal causation** for several reasons. One reason is related to the **third variable problem** wherein an observed correlation between two variables is influenced by any number of variables that were not measured. Another explanation lies in the **directionality problem** in which it may be unclear which variable is influencing the other.

When Are Predictive Studies Indicated?

With a little statistical legwork, you can reveal some very helpful information about aspects of participant experiences or program participants that predict a variable of interest. This makes sense, and it probably feels pretty great to play the role of fortune teller once in a while. However, predictive designs rely on a few very important assumptions that will make or break a project (Lenz et al., 2026). First, predictive designs are typically nested within the concept of *linearity*; you will be attempting to depict a direct relationship between variables. Examples of linear relationships may include hours of studying and a score on a test, classroom size and teacher burnout, or amounts of social anxiety and intimacy. In each case, as one variable changes, so does the other. Second, variables should be theoretically linked in some important ways (Vigen, 2015). After all, you do not really believe that the number of films Nicolas Cage stars in will help you better understand the number of drowning deaths in the United States. Similarly, predictive studies test thoughtful, theoretically driven hypotheses associated with your criterion of interest. Finally, because predictive designs are often reliant upon data depicting constructs, all measures used should have psychometric reliability and validity for *your* participants, not just *any* participants (more on this in Chapters 5 and 15). Therefore, it is important to make sure that validity and reliability evidence for your participants is robust, especially in cases that have high stakes for your reporting such as programming decisions or allocation of funding.

When these assumptions are met, you may consider using a predictive design for one of three different purposes: (a) demonstrating simple links between two variables, (b) testing hypotheses about clusters of variables that predict a phenomenon, or (c) predicting the occurrence of an event happening. In each case, you will be able to portray associations that can be used to understand relationships between complex phenomena, develop and test theories, and predict behavior or outcomes.

Research and evaluation questions associated with predictive designs center around explaining shared and unique variance. Questions related to *shared variance* depict the correlation between two variables, whereas *unique variance* illustrates the amount of change in a criterion or outcome that is accounted for by one predictor within a model using multiple predictor variables. Predictive research questions will commonly test the statistical significance of relationships and lead one to interpret practical significance using estimates of effect size. Next, we describe the three identified purposes of predictive studies using the case study as a framework. In each case, we provide examples of research and evaluation questions. In each example, we italicize a functional component indicating the purpose of the research/evaluation to serve as a bridge to later analyses. Additionally, each question contains a specific reference to predictors and criteria of interest.

Demonstrating Simple Links Between Two Variables

At the foundational level, predictive designs help demonstrate a statistical relationship between two variables using *bivariate correlations*. Given the many complexities associated with human development across the lifespan, there are many possibilities for exploration. Therefore, it can be helpful to begin with identifying a criterion of interest and working backward to develop assumptions about which personal or program characteristics have a positive or negative influence. We might ask questions such as:

- Is there a *statistically significant* relationship between *participant age* and *symptom improvement* when completing the six-week DBT-A program?
- What are the *direction and magnitude* of association between *participant age* and *symptom improvement* when completing the six-week DBT-A program?

Testing Hypotheses about Groups of Variables That Predict a Phenomenon

It does not take a behavioral scientist to know that many of the phenomena we represent as criterion variables are not influenced by just one predictor. Instead, the synergy among characteristics and constructs tends to explain a greater proportion of the criterion variable. Consequently, you can use predictive designs to test ideas about the degree to which two or more variables predict a phenomenon. Multiple predictors can be associated with a theory of change, your clinically based anecdotes, or program reporting requirements. These designs may also help test differential associations for the same cluster of predictor variables across multiple criteria. We might ask questions such as:

- Are changes among *hypothesized mechanisms of change* (mindfulness, distress tolerance, emotion regulation, interpersonal effectiveness, and parent–child communication) *statistically significant predictors* of *symptom improvement* when completing the six-week DBT-A program?
- To what *degree* do *hypothesized mechanisms of change* (mindfulness, distress tolerance, emotion regulation, interpersonal effectiveness, and parent–child communication) predict *symptom improvement* when completing the six-week DBT-A program?

Predicting the Occurrence of an Event Happening

Of course, not everything of interest to practitioners, researchers, and evaluators is continuous in nature. For example, predicting educationally and clinically relevant categorical criteria such as first-time passing of the National Counselor Examination or participants no longer meeting diagnostic criteria following intervention is of great interest to many. Thus, predictive designs can be used to statistically model associations with categorical outcomes based on bivariate correlations and multiple variable associations. We might ask questions such as:

- Are changes among *hypothesized mechanisms of change* (mindfulness, distress tolerance, emotion regulation, interpersonal effectiveness, and parent–child communication) *statistically significant predictors* of *diagnostic remission* when completing the six-week DBT-A program?
- To what *degree* do *hypothesized mechanisms of change* (mindfulness, distress tolerance, emotion regulation, interpersonal effectiveness, and parent–child communication) predict *diagnostic remission* when completing the six-week DBT-A program?

BOX 9.3 CHECKLIST OF INDICATORS OF A QUALITY PREDICTIVE DESIGN

- Model for predictive relationship among variables is well defined and logically connected.
- Logical connection between the purpose of study/evaluation with related research/evaluation questions and analytic strategy.
  - Clear alignment between the measures selected as the basis for analyses
  - Reporting and interpretation of sample-specific reliability estimates
  - Data meet statistical model assumptions required for analyses.
- Estimates of statistical significance are reported and interpreted.
- Estimates of effect size such as Pearson's r, R^2, or β are reported and interpreted.
- Tables and visual depictions support reporting of findings.

TYPES OF PREDICTIVE DESIGNS

Bivariate: Correlations between Two Variables

Core Features

Correlations between two variables are represented by a class of designs known as bivariate designs. When implementing bivariate designs, you will collect information about two variables and statistically correlate their scores with one another to determine the magnitude and direction of their relationship (see Figure 9.1). There are instances where you may be interested in correlating two sets of categorical data. However, we will focus on designs that feature interval–ratio data such as scores on a psychological measure or age.

Intended Uses and Design Considerations

Bivariate designs are intended to answer research questions that demonstrate links between two phenomena. Given the degree of parsimony inherent within this design, you will want to assure that your variables are logically linked and linear. Your predictor variable should

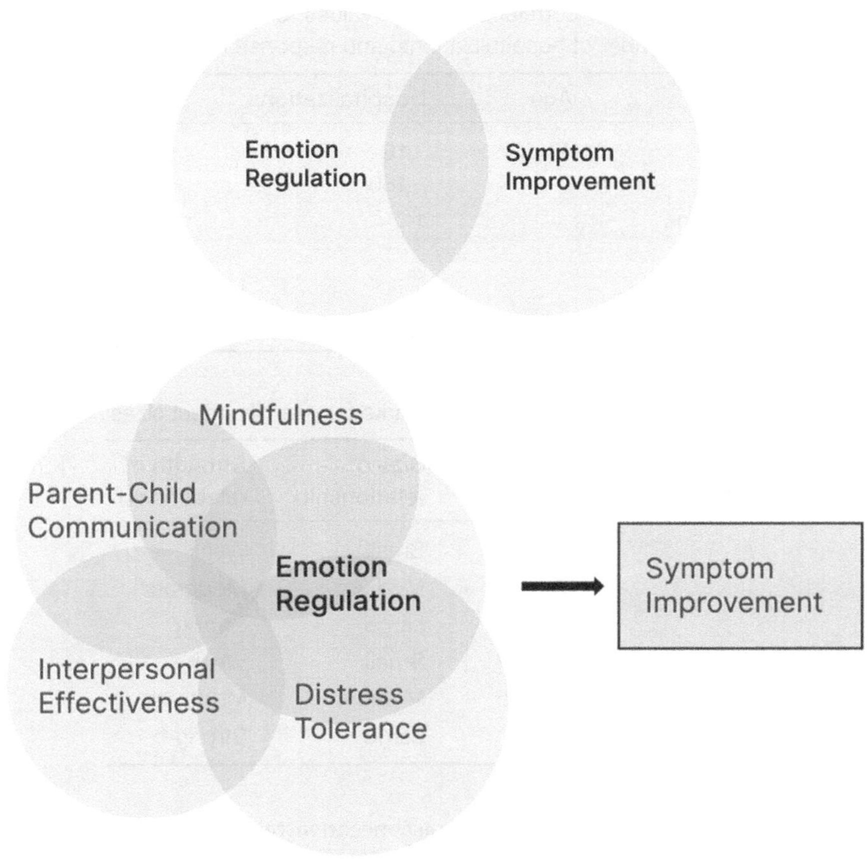

Figure 9.1 Visual Depictions of Bivariate and Multiple Variable Models for Predictive Designs

be reasonably expected to have an incremental relationship with the other variable. Additionally, the range of values for measures should be consistent across measures.

Data Analysis and Interpretation

The magnitude of bivariate relationships can be depicted using the Pearson product–moment correlation coefficient, which is noted by the statistical symbol r and associated with a p-value testing the null hypothesis that there is no relationship between scores. These values are typically situated in a matrix for interpretation (see Table 9.1).

In this scenario, r is a value representing the magnitude of association between variables *and* an effect size measuring practical significance of that relationship. The correlation coefficient will always be expressed in a value between 0 and 1 and may be positive (+) or negative (−) in nature. A value equal to 0 depicts no relationship between variables, whereas the value 1 represents a perfect match between variables. Positive relationships indicate situations when scores representing two variables tend to move together in the same direction. For example, Table 9.1 indicates a positive relationship between age and treatment response, meaning that older participants tended to report a greater response to treatment

TABLE 9.1 Pearson's *r* correlations and *p*-values for bivariate relationships between age, number of hospitalizations, and response to intervention

Variable	Age	Hospitalizations	Response
Age	1	.16	.72
p-value		.280	.001
Hospitalizations		1	–.42
p-value			.018
Response			1
p-value			

TABLE 9.2 Interpretive benchmarks for *r*-family effect sizes

r-Family Effect Size	Effect size value	Size of relationship	Strength of relationship
r	.10 – .29	Small	Weak
	.30 – .49	Medium	Moderate
	≥ .50	Large	Strong
R^2	.02 – .12	Small	Weak
	.13 – .25	Medium	Moderate
	≥ .26	Large	Strong

when compared to younger ones. By contrast, negative relationships indicate situations when scores representing two variables tend to move in opposite directions. In Table 9.1, there is a negative relationship between number of previous psychiatric hospitalizations and treatment response. Participants with fewer previous hospitalizations had a greater response to treatment than those who had been hospitalized a greater number of times.

Now that you have interpreted the statistical significance and nature of relationships between two variables, it is time to characterize the practical significance of the association. Best practice suggests identifying reference benchmarks for size and strength of relationships such as those proposed by Cohen (1988) and Rosenthal (2001) as depicted in Table 9.2. These are just starting places; there is no value in any correlational value whether outside or inside of its context. A good practice is to begin by characterizing the size and strength of your *r* values as small/weak (.1), medium/moderate (.3), or large/strong (.5) and proceed to provide situational context that accounts for participant experiences, intervention/program characteristics, sociopolitical context, and previous findings.

Multiple Variable: Predicting a Single Criterion with Multiple Variables

Core Features

Multiple variable designs use two or more predictor variables to explain shared and unique variance with a single criterion. When implementing these designs, you will be testing a model that you believe should explain the presence of your criterion (see

Figure 9.1). First you collect information about two or more predictor variables and a criterion that is continuous or discrete in nature. Next, make sure that data are usable and meet assumptions that (a) all participant scores only occur once [*independence*], (b) predictors reflect different constructs [*multicollinearity*], (c) scores for the criterion measure are normally distributed [*normality*], and (d) differences in variances for the criterion variables are equal [*homoscedasticity*]. Then, you use a statistical technique known as regression to determine whether your model is statistically significant and, if so, how much change in the criterion can be accounted for through model predictors, both individually and together.

Intended Uses and Design Considerations

Multiple-variable predictive designs answer research/evaluation questions regarding the usefulness of a cluster of variables for predicting a phenomenon. When a well-defined, logically supported model exists, it is possible to explain a greater amount of relationships between variables. These models are well-suited to clusters of variables that predict a phenomenon. After all, human experiences are complex and make complex pathways to your criterion of interest. In these instances, your approach to prediction should be too. With greater complexity comes additional responsibility in design considerations. Whereas bivariate designs were simple, multiple-variable designs require that scores on the criterion variable meet additional assumptions. There is a little more leg work required on your end, but greater effort may lead to greater quality of information to inform counseling interventions, program efficiency, and accountability efforts.

Data Analysis and Interpretation

Researchers and evaluators use several analyses to understand the influence of multiple predictors on one criterion variable; however, we will focus on linear multiple regression as a practical tool most researchers and evaluators can use in a prudent way. These analyses require you to (a) test and verify model assumptions (linearity, independence, multicollinearity, normality, homoscedasticity) and (b) statistically regress scores for your criterion variable onto scores for your predictors.

Your results will provide some basic output related to the statistical significance of your model (p), the overall proportion of variance (i.e., change) in scores on the criterion variable accounted for by all of the predictors (R^2), and information about the unique contributions of each predictor (t, p, β). If you are feeling overwhelmed, you might think of those outputs this way: Did your ingredients contribute to baking a cake or not ($p < .05$)? How big of a piece of cake do your ingredients account for (R^2)? Of that piece of cake, how much does each ingredient contribute (t, p, β)?

By now, p-values are familiar. The size and strength of your R^2 values can be characterized as small/weak (.02), medium/moderate (.13), or large/strong (.26), but will require some clarifying information about contributions from individual model predictors to be fully appreciated (see Table 9.2). The contributions from individual predictors are tested in multiple regression analyses through t-tests, each with its own *p*-values and depiction of how much of the R^2 can be accounted for through its inclusion (sr^2).

Predicting an Event with Multiple Variables

Core Features

Multiple-variable predictive designs can also explain shared and unique variance with a categorical outcome. When implementing multiple-variable predictive designs, you will test a model you believe should explain the presence or absence of an event. First you collect information about two or more predictor variables, as well as an educationally or clinically relevant criterion that is categorical in nature. Next, you make sure data are usable and meet assumptions for independence, multicollinearity, normality, and homoscedasticity. Then, you statistically regress scores with a criterion to determine whether the model is statistically significant and, if so, how much change in the criterion can be accounted for through model predictors as a cluster and individually.

Intended Uses and Design Considerations

Multiple-variable predictive designs are best suited to answer research/evaluation questions related to using multiple variables to predict an event or outcome happening. These designs share many similarities with those previously discussed, with the main distinction being the nature of the criterion as an event occurring or not. Overall, this can be a wonderful addition to your toolkit for predicting key outcomes such as diagnostic remission, program completion, and other categorical benchmarks.

Data Analysis and Interpretation

Researchers and evaluators use several analyses to understand the influence of multiple predictors for one criterion variable; however, we will focus on binomial logistic regression as a useful tool most researchers and evaluators can use in a practical way. These analyses require you to (a) test and verify model assumptions (linearity, independence, multicollinearity, normality, homoscedasticity) and (b) statistically regress scores for a criterion variable onto scores for predictors.

Your results will provide some basic output related to the statistical significance of your model (p) and the odds that each predictor will increase the occurrence of the event occurring or not occurring. An odds ratio (OR) indicates the likelihood that each predictor will be associated with the event occurring or not. An OR value of 1 suggests a neutral scenario in which a predictor does not increase odds. However, any value above 1 represents a percentage increase in the odds of an event happening. Consider the multivariable design depicted in Figure 9.1. Let's imagine that we replaced the criterion variable with a categorical binomial one indicating whether or not a participant meets criteria for diagnosis at the end of a program. If your analyses detected an OR = 1.50 for the relationship between interpersonal effectiveness skills and not meeting criteria, you could infer that interpersonal effectiveness skills increase the odds of successful remission by 50%: (1.50–1) × 100 = participant odds.

PUTTING FINDINGS IN CONTEXT

Although you can describe the significance of findings in terms of statistical, practical, and clinical improvements, these changes are merely in *association* with an intervention or program, not necessarily *caused* by it. Therefore, putting predictive design findings into context begins with establishing that boundary. From that position you are well-situated to develop impact statements, interpret effect sizes, interpret clinical significance, and shape a summative conceptualization of intervention/program usefulness. Box 9.4 depicts a six-step guide to shape your process. You can modify capitalized words to suit your results, but only you can breathe life into your narrative and portray findings in a way that honors your project and participants' experiences (more on this in Chapter 17).

BOX 9.4 BASIC FRAMEWORK FOR REPORTING PREDICTIVE DESIGN FINDINGS IN CONTEXT

Step 1: Describe results of predictive analysis, including statistical and practical significance of model

The regression analysis estimating the influence of predictor variables on CRITERION scores DID/DID NOT result in a statistically significant model, F(df, df) = VALUE, p = p-VALUE, R^2 = R^2 VALUE, indicative of a SMALL, MEDIUM, LARGE effect size and WEAK, MODERATE, STRONG association between variables.

Step 2: Provide an interpretation of practical significance metric for the model

This finding suggests that model predictors account for approximately VALUE% of the change among scores predicting CRITERION.

Step 3: Report statistically significant predictors within the model first, including important elements such as standardized beta value, significance test, and measure of unique variance explained

Within the model, scores associated with PREDICTOR contributed a statistically significant proportion of variance to the model, β = VALUE, p = VALUE, sr^2 = VALUE.

Step 4: Provide a plainly spoken interpretation of each finding

This finding accounted for approximately VALUE% of change among participants' scores on the CRITERION and can be attributed to EXPLAIN THE MEANING OF FINDING.

Step 5: Report nonsignificant findings all together and use a similar format for significant findings

Statistically significant findings were not detected for scores related to PREDICTOR, β = VALUE, p = VALUE, sr^2 = VALUE and PREDICTOR, β = VALUE, p = VALUE, sr^2 = VALUE.

Step 6: Develop a summative statement about the findings

Constructively integrate all this information through your uniquely informed lens to make a conservative, even-handed summative statement about the usefulness of your model for understanding the criterion of interest.

Developing General Impact Statements

The impact statements you develop from predictive designs should be nested in an understanding of amounts of change in a criterion that were associated with your model and its constituent variables. You should take care to avoid causal language, instead opting for expressions such as *were associated with* and *tended to predict*. This provides an authentic depiction of results that acknowledges that predictive modeling is just that—modeling. Because all predictive designs convey information about viability of a model and proportions of variance, a technical statement followed by plainly spoken interpretations tend to be a good place to start.

Interpreting Significance

Following this general statement, provide support based on some metrics that can be communicated from one service clinician, educator, researcher, or evaluator to another. For multiple-variable designs relying on linear regression, report values for your overall model (F, R^2) and predictors (standardized beta (β), t, p, and sr^2). For designs intended to predict a binomial criterion or probability using logistic regression, report values for the overall model (X^2, p) and the influence of individual predictors using OR, related confidence intervals, and p-values.

Shaping Summative Findings

In the end, aim to integrate all of this information through your uniquely informed lens to make a conservative, even-handed statement about the usefulness of your model for understanding the criterion of interest. Develop your summative statement of findings in reference to strengths and limitations of predictive studies, your ability to explain the nature of statistical correlations, and an understanding of the meaning of scores within your unique context. This statement will rely on you to synthesize findings through your unique lens and meaning-making processes, and you will use evidence of statistical and practical significance to support your conclusions.

DISPLAYING RESULTS

As with other designs, you may find descriptive tables and easily understood graphics helpful for depicting results. Because these projects rely heavily on depicting proportions of variance explained by variables, modified Venn diagrams, pie charts, and partially filled vertical bar graphs lend themselves well to conveying relationships.

Transparency in reporting the statistical output of predictive designs is imperative when considering that the concept of statistical correlation usually relies on measurement of constructs. Therefore, reporting means, standard deviations, and reliability information for your measures within tables can promote transparent reporting.

A Venn diagram is composed of at least two circles or ovals that represent the data for unique variables, which overlap to some degree to represent a relationship. In this case, the overlap represents shared variance among scores. This is perfect for demonstrating relationships in bivariate and multiple-variable designs. Venn diagrams can be seen in Figure 9.1.

Pie charts can be used to depict unique and shared variance for multiple-variable models. When using these charts, the overall shape reflects 100% of variance explained for your criterion variable (i.e., a correlation coefficient or R^2 value of 1). Therefore, each slice of the pie represents the unique amount of variance explained by each predictor, and their collective presence represents the influence of your predictive model. Using our case study as an example, this includes the relative associations of the predictors (mindfulness, distress tolerance, emotion regulation, interpersonal effectiveness, and parent–child communication) with the criterion variable (symptom improvement). When developing these charts, be sure to provide a slice of the pie that depicts unknown contributors to your model. This provides an element of transparency when presenting findings and impact statements related to the boundaries of your findings and priorities.

Finally, stacked bar graphs are another resource for displaying proportions of variance explained by your predictive model. The concept is similar to that of a pie chart; however, data will be presented linearly rather than circularly. Often, we present data in a manner of accumulating variance from smallest to largest, with the unknown proportion coming last. Stacked bar graph depictions may be most clear when only a few variables exist within the predictor model.

BOX 9.5 CASE STUDY REVISITED

The clinical director developed a multiple-variable predictive design to evaluate relationships between hypothesized mechanisms for change within a DBT-A framework and therapeutic change. The model was tested using a multiple regression analysis. This section will provide a brief application of chapter content to illustrate single-group principles and practices you can replicate in your work.

Purpose of Evaluation

- Testing contributions of constructs associated with the DBT-A framework for therapeutic change.

Related Questions Guiding the Evaluation

- Are changes among hypothesized mechanisms of change (mindfulness, distress tolerance, emotion regulation, interpersonal effectiveness, and parent–child communication) statistically significant predictors of symptom improvement when completing the six-week DBT-A program?
- To what degree do hypothesized mechanisms of change (mindfulness, distress tolerance, emotion regulation, interpersonal effectiveness, and parent–child communication) predict symptom improvement when completing the six-week DBT-A program?

Selected Predictive Design

- Multiple-variable predictive model with one criterion (therapeutic change) and five predictors (mindfulness, distress tolerance, emotion regulation, interpersonal effectiveness, and parent–child communication).
- Statistical and practical significance for model predictors tested using a simultaneous multiple regression analysis.

Putting Findings into Context

The regression analysis estimating the influence of predictor variables on therapeutic change in psychiatric symptoms resulted in a statistically significant model, $F(4, 98) = 23.31$, $p < .01$, $R^2 = .68$, indicative of a large effect size and strong association between variables. This finding suggests that model predictors account for approximately 68% of the change among scores predicting therapeutic change among participants. Within the model, associated scores were Distress Tolerance ($\beta = .39$, $p < .05$, $sr^2 = .15$), Emotion Regulation ($\beta = .43$, $p < .05$, $sr^2 = .18$), Interpersonal Effectiveness ($\beta = .39$, $p < .05$, $sr^2 = .15$), and Parent–Child Communication ($\beta = .31$, $p < .05$, $sr^2 = .14$). This finding accounted for approximately 62% of change among participants' scores associated with psychiatric symptoms and can be attributed to the ability of participants to mobilize DBT-A skills associated with managing distress, positively modulating affect, interacting with others in ways that preserve self-respect, and negotiating middle ground with parents. Statistically significant findings were not detected for scores related to Mindfulness ($\beta = .02$, $p = .12$, $sr^2 = .06$). These findings suggest that the greatest proportions of therapeutic change were associated with mastery and implementation of skills associated with DBT-A modules teaching distress tolerance, emotion regulation, interpersonal effectiveness, and parent–child communication. Although mindfulness skills contributed some proportion of change within the model, scores reflecting this construct were not a statistically significant predictor of therapeutic change within this sample of adolescents.

Displaying Findings

Relevant information depicting statistical and practical significance of the predictive model and amounts of variance associated with each predictor variable can be depicted in a table.

Variable	β	t	sr^2	F	R^2
Therapeutic Change in Psychiatric Symptoms				23.21	.68
Mindfulness	–.02	–1.18	.06		
Distress Tolerance	–.39	–3.54*	.15		
Emotion Regulation	–.43	–3.89*	.18		
Interpersonal Effectiveness	–.39	–3.55*	.15		
Parent–Child Communication	–.31	–3.31*	.14		

Note. *= statistically significant at the.05 level.

Unique and shared variance for model predictors can be displayed using a stacked bar graph:

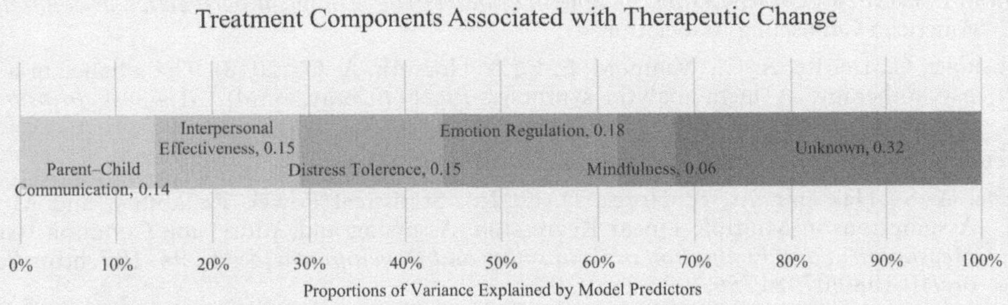

Figure 9.2 Visual Depiction of Unique and Shared Variance for Model Predictors

CHAPTER SUMMARY

This chapter has presented initial concepts and tools to design, develop, and implement predictive designs. With this information, you are ready to clarify your purpose and begin developing your own project based on logically connected research/evaluation questions, design selection, analyses, and reporting practices. These concepts and tools were illustrated with a case example of a DBT-A program delivered in a partial hospitalization program for adolescents. By referencing the checklist presented in this chapter, you are prepared to begin evaluating programs that have potential to stimulate meaningful changes in your community. We hope the resources in this chapter will help you describe the many relationships between variables which will support best practices for program design, implementation, and evaluation, and also empower your academic community, stakeholders, and relevant policy makers.

RESOURCES

- American Educational Research Association. (2006). Standards for reporting on empirical social science research in AERA publications. *Educational Researcher*, *35*, 33–40. https://10.3102/0013189X035006033

- Hosmer, D. W., Lemeshow, S., & Sturdivant, R. (2013). *Applied logistic regression* (3rd ed.). Wiley.
- *Educational Research Basics by Del Siegle*, University of Connecticut. https://researchbasics.education.uconn.edu
- Keith, T. Z., Reynolds, M. R. & Caemmerer, J. M. (2025). *Multiple regression and beyond: An introduction to multiple regression and structural equation modeling* (4th ed.). Routledge.
- *Spurious Correlations*, Tyler Vigen. www.tylervigen.com

REFERENCES

Adler, A. (1927/2014). *Understanding human nature*. One World Publications.

Cohen, J. (1988). *Statistical power analysis for the behavioral sciences* (2nd ed.). Lawrence Erlbaum.

Cook, E. P. (2015). *Understanding people in context: The ecological perspective in counseling*. American Counseling Association.

Flückiger, C., Del Re, A. C., Wampold, B. E., & Horvath, A. O. (2018). The alliance in adult psychotherapy: A meta-analytic synthesis. *Psychotherapy*, *55*(4), 316–340. *https://doi.org/10.1037/pst0000172*

Freud, S. (1905). *Three essays on the theory of sexuality*. Verso.

Lenz, A. S., Haktanir, A., & Flores, D. (2026). Statistical Power, Reliability, and Model Assumptions in Multiple Linear Regression: Assessing and Addressing Common Issues. *Measurement and Evaluation in Counseling and Development*, *59*(1), 94–107. https://doi.org/10.1080/07481756.2025.2589207

Lenz, A. S., & Oliver, M. (2017). Predictive associations between family system characteristics and emergent protective factors. *The Family Journal*, *26*, 40–47. https://doi.org/10.1177/1066480717731343

McLaren, L., & Hawe, P. (2005). Ecological perspectives in health research. *Journal of Epidemiology and Community Health*, *59*, 6–14. https://doi.org/10.1136/jech.2003.018044

Rathus, J. H., & Miller, A. L. (2015). *DBT skills manual for adolescents*. Guilford.

Rosenthal, J. A. (2001). *Statistics and data interpretation for the helping professions*. Wadsworth.

Vigen, T. (2015). *Spurious correlations: Correlation does not equal causation*. Hachette.

CHAPTER 10

Evaluating Change within an Individual

There is something very special about the power of one. As mental health professionals, we see the unique, nuanced experiences of individuals receiving treatment. We measure their response to therapeutic interventions against their historical experiences rather than a large group of randomly selected participants. This is the hallmark of single-case research designs (SCRDs). With intentionality and some attention to detail, SCRDs provide a set of dynamic experimental strategies for evaluating cause-and-effect relationships between interventions and outcomes within an individual participant. When these *N of 1* experiments are replicated with data from other individuals and settings, it is possible to establish our practices or programs as empirically supported interventions. For these reasons, SCRDs have been regarded as the method of choice for counselors due to their responsiveness and practicality (Brown et al., 2024; Institute of Education Science (IES), 2022; Lenz, 2015, 2018).

This chapter introduces you to some essential activities associated with research and evaluation approaches with individual participants to demonstrate the course of treatment response and effect of interventions. Specific methods covered in this chapter include AB phase contrasts, replication designs, and multiple baseline designs. Elements of each method will be applied to a case study of a program designed to treat trauma among adolescents who have witnessed domestic violence.

BOX 10.1 CHAPTER LEARNING OUTCOMES

- Develop research questions consistent with use of single-case research designs
- Design, plan, carry out, record, and analyze results of single-case research designs
- Communicate findings from single-case research designs using a variety of methods
- Identify and critique data associated with single-case research designs

DOI: 10.4324/9781003586210-12

BOX 10.2 CASE STUDY

Consider a scenario wherein you are a counselor supervisor for the small trauma arm of a large behavioral health agency; your focus is on treating children who have been victims of crime in an urban city. Recently, your external funding source has received a legislative mandate that prioritizes reimbursement for a *priority population* which consists of individuals who have a primary behavioral health diagnosis of major depressive disorder, bipolar disorder, or schizophrenia. Although your administration recognizes that your trauma clinic fills an important gap within the local public mental health infrastructure, they are requesting data depicting the efficacy of your clinic's services. In the absence of efficacy data, it is possible that client care will be coordinated with other agencies, you will be reassigned to another unit within the agency, and the facilities you occupy will be repurposed to expand capacity to treat the priority population.

You decide that a single-case research design may provide you with an evaluation framework for demonstrating clinical outcomes for your trauma-focused cognitive behavior therapy (TF-CBT; Cohen et al., 2017) program that has been delivered at your clinic for years. You select the Child PTSD Symptom Scale for DSM-5 (CPSS; Foa et al., 2017) to administer weekly to clients. Scores on the CPSS range from 0 to 80, with a score of 31 representing a critical cut score in which severity of symptoms may meet clinical criteria for diagnosis of PTSD, and good test-retest reliability ($r = 0.80$).

OVERVIEW OF SINGLE-CASE RESEARCH DESIGNS

What Are Single-Case Research Designs?

SCRDs are a class of experimental methods that have the potential to demonstrate causal relationships between an intervention and an outcome within an individual participant. Well-designed SCRDs allow us to make inferences about the efficacy of an intervention outside constraints associated with between-groups studies which require large sample sizes, high costs, complex logistics, comparisons to alternative treatments, and sophisticated data analyses (Lenz, 2015). Instead, researchers and evaluators who implement SCRDs determine how well an intervention works by comparing participants to themselves, a concept called **self-as-control**. This strategy, along with requiring a minimal sample size, ease of data analyses, and logistical practicality, makes SCRDs a great alternative for depicting response to intervention in the real world (Brown et al., 2024; Lenz, 2025).

Core Features of Single-Case Research Designs

Many researchers hear "you only need a few participants" and tend to assume SCRDs can or should be used any time someone is working with a small sample size. However, for findings to be regarded as defensible, we must account for several characteristics and assumptions (Ray, 2015). First, SCRDs all have a minimum of one **AB phase contrast** wherein a baseline phase when no treatment is present (denoted as the letter A) is compared to one intervention phase (denoted as the letter B). If an intervention is withdrawn, we go back to an A phase (ABA); if another intervention is introduced, it is denoted by the letter C (ABC). Second, all SCRDs rely on **continuous measurement of outcome variables** in a way that is systematic and stable across all phases which has implications for test-retest reliability and appropriate use of measures. Third, inferences about an intervention's efficacy can only be inferred when baseline data show a degree of **stability** across observations and thus accurately represent participant experiences. Finally, baseline data that are stable prior to an intervention may support the most defensible **cause-and-effect inferences** related to associations between an intervention an outcome when replicated across multiple AB phases or when compared to other interventions. Therefore, the independent variable in SCRDs is often the intervention or program and the dependent variable is the outcome of interest. To summarize, all SCRDs will feature a common language, at least two phases (baseline and intervention), continuous measurement of the outcome variable, and stability within the baseline phase prior to introducing an intervention.

In addition to these characteristics, the degree to which SCRD results are defensible is a function of the point to which certain assumptions are met. Foremost, is the issue of ***caseness***; because the number of participants will be few, they should be similar in important ways such as age, gender, ethnicity, held identities, location, and presenting issue. Next, the study should feature **intervention fidelity** to assure that the type/amount of an intervention received by participants is equivalent. Although SCRDs can be used to evaluate novel practices, those practices should be manualized or standardized to a reasonable degree. Additionally, reliance on continuous assessment can be confounding for SCRDs because many assessments are not designed to be administered daily, biweekly, or weekly (but some are!). Therefore, we must account for related **test-retest reliability** considerations when selecting measures to represent outcome variables in any SCRD. Finally, results of SCRDs rest on the assumption that an earnest effort was made to demonstrate **replication of intervention effects** across at least three participants, but ideally more (IES, 2022; Lenz 2024).

When Are Single-Case Research Designs Indicated?

SCRDs are a helpful framework for demonstrating causal relationships between interventions and outcomes, and they are particularly well-suited for some purposes. First, SCRDs can be helpful for understanding whether the efficacy of an already established intervention can be replicated with samples similar to those identified in the literature or extended to a new population of intervention or program recipients. Second, SCRDs may be prudent to investigate the preliminary support for novel counseling services and programs when general effectiveness and the factors contributing to treatment success may be unclear such as dosage-response interactions, adherence to measurement, and completeness of the intervention protocol. Third, SCRDs can provide a strong scientific foundation for assessing applications of treatments with low incidence or understudied groups (Lenz, 2015; Lenz, 2025).

Understanding the Efficacy of an Intervention

Generally speaking, SCRDs can be implemented when attempting to understand how efficacious an intervention is for meeting a particular outcome with a sample of participants. By comparing an individual's performance on an outcome measure before and after intervention, apparent changes can be readily observed with the naked eye or a range of statistical methods, some requiring little more than basic addition and division. The contrasting of outcome observations across baseline and intervention phases will not provide a *yes/no* understanding about whether an intervention or program is *effective*. Instead, SCRDs can depict the amount and type of efficacy that can be experienced by participants.

Establishing Preliminary Support for Novel Practices

Ever have a novel idea for solving a problem? Most counselors do; we are a creative group always pushing ourselves to help others in the best, most efficient ways possible. New ideas are rarely accompanied by 100 participants who can be randomized into at least two groups. SCRDs can be a great strategy for determining preliminary support for novel or modified counseling practices. If evidence from initial interventions is strong, larger, more logistically challenging evaluations may be warranted. As clinicians, educators, and administrators continue to innovate new ways to meet client needs, SCRDs will continue to be a viable option.

Assessing Applications of Treatments with Low Incidence or Understudied Groups

There is a high probability that if you picked up an article about an intervention study or Googled "evidence-based practices" they would detail interventions with commonly occurring disorders or developmental issues. Highly occurring disorders tend to be studied the most because they affect the largest number of individuals, and their treatment is associated with broad efforts for mental health care. By contrast, rarely occurring but serious disorders such as Munchausen syndrome or the emergence of obsessive-compulsive disorder symptoms among caregivers following a child's tracheotomy can interfere with well-being and warrant their own evidence-supported interventions. In such instances, SCRDs can provide a framework for understanding best practices and support groups that are underrepresented or understudied in the professional literature.

What Types of Questions Can Be Answered Using SCRDs?

In all three scenarios, SCRDs are well-suited to answer two categories of research and evaluation questions: those about the degree of treatment effect and those about the course of treatment response.

Depicting Degree of Treatment Effect

Studies about treatment effects facilitate understanding about the amount or magnitude of changes observed across baseline and intervention phases. In many cases, this question will be addressed through one of two methods: (a) nonoverlap of data between baseline and intervention phases and (b) computation of an effect size which depicts direction and magnitude of the change in scores between phases. When used in tandem, you will be poised to explain how much of your intervention was associated with a desired outcome (e.g., 75%), and you will be able to represent a standardized outcome that can be compared to results of other sites, projects, or interventions. Examples of questions related to depicting the amount and degree of treatment effect include:

- *How effective* is a 12-week TF-CBT intervention for decreasing the symptoms of PTSD among adolescents who have witnessed long-term domestic violence?
- *To what degree* is a 12-week TF-CBT intervention effective for decreasing the symptoms of PTSD among adolescents who have witnessed long-term domestic violence?

Depicting Course of Treatment Effect

You can also use SCRDs to understand the trajectory of someone's response to intervention. This is an invaluable resource for using data trends from repeated measurement of outcomes to understand how participants experience your intervention or program. For example, sessions 1 to 8 of TF-CBT are dedicated to developing coping skills, and sessions 9 to 12 are associated with trauma narration, processing, and enhancing future safety. If all participants demonstrate a noticeable jump in trauma symptoms after session 9, when trauma narration and processing are introduced, that information may be helpful to clinicians as they prepare families during the therapeutic process. Similarly, if all participants demonstrate a levelling off from therapeutic progress following skills training (i.e., no additional improvements were noted during sessions 9 to 12), it may be reasonable to suggest that families decide whether addressing the trauma narrative would add value to their experience and outcome. An example question related to depicting the amount and degree of treatment effect includes:

- *What is the course of treatment response* for a 12-week TF-CBT intervention for decreasing the symptoms of PTSD among adolescents who have witnessed long-term domestic violence?

TYPES OF SINGLE-CASE RESEARCH DESIGNS

A-B Phase Contrasts

Core Features

All SCRDs are grounded in the basic contrast between data gathered during the baseline (A) and intervention (B) phases. This framework is depicted in Figure 10.1 and is representative of the premise that when reasonable threats to validity have been accounted for, the differences or *contrast* between A and B phases can be attributed to the influence of an intervention or program. Contrasting of A and B phases relies on

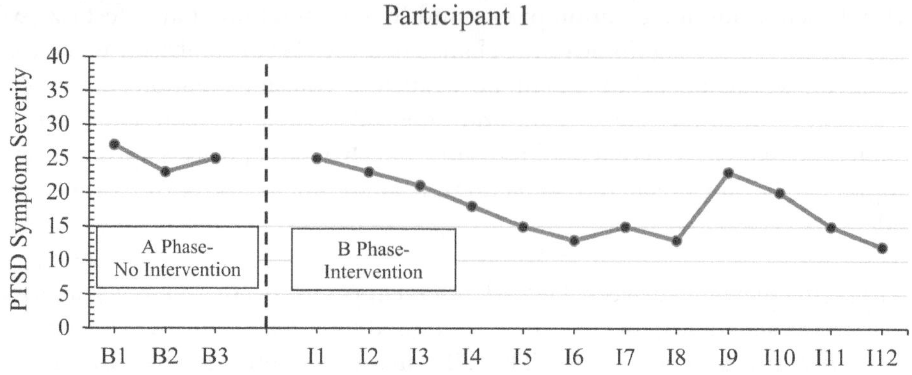

Figure 10.1 Visual Depiction of Data Associated with an A-B Phase Contrast Design

consistent measurement of the dependent variable over time. As seen in Figure 10.1, data representing the dependent variable (PTSD Symptom Severity) are noted on the ordinate (vertical) axis, time is presented on the abscissa (horizontal) axis, and data are separated across A and B phases.

Intended Uses and Design Considerations

A-B phase contrasts are intended to depict the interaction between an intervention and an outcome. Oftentimes, this design is a useful strategy because contact with participants almost always includes knowing them just before and during an intervention. Conveniently, many treatments and program procedures involve some degree of assessment during these periods. With some careful attention to detail, you are able to illustrate some preliminary evidence for an intervention or program.

You may have noticed the word *preliminary* in the preceding sentence. The simple contrasting of A-B phases is limited due to an inability to account for threats to internal validity such as history and time (Ray, 2015; Vannest & Ninci, 2015). The causal relationship between intervention and outcome is most defensible when a few characteristics are present. First, baseline data (A) have been relatively stable over time, as noted by enough observations recorded to represent the presence of a construct over time. Kratochwill et al. (2013) identified five observations as the standard for practice, yet others such as Kennedy (2005) suggested that three observations may be the most that can be reasonably expected due to ethical or practical considerations in some cases. Although some counseling researchers have capitalized on baseline datasets composed of three data points (Callender et al., 2019; Cox et al., 2015; Hollenbaugh & Lenz, 2018; Schmidt et al., 2022), this strategy is only defensible if data are stable over time. Second, intervention-phase data (B) should demonstrate a convincing, persistent trend toward the desired effect. It is unreasonable to expect that all interventions will have an immediate or stable effect, but treatment responses that are erratic may indicate issues related to extraneous variables. Ideally, the pattern of intervention-phase data would be apparently convincing. However, some interventions take time to be efficacious, and participants' life events may present challenges that move data outside the desired range during intervention. If these trends are noted across participants, they may represent the nature of the functional relationship between intervention and outcome; if they are not consistent, the issue may lie in threats to experimental validity within the design.

Replication Designs

Core Features

We can overcome limitations of A-B phase contrast designs by inspecting the outcome variable during a withdrawal phase (A-B-A design), but we can draw more robust inferences from a replication design. Replication designs feature an initial A-B phase, followed by a withdrawal phase and reintroduction of the intervention. Figure 10.2 represents the framework for an A-B-A-B replication in which data were continuously collected during baseline, a six-session intervention, withdrawal phase, and reintroduction of intervention. Although it is difficult to make too many assumptions regarding activity within the withdrawal phase, if participant performance is similar or shows greater improvement in the second B phase, we can make strong inferences about the functional relationship between intervention and outcomes.

Intended Uses and Design Considerations

Replication designs account for several threats to internal validity such as history, maturation, and concurrent exposures to other interventions through repeated illustrations of outcomes in the presence versus absence of an intervention (Vannest & Ninci, 2015). This strategy is particularly well-suited for interventions such as dialectical behavior therapy (Linehan, 2025) or the Adult Recidivism Reduction Alternatives program (Cox et al., 2017) intended to be delivered in multiple iterations;

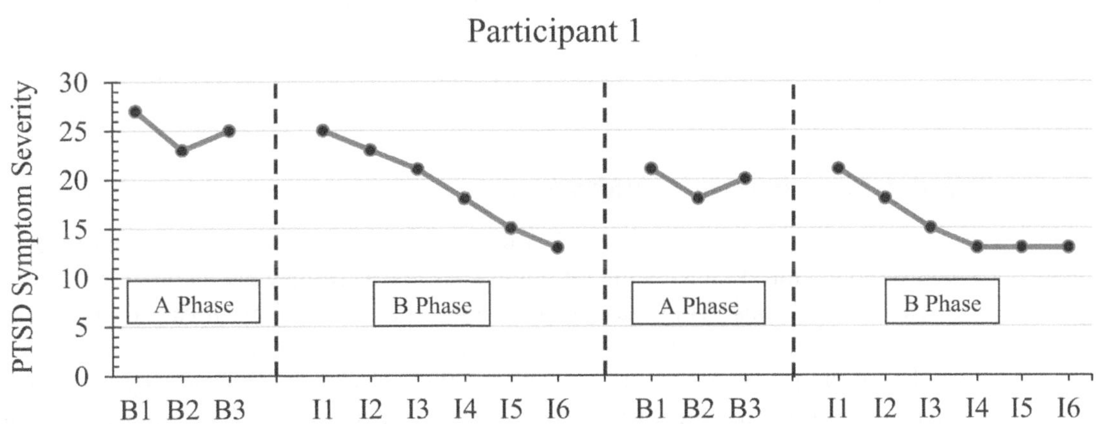

Figure 10.2 Visual Depiction of Data Associated with an A-B-A-B Replication Design

in both cases, participants complete the program the first time to learn skills and then again to master the skills. In these cases, replication designs are a great strategy for developing defensible, robust inferences about treatment effect (Liu et al., 2019; Toomey et al., 2023).

However, implementing replication designs and interpreting their data may be a challenge for two reasons. First, the objective of many interventions or programs is lasting effect. Therefore, non-replication or non-magnification of an intended outcome in the second B phase may be because the intervention worked the first time. Second, withdrawal of an intervention from a client may be antithetical to the premise of an intervention, or even unethical. For example, when evaluating an intervention that relies on the counselor–client relationship as the curative factor, withdrawing the relationship in the name of science does not make much sense. Similarly, when an individual is just beginning to make progress or appears to be destabilizing, removing an intervention may not be safe for the participant. Taken together, replication designs overcome several limitations of simple A-B phase contrasts and provide robust findings that inform evidence-supported practices. Nevertheless, they should be used only in a context that is logically sound and ethically responsible. Fortunately, when replication designs are not possible, we have alternatives to draw upon within our toolbox.

Multiple-Baseline Designs

Core Features

Multiple-baseline designs help us evaluate the functional relationships between interventions and outcomes across participants. Multiple-baseline designs feature A-B phase contrasts across at least three participants that are noted by different lengths of baseline phases. In these designs, the functional relationship is demonstrated through replication of treatment effect across staggered introduction of the intervention and multiple lengths of baseline phases. Figure 10.3 represents the framework for a multiple-baseline design in which all participants received a 12-week intervention, yet baseline lengths were staggered at 3-, 5-, and 6-week intervals. In cases where treatment responses and amount of treatment effect are similar despite differing baseline phase lengths, we can make strong inferences about the functional relationship between intervention and outcomes.

Intended Uses and Design Considerations

Multiple-baseline designs are a wonderful strategy for overcoming the limitations of A-B and replication designs while retaining a sufficient framework for making cause-and-effect attributions. As alluded to previously, the defensibility of causal inferences will depend on the degree to which you are able to provide evidence of a stable baseline. The truest understanding of intervention effect may be based upon all participants receiving the same amount, format, and duration of treatment. This latter point can be challenging in some settings where there is a fixed time period for collecting data.

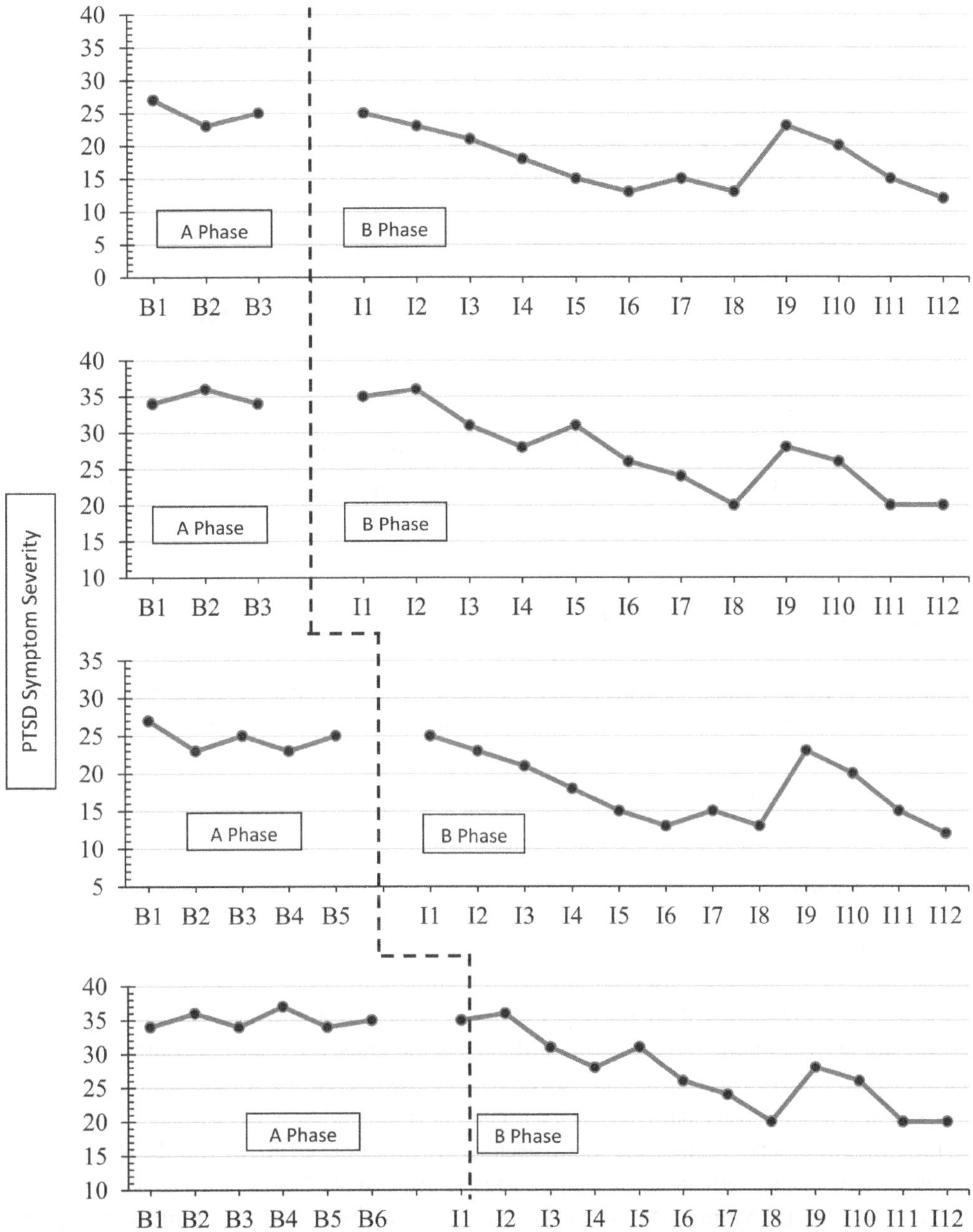

Figure 10.3 Visual Depiction of Data Associated with a Multiple-Baseline Design

However, we may make some viable inferences from partially collected data that are collected in an ethical manner and do not deny treatment to someone in need. In the end, you will have to balance the benefits and limitations of all designs to understand whether an A-B, A-B-A, replication, or multiple-baseline design is most appropriate for your needs.

BOX 10.3 INDICATORS OF A QUALITY SINGLE-CASE RESEARCH DESIGN

- Caseness of participants.
- Fidelity of intervention delivered across participants.
- Timing of intervention is pre-established and reasonable considering participant experience.
- Evidence of test-retest reliability and appropriateness of measure use for repeated data collection
- Repeated measurement of outcome variable is consistent and sensitive to multiple administrations.
- Baseline data are stable over time.
- Estimates of treatment course and effect are provided.
- Findings are situated in context of design limitations.
- Tables and visual depictions support reporting of findings.

DATA ANALYSES AND INTERPRETATION

Data analyses and their related interpretations tend to fall into three broad categories: (a) visual analyses, (b) estimates of treatment effect, and (c) estimates of practical significance based on effect size. Each strategy is associated with a certain utility, but findings are most meaningful when we integrate all three categories into meaningful clinical and social contexts.

Visual Analyses

Practices for completing visual analyses are based on graphing the data for each participant across baseline and intervention phases, similar to those depicted in Figures 10.1, 10.2, and 10.3. Once we make these graphs, four steps can support our analyses and interpretation: (a) document a predictable, stable baseline phase; (b) examine data within each phase to characterize within-phase patterns; (c) compare data with adjacent and similar phases; and (d) integrate data across all phases and participants (IES, 2022). To examine data within and between phases, we inspect six features: (a) level, (b) variability, (c) trend, (d) immediacy of the effect, (e) overlap, and (f) consistency of data patterns across similar phases (Ray, 2015; Vannest & Ninci, 2015). The first three of these features (level, variability, trend) are helpful for estimating whether an intervention was effective; the latter three features (immediacy, overlap, and consistency) are helpful for describing the course of the intervention effect. We should consider each feature individually and together to form a general impression that characterizes participants' responses to intervention.

Level

Level refers to the average score for data within each phase and represents participants' mean performance. Once the arithmetic average is identified for each phase, comparing the differences of these levels can support inferences regarding clinically significant amounts of change.

Trend

Trend of data is noted by a best-fitting line drawn through a series of graphed data points that shows the overall trend in the data. When using trend lines, we assume that if participant conditions remained unchanged (no intervention, intervention), participants would perpetually continue in this manner. Trend lines can be generally characterized as therapeutic, therapeutically neutral, or contra-therapeutic; we may also consider them as desired or undesired.

Variability

Variability is indicated by the absence of stability among data with phases and ranges of score differences surrounding trend lines. These metrics are helpful for depicting the stability of performance within phases. In some phases, such as baseline observations, minimal variability may be preferable. In other instances, such as longer intervention protocols, it may be preferable to have more variability that reflects greater amounts of change over time.

Immediacy of Effect

Immediacy of effect refers to the degree of change in the level between the last three observations of a baseline phase and the first three observations of an intervention phase. In some cases, more immediate changes provide more convincing evidence of intervention effect. On the other hand, many counseling interventions do not produce clinically significant changes immediately. Instead, they rely on skill development, rehearsal, and mastery over time. When delayed or gradual effects are predicted, you will want to account for this consideration when making decisions about length of phases.

Overlap

Overlap is the ratio of data in one phase (e.g., baseline) that overlaps with data in another phase (i.e., intervention). Although some overlap may be expected for interventions, especially when delayed or gradual effects are predicted, we can make the most convincing inferences from instances of minimal overlap.

Consistency of Data Patterns across Similar Phases

Consistency of data is indicated by the degree that data within similar phases (e.g., all intervention phases) share the same characteristics. When individual and overall participant data are consistent across similar phases, we can make stronger inferences about treatment effect.

Estimates of Treatment Effect

Estimates of treatment effectiveness are measured by analyzing nonoverlap. Nonoverlap is a term used to refer to the ratio of data points in the treatment phase that do not overlap with data points prior to the introduction of an intervention. We can represent a feature of visual analysis (overlap) in a way that is quantifiable and replicable. When a procedure can be reliably replicated, it will allow us to compare results to those of other investigators in an apples-to-apples manner.

Although several methods are available, two procedures require little more than a straight edge and some light arithmetic: percent of nonoverlapping data (PND; Scruggs et al., 1987) and percent of data exceeding the median (PEM; Ma, 2006). In both cases, a meaningful data point in the baseline phase is used as an **anchor** to reference a participant's most representative symptom severity (see Figure 10.4). For PND, that anchor is indicated by the baseline value representing the most therapeutic effect or favorable data point; for PEM, the anchor point is the median data point within the baseline phase. In both cases, the number of intervention-phase data points above or below that line on the therapeutic side is divided by the total number of observations in the intervention phase and multiplied by 100. Scruggs and Mastropieri (2001) suggested that the resulting percentage can be characterized as ineffective (0–50%), debatable (50–70%), effective (70–90%), or very effective (90–100%).

These estimates of the amount of treatment within the effective range can be a helpful accompaniment to visual analyses. Nonoverlap indices are not all created equal, and each has its strengths and limitations, which should be carefully considered in higher-stakes situations (Lenz, 2013). A primary consideration is the placement of the anchor point that establishes the nonoverlap line. As seen in Figure 10.4, this choice can result in different percentages of treatment experiences that were within the effective

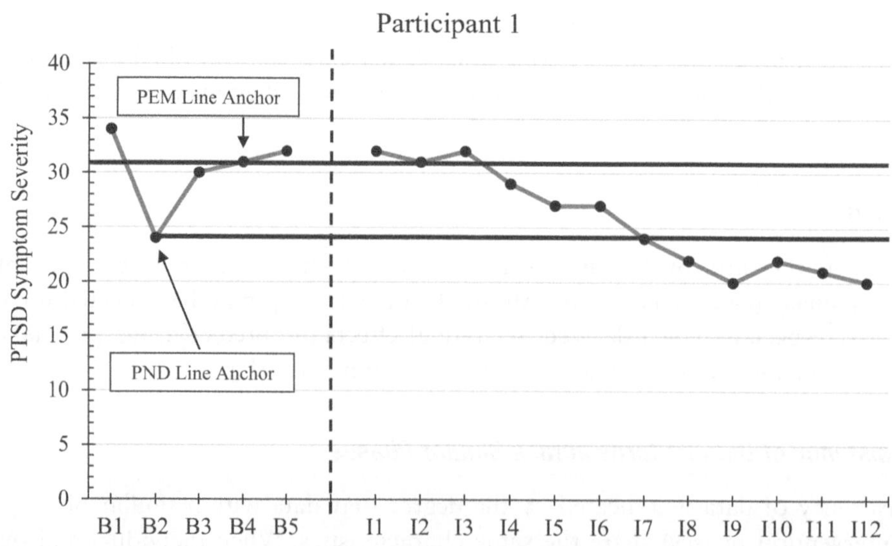

Figure 10.4 Representation of Percentage of Nonoverlapping Data (PND) and Percentage of Data Points Exceeding the Median of Baseline Phase (PEM) Reference Anchors With Associated Lines

range for PND (5/12 * 100 = 41%) and PEM (9/12 * 100 = 75%). In general, PND may be a more conservative selection when baseline data are stable, and PEM may be more appropriate when baseline data include an outlier (Lenz, 2013; Vannest & Ninci, 2015).

Estimating Practical Significance Using Effect Sizes

Although nonoverlap approaches are a wonderful addition to our toolkit, they do not detect statistically significant changes or provide a standardized metric of practical significance like those available through use of effect sizes. Scholars have proposed several effect size metrics for SCRD data, including those described in other chapters, but many can be negatively influenced by use of parametric statistics for nonparametric data. One promising alternative appears to be *Tau-U* (Parker et al., 2011), which accounts for many limitations of nonoverlap and parametric methods. As a welcome bonus for most practitioners, the developers have provided a free online calculator (www.singlecaseresearch.org), and effect sizes can be readily interpreted as small (0 to.20), moderate (.20 to.60), large (.60 to.80), or very large (.80 to 1). As with visual analyses and measures of non-overlap, these effect size conventions are valuable when situated into a context that is meaningful for participants.

PUTTING FINDINGS IN CONTEXT

Given that the results of your SCRDs will represent the experiences of a small number of individuals, it is critical that we situate their findings into context when conveying utility and practicality of an intervention. Within the realm of SCRDs, this context tends to center around the concept of *social validity*, which refers to the degree to which clients are satisfied, the feasibility of implementing intervention processes, and the relevance of outcomes for society (Hott et al., 2015).

Two strategies for situating findings into a socially valid context rely on subjective accounts and comparisons to others. First, given the intimate connection of clinicians, investigators, and participants within SCRDs, it is possible to accurately portray participants' subjective experiences with the intervention. You can draw these perspectives from participants themselves or through your own observations. Second, you can compare participants' responses to the intervention with those who have or have not received an intervention. In either case, we can answer useful questions related to clinical significance, such as: (a) Did participants tend to respond similarly across cases? and (b) Are there any discernible differences between participants and individuals without similar presenting issues? Although there are no guidelines or templates for estimating social validity, this concept should establish the boundaries of outcome reporting as you convey the impact of your intervention or program.

Developing General Impact Statements

Strategies for conveying the impact of an intervention or program will be informed by the project purpose, research questions, and arc of project activities. Next, you will need to decide which categories of impact are most important to you: individual participant response, implications for outcomes across participants, or response to hypotheses or evaluation questions. There is no right way for presenting your findings, and guidance from professional standards is scant (Appelbaum et al., 2018; Hott et al., 2015). However, we recommend at least including information related to the course of treatment response and estimations of treatment effect.

Reporting Course of Treatment Response

You can rely heavily on visual analyses when reporting participant response to treatment. Generally speaking, you will also want to provide specific quantitative metrics while including relevant qualitative details. With these considerations in mind, we make the following recommendations:

1. Provide visual depictions of each participant's data using a basic line graph. A picture is worth a thousand words; oftentimes, this visual will be needed to contextualize your commentary.
2. Explore level and variability for data through identifying and contrasting means and standard deviations in adjacent A-B phases. This activity will support inferences and can be strengthened in instances when an outcomes measure provides benchmarks for meaningful change, clinical change, or level of concern warranted (e.g., mild, moderate, severe).
3. Characterize the trend of data in adjacent A-B phases using a straight line depicting the trajectory. We may characterize trends as therapeutic, contra-therapeutic, or therapeutically neutral; alternatively, we may describe them as desired, undesired, or level using trend lines based on more sophisticated statistical procedures. It can also be helpful to describe trends across meaningful phases of treatment such as first versus second half, or before versus after a shift of intervention emphasis.
4. Portray the degree of immediacy for intervention response. This can be done in a traditional way by describing differences in level between the last three observations in an A phase compared to the first three in the B phase. However, you will want to account for planned or delayed effects associated with your intervention.
5. Identify and describe onset and/or reversal of data overlap. These descriptions support understanding about how long it takes for outcomes to emerge into the desired range, when the desired effect stops increasing, or any other meaningful patterns of response.

BOX 10.4 BASIC FRAMEWORK PUTTING SINGLE-CASE RESEARCH DESIGN FINDINGS INTO CONTEXT

Step 1. Provide visual depictions of each participant's data using a basic line graph

Data for PARTICIPANT IDENTIFIER are presented in Figure NUMBER.

Step 2. Explore level and variability for data through identifying and contrasting means and standard deviations in adjacent AB phases

Comparison of level across baseline (*M* = VALUE) and intervention phases (*M* = VALUE) indicated MINIMAL/MODERATE/NOTABLE changes in participant scores noted by DECREASE/INCREASE in mean DEPENDENT VARIABLE scores over time. Variation between scores in baseline (*SD* = VALUE) and intervention (*SD* = VALUE) INDICATED/DID NOT INDICATE differential range in scores before and after intervention.

Step 3. Characterize the trend of data in adjacent AB phases

Data in the baseline phase trended UPWARD/DOWNWARD/LEVEL toward a THERAPEUTIC/CONTRA-THERAPEUTIC/THERAPEUTICALLY NEUTRAL effect over time. SIMILARLY/DISSIMILARLY, data in the intervention phase trended UPWARD/DOWNWARD/LEVEL toward a THERAPEUTIC/CONTRA-THERAPEUTIC/THERAPEUTICALLY NEUTRAL effect over time.

Step 4. Portray the degree of immediacy for intervention response

Comparison of baseline level and trend data with the first three observations in the intervention phase DID/DID NOT suggest immediacy of treatment response for the participant.

Step 5. Identify and describe onset and/or reversal of data overlap

Data in the intervention phase DID/DID NOT move into the desired range of effect for scores representing DEPENDENT VARIABLE.

Step 6. Report and interpret metrics of treatment effect

NONOVERLAP INDEX values indicated that VALUE of the overall intervention data points (VALUE) did not overlap with the DESCRIPTION OF BASELINE DATA POINT. This finding indicates that VALUE% of intervention-phase data were associated with the desired effect and suggests that the intervention was NOT EFFECTIVE/DEBATABLE/EFFECTIVE/VERY EFFECTIVE for the participant.

Step 7. Provide summative statement of practical impact and social validity

Constructively integrate all of this information through your uniquely informed lens to make a conservative and even-handed summative statement about the usefulness and social validity of your intervention/program for participants.

Reporting Measures of Treatment Effect

Each measure of treatment effect or effect size has a feature that makes it unique. For nonoverlap metrics such as PND and PEM, baseline data serve as a critical anchor for the analysis. When reporting these metrics, start with identifying this baseline value, the total number of baseline versus values, and the resulting nonoverlap ratio.

Furthermore, provide an interpretation of the nonoverlap ratio within the context of your visual analysis data. For example, a PND value of 100 would mean that all of the intervention data were more therapeutic than any baseline value. Yet if variability were low, such as a baseline level of 28 and intervention level of 29, it may be difficult to defend suppositions about meaningful amounts of impact. In cases when using true effect size metrics, it is standard practice to report and interpret values with related confidence intervals.

Shaping Summative Findings

So far, our conversation about communicating impact has been on the individual level. To convey the overall impact of your intervention or program, we recommend using a summative synthesis across participants. Through this statement, you will identify and describe similarities and differences across participants. In addition, you will present an evidence-supported position about the degree of social validity associated with your intervention or program. Summative statements should be inclusive and constructed in the same feature-by-feature format as individual reporting. The chief distinction between this summative statement and individual reporting lies in the communication of value and potential for impact on a broader scope.

DISPLAYING RESULTS

The elegant simplicity of SCRDs may be best represented by the nature of their requisite displays: traditional data tables and line graphs. You can complete the majority of SCRD analyses and reporting with these two resources.

Use traditional data tables to describe participant characteristics and phase protocols across participants. These tables can also be a helpful resource for displaying important information about treatment response such as values for phase means, standard deviations, and medians. Nonoverlap and effect sizes data are also well-situated here.

Line graphs such as those presented throughout this chapter provide visual depictions of participant data with dependent variables situated on the vertical (ordinate) axis and measurement intervals such as time or number of interventions on the horizontal (abscissa) axis. These depictions can be enhanced through inclusion of text boxes that indicate important features such as trend lines, nonoverlap anchor points, and areas of nonoverlap in the intervention phase.

BOX 10.5 CASE STUDY REVISITED

Using our case study as an example, we developed an SCRD using an A-B design with a single participant to estimate preliminary support for the efficacy of a 12-session intervention for an adolescent who witnessed long-term domestic violence. This section provides a brief application of SCRD principles and practices you can replicate in your work.

Purpose of Evaluation

- Understanding the efficacy of an intervention.

Related Questions Guiding the Evaluation

- To what degree is a 12-week TF-CBT intervention effective for decreasing symptoms of PTSD among a pre-adolescent who witnessed long-term domestic violence?
- What is the course of treatment response for a 12-week TF-CBT intervention for decreasing the symptoms of PTSD among a pre-adolescent who witnessed long-term domestic violence?

Selected SCRD

- Based on logistics associated with screening, intake, and admission, we utilized an A-B design featuring 3 baseline (A) and 12 intervention (B) phase assessments using the CPSS.

Putting Findings Into Context

Data for Romero are presented next. Comparison of level across baseline ($M = 31.33$) and intervention phases ($M = 22.66$) indicated notable changes in participant scores, as evidenced by a decrease in mean PTSD symptom scores over time. Variation between scores in baseline ($SD = 1.15$) and intervention ($SD = 7.73$) indicated differential range in scores before and after intervention. Data in the baseline phase trended upward toward a contra-therapeutic effect over time. Dissimilarly, data in the intervention phase trended downward toward a therapeutic effect over time. Comparison of baseline level and trend data with the first three observations in the intervention phase did not suggest immediacy of treatment response for the participant. However, the percentage of nonoverlapping data (PND) value for Romero indicated that 9 of the overall intervention data points (12) did not overlap with the most therapeutic data value prior to intervention (30). This finding indicates that 75% of intervention-phase data were associated with the desired effect and suggests that the intervention was effective for the participant. This finding is corroborated by the associated Tau-U value ($\tau_U = -.64$), which is suggestive of a large degree of change in which the null hypothesis about intervention efficacy for Romero can be rejected ($p = .03$).

Romero's response to the TF-CBT intervention was characterized by a delayed but meaningful efficacy. During the initial psychoeducation and skills training sessions, PTSD symptoms remained unchanged. Over time, increases in skill mastery, caregiver buy-in, and therapeutic rapport with his counselor were associated with steady decreases in symptom severity. The exception to this therapeutic trend was associated with transitioning from skills training alone to implementing those skills within processing of Romero's trauma narrative in week 9. With an increase in caregiver support and additional check-ins, Romero's treatment response resumed course. The degree of treatment response was clinically meaningful, with his final three weeks of treatment being associated with symptom severity below clinical thresholds for concern. This finding suggests that after completing the 12-week intervention, Romero's amount and severity of PTSD symptoms were indistinguishable from nonclinical samples.

Displaying Findings

Data representing repeated measurement of the outcome variable across baseline and intervention phases can be represented using a line graph

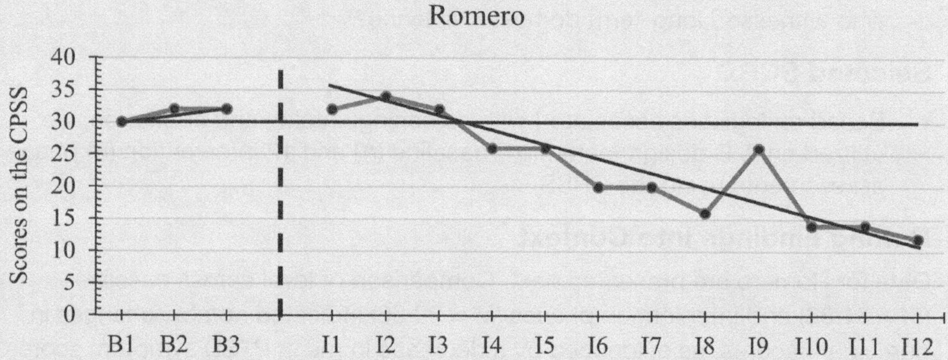

Figure 10.5 Visual Depiction of Repeated Measurement of Outcome Variable

Data representing individual participant characteristics, trend, level, and treatment effect data can be presented using a table.

	Age	Ethnicity	Gender	Baseline data		Intervention data		PND	τ_U (p)
				M	*SD*	*M*	*SD*		
Romero	12	Hispanic	Boy	31.33	1.15	22.66	7.73	75%	–.64 (.03)

CHAPTER SUMMARY

This chapter presented you with foundational concepts and tools to implement SCRDs. With this information, you are ready to begin completing experimental studies with just one or a few participants. These concepts and resources were illustrated with a case example of a 12-week TB-CBT program delivered in a community mental health clinic to a unique population. By referencing the checklist presented in this chapter, you are equipped to begin conducting your own applied research and demonstrating outcomes for activities that mean the most to you and your participant population. We encourage you to share these findings within your academic community, among stakeholders, and with relevant policy makers as applicable.

RESOURCES

- *Journal of Counseling and Development*. (2015). *93*(4). Special Issue: Single-Case Research Design.
- Institute of Education Sciences (2022). *What works clearinghouse procedures and standards handbook, version 5.0*. U.S. Department of Education. https://ies.ed.gov/ncee/wwc/handbooks
- *Single-Case Research Webpage*, Online Resource Repository and Free Effect Size Calculators. http://singlecaseresearch.org
- *What Works Clearinghouse*, Single-Case Design Technical Documentation. https://ies.ed.gov/ncee/wwc/Document/229

REFERENCES

Appelbaum, M., Cooper, H., Kline, R. B., Mayo-Wilson, E., Nezu, A. M., & Rao, S. M. (2018). Journal article reporting standards for quantitative research in psychology: The APA publications and communications board task force report. *American Psychologist*, *73*, 3–25. https://doi.org/10.1037/amp0000191

Brown, C. L., Peltier, C., Smarinsky, E. C., Lewis, O. J., & Lee, D. Y. (2024). A review of counseling research using single-case research design. *Journal of Counseling & Development*, *102*, 334–349. https://doi-org/10.1002/jcad.12517

Callender, K. A., Trustey, C. E., Alton, L., & Hao, Y. (2019). Single case evaluation of a mindfulness-based mobile application with a substance abuse counselor. *Counseling Outcome Research and Evaluation*, *12*(1), 16–29. https://doi.org/10.1080/21501378.2019.1686353

Cohen, J., Mannarino, A., & Deblinger, E. (2017). *Treating trauma and traumatic grief in children and adolescents* (2nd ed.). Guilford.

Cox, R. M., Lenz, A. S., & James, R. K. (2015). A pilot evaluation of the ARRAY program with offenders who have mental illness. *Journal of Counseling and Development*, *93*, 471–480. https://doi.org/10.1002/jcad.12045

Cox, R. M., Skirius, M., Lenz, A. S., & James, R. K. (2017). The effects of repeated exposure to the ARRAY program with offenders with mental illness. *Journal for Addictions and Offender Counseling*, *38*, 98–114. https://doi.org/10.1002/jaoc.12033

Foa, E.B., Asnaani, A., Zang, Y., & Capaldi, S. (2017). Psychometrics of the Child PTSD Symptom Scale for DSM-5 for trauma-exposed children and adolescents. *Journal of Clinical Child & Adolescent Psychology*, *47*, 38–46. https://doi.org/10.1080/15374416.2017.1350962

Hollenbaugh, M. K. H., & Lenz, A. S. (2018). An examination of the effectiveness of dialectical behavior therapy skills groups. *Journal of Counseling and Development*, *96*, 233–242. https://doi.org/10.1002/jcad.12198

Hott, B. L., Limberg, D., Ohrt, J. H., & Schmit, M. K. (2015). Reporting results of single-case studies. *Journal of Counseling and Development*, *93*, 412–417. https://doi.org/10.1002/jcad.12039

Institute of Education Sciences (2022). *What works clearinghouse procedures and standards handbook, version 5.0*. U.S. Department of Education. https://ies.ed.gov/ncee/wwc/handbooks

Kennedy, C. (2005). *Single-case designs for educational research*. Pearson.

Kratochwill, T., Hitchcock, J., Horner, R. H., Levin, J. R., Odom, S. L., Rindskopf, D. M., & Shadish, W. R. (2013). Single-case intervention research design standards. *Remedial and Special Education*, *34*, 26–38. https://doi.org/10.1177/0741932512452794

Lenz, A. S. (2013). Calculating effect size in single-case research: A comparison of nonoverlap methods. *Measurement and Evaluation in Counseling and Development*, *46*, 64–73. https://doi.org/10.1177/0748175612456401

Lenz, A. S. (2015). Using single-case research designs to demonstrate evidence for counseling interventions. *Journal of Counseling and Development*, *93*, 387–393. https://doi.org/10.1002/jcad.12036

Lenz, A. S. (2018). Reconsidering the value assigned to counseling research paradigms and outcomes. *Counseling Outcome Research and Evaluation*, *9*(1), 1–4. https://doi.org/10.1080/21501378.2017.1423202

Lenz, A. S. (2025). Single-case research design. In C. A. Morris and K. L. Wester (Eds.), *Making research relevant: Applied research designs for the mental health practitioner* (2nd ed.). Routledge.

Linehan, M. M. (2025). *DBT skills training manual* (Revised Edition). Guilford.

Liu, V. Y., La Guardia, A., & Sullivan, J. M. (2019). A single-case research evaluation of collaborative therapy treatment among adults. *Counseling Outcome Research and Evaluation*, *11*(1), 45–58. https://doi.org/10.1080/21501378.2018.1531238

Ma, H. H. (2006). An alternative method for quantitative synthesis of single-subject research: Percentage of data points exceeding the median. *Behavior Modification*, *30*, 598–617. https://doi.org/10.1177/0145445504272974

Parker, R. I., Vannest, K. J., Davis, J. L., & Sauber, S. B. (2011). Combining nonoverlap and trend for single case research: Tau-U. *Behavior Therapy*, *42*, 284–299. https://doi.org/ 10.1016/j.beth.2010.08.006

Ray, D. C. (2015). Single-case research design and analysis: Counseling applications. *Journal of Counseling & Development*, *93*, 394–402. https://doi.org/10.1002/jcad.12037

Schmidt, C., Lenz, A. S., & Oliver, M. (2022). Effectiveness of TF-CBT with sex trafficking victims in a secure post-adjudication facility. *Journal of Counseling and Development*, *100*(4), 399–411. https://doi.org/10.1002/jcad.12438

Scruggs, T. E., & Mastropieri, M. A. (2001). How to summarize single-participant research: Ideas and applications. *Exceptionality*, *9*, 227–244. https://doi.org/10.1207/S15327035EX0904_5

Scruggs, T. E., Mastropieri, M. A., & Casto, G. (1987). The quantitative synthesis of single-subject research: Methodology and validation. *Remedial and Special Education*, *8(2)*, 24–33. https://doi.org/10.1177/074193258700800206

Toomey, T. M., Garrison, P., Waddington, A., Jefferson, L., & Jackson, T. (2023). Effectiveness of a well-being therapy protocol on sexual minority psychological well-being: A single-case research design. *Counseling Outcome Research and Evaluation*, *15*(2), 143–156. https://doi.org/10.1080/21501378.2023.2287243

Vannest, K. J., & Ninci, J. (2015). Evaluating intervention effects in single-case research designs. *Journal of Counseling & Development*, *93*, 403–411. https://doi.org/10.1002/jcad.12038

CHAPTER 11

Measuring Change within a Single Group

There is a unique beauty in data that can be garnered from a single group of individuals. When community advisory boards, program administrators, directors of school counseling, or policy makers are determining the usefulness of an intervention for their stakeholders, are they fixated on experimental control? Are they emphatic about the homogeneity of two equally sized, randomized samples? Probably not. Instead, they are trying to understand how well individuals are doing after they complete a counseling intervention or program compared to when they started. Likewise, the practicality and viability of counseling interventions and programs for your practice setting probably rest on whether your participants have met some important criterion for improvement. For example, have they improved meaningfully or experienced development that stimulates opportunity for increased well-being? All this information is available from well-designed single-group research and evaluation designs, which provide a practical addition to any scientist-practitioner's toolkit.

This chapter will introduce you to some essential activities associated with applied research and program evaluation approaches you can use with a single group of participants to demonstrate the degree and relevance of intervention effects over time. The specific methods covered in this chapter include (a) post-test-only designs, (b) pre-post evaluations, and (c) use of qualitative and predictive data to provide explanatory data within a single-group design. We will apply elements of each method to a case study of an intervention program to increase coping following a natural disaster.

BOX 11.1 CHAPTER LEARNING OUTCOMES

- Develop research questions consistent with use of single-group methods
- Design, plan, carry out, record, and analyze the results of single-group studies
- Communicate findings from single-group studies using a variety of methods
- Identify and critique data associated with single-group studies

DOI: 10.4324/9781003586210-13

BOX 11.2 CASE STUDY

A hospital-based mental health unit is providing an eight-week mindfulness-based stress reduction (MBSR) program for patients who have recently been diagnosed with cancer in an effort to help manage the stress and anxiety reported by patients in association with treatment. The hospital requires the mental health unit to report utilization outcomes, demographic data, and treatment effects. As the lead, you decide to use the Hamilton Anxiety Rating Scale (HAM-A) because it is brief, open access, and has a robust history of use in outcome research. Total HAM-A scores are interpreted within a total score range of 0 to 56, wherein values less than 14 indicate mild severity, 15–23 suggest moderate severity, and scores greater than 24 imply severe symptoms of anxiety (Matza et al., 2010). Previous meta-analyses by Khoury et al. (2015) have suggested average treatment effect sizes of.55 at post-test and.53 at follow-up. You administered the HAM-A one week prior to the program beginning, one week after program completion, and six months later.

OVERVIEW OF SINGLE-GROUP METHODS

What Are Single-Group Studies?

Single-group studies are formal investigations of one group of individuals that share a common therapeutic or educational experience. When implementing single-group designs, your chief concern will be to estimate participant outcomes, and thus intervention effect, by comparing the group performance to itself at reasonable intervals for measurement. As you will see in the following sections, types of designs can vary. Ultimately, they all share some common elements of identity: one group of people who are like one another in meaningful ways that receive the same intervention, for the same amount of time, and whose outcomes are assessed and evaluated in a systematic way.

Core Features of Single-Group Studies

Single-group studies have many aliases including pre-experimental designs and open trials. The design and implementation of single-group studies feature a high degree of **control** over elements such as sampling, intervention delivery, and assessment procedures. As with single-case and experimental research designs, there remains an emphasis on the ***caseness*** of participants across meaningful characteristics, **fidelity** associated with the delivery and monitoring of an intervention, and equivalent **timing** when measuring the dependent variable. However, there is also a distinct **absence of experimental manipulation** that renders even the most robust efforts unable to support cause-and-effect inferences about the relationship between an intervention and the observed outcomes. Therefore, within single-group studies, the quasi-independant variable is often time while the dependent variable remains the outcome that is intended to be influenced by the intervention or program. Because of the related **vulnerabilities to history effects and selection bias**, researchers and evaluators are limited to **inferences about change over time**. Within these boundaries, the simple pre-post contrasts afforded by single-group studies provide a powerful tool to cultivate preliminary evidence of treatment gains that is often sufficient for pilot studies, program evaluation, and reporting to stakeholders.

When Are Single-Group Methods Indicated?

There are several instances in which single-group methods are indicated (Balkin & Kleist, 2022; Linfield & Kniffley, 2025; Lenz et al., 2024). Linfield and Kniffley suggested four uses for this category of methods: (a) measuring whether participants improved in association with the intervention/program, (b) measuring whether participants improved enough to exhibit a practical effect on their well-being, (c) identifying whether participants have met a criterion associated with successful completion of the intervention or program, and (d) relating improvement to participant characteristics or features of an intervention. We offer a fifth suggestion that single-group designs are well-suited to complete pilot inquiries regarding whether an intervention or program and setting are ready for more complex evaluation.

With these suggestions in mind, let's take a deeper look into how single-group methods may be helpful to you. After we discuss specific uses of this method, we provide examples of questions we might ask using our case study as a framework. In each example, we italicize the distinguishing component that links the evaluation purpose to the question content.

Measuring Improvement

We develop interventions and programs under the assumption that they will influence participants in developmental and growth-fostering ways. In the case of innovative practices, it is hard to know for certain if that assumption is met. Likewise, using tried-and-true practices with participants, settings, or formats that are outside of the evidence base may not be associated with improvement. Fortunately, the pre-intervention and post-intervention measurement intervals inherent within most single-group methods can be a great way to detect whether your participants have improved over time. We can make additional inferences through comparisons of pre- and post-scores obtained at reasonable follow-up intervals. For our case study, we might ask:

- Do participants report *statistically significant decreases* on the HAM-A Scale following a ten-week MBSR intervention following a diagnosis of cancer?

Measuring Meaningful Improvement

Let's be honest—not all improvement is meaningful improvement. Does a 20-point change on a symptom inventory represent enough change for clients to feel better?

Does a 20% change in the frequency of office referrals make a difference for school counselors to experience less work-related exhaustion? Is a 20% decrease in juvenile recidivism enough to sufficiently decrease the cost to society? In all cases, the answer is resounding-maybe. Oftentimes, what is meaningful is socially constructed in intersections of participants' ecological contexts where value systems and culture indicate what is typical of personal development and functioning. Other times, well-established biopsychosocial markers such as positive health status, absence of psychological distress, or relationship satisfaction can be convenient guides. In either case, you can measure meaningfulness of impact associated with your intervention or program through various strategies described in this chapter. For our case study, we might ask:

- Do participants report *clinically significant change* in scores on the HAM-A following a ten-session MBSR intervention following a diagnosis of cancer??

Relating Improvement to Participant and Intervention or Program Characteristics

So far, we have discussed the usefulness of single-group studies for detecting improvement and meaningful impact associated with interventions and programs. That information can be very useful, but it is also flawed in the assumption that effects are ubiquitous among participants. Although single-group studies are grounded in caseness, intervention fidelity, and the timing of outcome measurement, common sense tells us that not every participant will experience the same amount of improvement. Luckily, we can easily compare differences in scores before and after interventions or programs across categorical groups or correlated with continuous variables. This allows us to relate improvement to participant and intervention characteristics. Typically, relating improvement to categorical variables such as participant gender, ethnicity, or diagnosis will rely on subgroup analyses. By contrast, continuous variables such as age, scores on related measures, or number of sessions can be related to improvement using approaches ranging from simple bivariate correlations to advanced predictive modeling. For our case study, we might ask:

- *To what degree* does participant age *predict changes in HAM-A scores* for participants receiving a ten-session MBSR intervention following a diagnosis of cancer?
- Are there *statistically significant differences between groups* of men, women, and nonbinary participants for changes in HAM-A scores after receiving a ten-session MBSR intervention following a diagnosis of cancer?

Meeting a Criterion Representing Success

Although many interventions and programs are intended to change the presence of a construct such as depression, others are situated around meeting an important criterion or standard that represents success. For example, which is likely to provide more relief for participants: a decrease in scores on the HAM-A, or absence of panic attacks during the program? The former outcome represents a construct, the latter a criterion.

As someone who is invested in promoting optimal development and well-being over the lifespan, the number of meaningful criteria to you, your participants, and the community is innumerable. On one hand, criteria can be the categorical presence or absence of an event such as obtaining employment, recidivation, abstinence from substance use, or no longer meeting criteria for a diagnosis. On the other hand, criteria can be represented by meeting a benchmark representing a standard for success. For our case study, we may ask a question such as:

- Do participants *meet clinically significant symptom thresholds* as measured by the HAM-A following a ten week MBSR intervention delivered in a primary care setting during the community rebuilding phase following a major hurricane event?

Understanding Readiness for More Complex Evaluations

Each of the previously described indications is situated around detecting how your participants improved following your intervention or program. Single-group methods also provide a great platform for understanding how ready you, your colleagues, and the setting are to complete evaluation activities. In our experience, applied research and program evaluation activities are typically organized by a few enthusiastic individuals within a system. That may be someone like yourself, who believes greatly in the impact experienced by clients or students, and who also believes that there is an opportunity to magnify these effects. At the other end of the spectrum are individuals spearheading a project to meet accreditation requirements for periodic or continuous improvement cycles. In these cases, and all those in between, it is easy to overlook the importance of establishing a culture of comfort with evaluation, understanding among staff roles in the larger picture, and instituting logistical considerations. Single-group methods in the form of low-risk pilot projects can provide opportunities to help colleagues understand how their activities and roles fit within the greater project. These pilot projects support the onboarding of logistical activities such as the flow of data collection and bringing interventions to acceptable fidelity, while providing opportunities to revise activities to be evaluative in nature. For our case study, we may ask:

- What are the *strengths and barriers among logistical aspects* of a primary care setting delivering a ten-week MBSR intervention following a diagnosis of cancer?

With these questions in mind, you are ready to begin conceptualizing your single-group study by matching the purpose and related questions to designs that support you closing the information loop.

TYPES OF SINGLE-GROUP DESIGNS

So far, we have described the purposes for using single-group designs and the types of questions they are suited to answer. With these considerations in mind, we will move on to identifying and describing specific types of single-group designs that can be

TABLE 11.1 Assessment Intervals and Adjunctive Components for Types of Single-Group Designs

	Assessment intervals			Adjunctive components
Design type	**Pre-test**	**Post-test**	**Follow-up**	
Post-test only	⊘	✓	⊘	⊘
Pre-test-Post-test	✓	✓	Maybe	⊘
Explanatory	✓	✓	Maybe	Qualitative
Multimethod	✓	✓	Maybe	Quantitative

paired with each purpose–question dyad. Most researchers and evaluators can work very well with just a few types of designs in their toolbox. We will introduce you to (a) post-test-only, (b) pre-test and post-test, and (c) mixed explanatory designs and multimethod designs. Each has its virtues and limitations; Table 11.1 includes details regarding assessment intervals and adjunctive components inherent in each type of single-group design.

Post-test-Only Designs

Core Features

In post-test evaluations, participants are only assessed after completion of the intervention or program. Post-test assessments are typically only completed with those who finished the intervention or program as they represent the group of individuals for whom the independent variable may have had a salient influence.

Intended Uses and Design Considerations

With post-test-only designs, researchers and evaluators are able to make statements about the presence of terminal outcomes following completion of an intervention or program. As you can imagine, this is problematic when using continuous variables such as symptom severity or the degree to which a construct is present. For example, knowing HAM-A scores only after program termination will provide negligible insight into the degree of program usefulness or overall change. However, post-test-only design becomes more defensible when used to explain proportions or frequencies of participants meeting a categorical criterion or universally accepted benchmark following participation.

Among the single-group methods, post-test-only lacks any rigorous attempt to control for the influence of error from all sides of your project. For this reason, academics and individuals with an interest in considering changes over time may offer criticisms. However, if the nature of your outcomes is concrete and has inherent meaning, such as obtaining gainful employment or not recidivating, this strategy may appeal to policymakers and be sufficient for stakeholder reporting.

Analysis and Interpretation

Analysis of post-test-only designs is relatively simple, with researchers and evaluators relying primarily on frequency distribution of occurrences versus nonoccurrences of the outcome. By inspecting frequencies and related percentages, you will be able to interpret two aspects of your intervention or program's success: proportions of completers versus noncompleters and how many completers met your intended purpose or benchmark.

Pre-test-Post-test Designs

Core Features

In pre-test-post-test designs participants are assessed no less than before and after completion of the intervention or program. This paradigm may also use follow-up assessments to approximate persistence of changes over time. All assessments should be collected from participants in a systematic way that accounts for considerations of timing, setting, and opportunity.

Intended Uses and Design Considerations

Pre-test-post-test designs will allow you to make statements about whether participants improved meaningfully. Your outcome types can be categorical (e.g., meets diagnostic criteria or not) or continuous (e.g., decreased scores on the HAM-A). Among single-group methods, pre-test-post-test design is a bit more rigorous in its attempt to control for the influence of error. Although you will be unable to make causal attributions about the relationship between the intervention or program and observed changes over time, your argument of usefulness will be a bit more defensible, especially if positive results are maintained or magnified over time. Therefore, findings based on pre-test-post-test designs are often sufficient for conservative reporting in the professional literature and are usually sufficient for discussions with policymakers and stakeholder reporting.

Data Analysis and Interpretation

Analysis of pre-test-post-test designs is based on changes in means and standard deviations over time. You can answer the question of improvement with a simple bar graph of means before and after the intervention or program; you can use follow-up data to infer whether improvement was maintained or magnified over time. However, you may wish to demonstrate that these changes were large enough or important in some way. A simple paired samples *t*-test will let you test the null hypothesis that the difference between your measurement intervals is zero. Next, you will want to interpret the practical significance of your findings based on the standard deviation of improvement with a metric such as Cohen's *d*. Finally, you will want to situate your findings in terms of clinical significance. Using our case study as an example, decreased scores of

10 or greater on the HAM-A represent clinically relevant change. It can be helpful to describe changes over time with such benchmarks in mind. We discuss these analytic and interpretive procedures in later chapters. For now, just take a mindful breath and let's move on to the final design for this chapter.

Mixed Explanatory and Multimethod Designs

Core Features

In exploratory and explanatory designs, you can capitalize on strengths inherent within the pre-test-post-test paradigm, yet expand your findings to include more impactful, nuanced considerations of participant experiences. Explanatory designs will allow you to interpret quantitative results using qualitative data regarding participants' narratives. By contrast, multimethod designs allow you to use several quantitative methods to create a more specific depiction of improvements over time. In either case, the inclusion of additional information will augment your single-group study from solely depicting improvement that may have happened to portraying for whom, how, and under what circumstances it occurred.

Intended Uses and Design Considerations

Mixed explanatory and multimethod designs offer you two avenues to move beyond demonstrating the impact of quantitative findings alone toward a more representative depiction of the true potential of your intervention or program for others. In both cases, these designs offer a variety of options for understanding impact and relating improvement to participant and intervention or program characteristics.

Explanatory designs provide you with an opportunity to add context and complexity alongside simple pre-test–post-test contrasts of means and standard deviations. Sure, it may be helpful to include effect size and clinical significance interpretations, but those interpretations come from the evaluator rather than those the intervention or program is intended to benefit. It seems logical that we take our data to a representative group of participants and attempt to understand context-shaping information such as (a) what about the intervention or program was most helpful or least salient; (b) how do participants experience [outcome]; (c) how has [outcome] been associated with relationships with self, others, and community; and (d) what about the intervention or program could be modified to create an impact? Newly emerging frameworks and strategies for qualitative inquiry make the use of explanatory designs incredibly flexible and trustworthy (see Chapter 13). The impact statements that emerge from these interviews will help you interpret your findings and are well-suited for reporting within the academic literature, program reports, and policy briefs (see Chapter 17).

Multimethod quantitative designs represent an opportunity to tease out who your findings apply to most by providing a framework for understanding which participant and study characteristics are associated with improvements over time.

These designs allow us to parse out findings between categories of participants and relate improvement to continuous variables. As mentioned earlier, relating improvement to categorical variables such as gender identity, ethnicity, or diagnosis will rely on comparing subgroup means visually or through hypothesis testing. Alternatively, continuous variables such as age, scores on related measures, or number of sessions can be used to portray relationships with improvement using approaches ranging from simple bivariate correlations to advanced predictive modeling approaches.

For example, the group receiving MBSR in our case study was composed of participants who identified as men, women, and nonbinary. A comparison of means for those groups within our sample can help us understand gender differences in improvement over time. Likewise, we may notice that age was dispersed over a broad range among our participants. A simple bivariate correlation of participant age and amount of improvement may reveal trends in degree of response to MBSR. In both cases, non-statistically significant findings may suggest that the effect is ubiquitous and applies to participants in even-handed ways. However, if statistically significant findings are present, you will be able to portray findings more accurately within the academic literature, stakeholder reports, and policy briefs.

BOX 11.3 INDICATORS OF A QUALITY SINGLE-GROUP DESIGN

- Caseness of participants.
- Fidelity of intervention delivery and monitoring.
- Timing of measurement pre-established and reasonable considering hypothesized improvements among participants.
- Sample-specific reporting of psychometric reliability
    - Estimates of statistical, practical, and clinical significance provided.
- Findings situated in context of design limitations.
- Tables and visual depictions support reporting of findings.

PUTTING FINDINGS INTO CONTEXT

Although you can describe the significance of findings in terms of statistical, practical, and clinical improvements, these changes are merely in *association* with your intervention or program, not necessarily *caused* by it. Putting your single-group design findings into context begins with establishing that boundary. From that position you are well-situated to develop impact statements, interpret effects sizes, interpret clinical significance, and shape a summative conceptualization of intervention or program usefulness. Box 11.4 depicts a six-step guide you can use for reporting. You can modify capitalized words to suit your results, but only you can breathe life into your narrative and portray findings in a way that honors your project and participants' experiences.

BOX 11.4 BASIC FRAMEWORK FOR REPORTING SINGLE-GROUP DESIGN FINDINGS

Step 1: Characterize the general impact of your findings

The findings from our evaluation indicated MINIMAL/MODERATE/MIXED/STRONG support of changes in OUTCOME VARIABLE over time for participants who completed the INTERVENTION/PROGRAM NAME delivered in SETTING NAME.

Step 2: Report the findings of your statistical significance test and practical significance estimates

Findings from a paired samples *t*-test revealed that participants REPORTED/DID NOT REPORT statistically significant INCREASE/DECREASE in OUTCOME VARIABLE at END POINT when compared to BEGINNING POINT, *t*(df) = *t*-VALUE, *p* = *p*-VALUE.01, *d* =.*d VALUE* indicative of a SMALL/MEDIUM/LARGE effect size.

Step 3: Interpret the meaning of your effect size

These findings illustrate an improvement over time of about *d* VALUE CONVERTED TO PERCENTAGE standard deviation units among participants completing the INTERVENTION.

Step 4: Compare your findings to previous studies

This outcome WAS/WAS NOT consistent with previous studies of INTERVENTION that detected effect sizes ranging within the SMALL/MEDIUM/LARGE range.

Step 5: Situate your findings into clinical/educational context

The difference in mean scores from admission to termination of VALUE INDICATES/DOES NOT INDICATE a clinically significant degree of improvement among the severity or frequency of the symptoms representing OUTCOME VARIABLE.

Step 6: Develop a summative statement about your findings

Constructively integrate this information through your uniquely informed lens to make a conservative, even-handed summative statement about the usefulness of your intervention or program for participants.

Developing General Impact Statements

The impact statements you develop from single-group studies should be void of causal language, instead opting for phrases such as *over time* and *following completion*. This provides an honest, even-handed depiction of results while being transparent about the nature of your findings. It is important to consider that findings can cover outcome categories ranging from no evidence to strong evidence for occurrence of an event or changes over time. Thus, findings should be conceptualized along a continuum with you deciding where the general nature of your findings falls; overall impact may include minimal, moderate, mixed, or strong support.

Interpreting Significance

Following this general statement, provide support based on some metrics that can be communicated from one service clinician, educator, researcher, or evaluator to another. With single-group designs, we are most interested in reporting results of null hypothesis statistical testing (p-values), estimates of effect size (d-values), and clinical significance (benchmarks for success). Statistical significance can be inferred for p-values less than.05. Practical significance of participant improvement can be inferred from interpreting Cohen's d values as small (d =.20), medium (d =.50), or large (d =.80). Clinical significance can be inferred from comparing differences in mean scores from pre-test to post-test, with reference to benchmarks representing success or use of easy to calculate metrics such as reliable change index or percent improvement (see Blampied, 2022; Lenz, 2020). Although post-test-only designs will not yield enough information to complete these analyses, and explanatory designs will require the use of qualitative data, these are the typical standards for single-group designs.

Shaping Summative Findings

Your summative statement of findings will be grounded in awareness of the strengths and limitations of single-group studies, familiarity with project processes, and an understanding of limitations of statistical measures. You must also view this interpretation through the ecological context in which your study was completed. Although interpreting significance of statistical, practical, and clinical significance is easily completed with reference to the conventions named earlier, you'll need to bring science and humanness together in a way that communicates findings plainly and clearly.

DISPLAYING FINDINGS

You can easily display the results of your single-group design using bar graphs and tables reporting descriptive statistics. Each will provide you with visual support for the narratives you provide to academic audiences, stakeholders, or policymakers.

Using Bar Graphs

Bar graphs can be used to display comparisons between categories such as pre-test, post-test, and follow-up scores or the proportion of participants who met a criterion. In a pre-test–post-test design, the values of scores will be situated on the Y-axis (vertical) and the categories on the X-axis (horizontal). These visual aids can support your general impact statement and statements about clinical significance. Simple tools in most word processing and data management systems will allow you to create and edit graphs to communicate about data.

Using Descriptive Statistics Tables

With so many statistics provided by most software or web-based programs, it can be hard to know what is important to include in tables. For most smaller or local projects, it is sufficient to include sample size, frequencies, means, and standard deviations. Larger or higher-stakes projects may require a bit more information, including information related to statistical significance testing, effect size, and measurement reliability. In either case, tables are readily accessible and should only include information that supports your dialogue about group performance.

Some standards for reporting encourage the use of supplemental illustrations that organize and display themes and supportive statements for mixed-method designs (Levitt et al., 2018; Linfield & Kniffley, 2025). Similarly, you can supplement multimethod studies with a table portraying the relationship between continuous variables and statistical differences between categories of participant and study characteristics (Appelbaum et al., 2018). The case study revisited includes a presentation of results from the single-group evaluation.

BOX 11.5 CASE STUDY REVISITED

A basic pre-test–post-test single-group design can be enhanced with other data to describe program effectiveness alongside participant and study characteristics. This section provides a brief application of chapter content to illustrate single-group principles and practices that can be replicated in your work.

Purposes of Evaluation

- Measuring meaningful improvement.
- Relating improvement to participant and intervention or program characteristics.

Related Questions Guiding the Evaluation

- Do participants report *statistically significant change* in scores on the HAM-A following a ten-session MBSR intervention delivered in a primary care setting during the community rebuilding phase following a major hurricane event?
- Do participants report *clinically significant change* in scores on the HAM-A following a ten-session MBSR intervention delivered in a primary care setting during the community rebuilding phase following a major hurricane event?
- *To what degree* do participant age and number of sessions attended *predict changes in HAM-A scores* for participants receiving a ten-session MBSR intervention in a primary care setting during the community rebuilding phase following a major hurricane event?

Selected Single-Group Design

- Pre-test–post design with a quantitative multimethod component.

Putting Findings Into Context

The findings from our evaluation indicated strong support for changes in anxiety over time for participants who completed the ten-week MBSR program delivered in primary care. Findings from a *t*-test revealed that participants reported significantly fewer anxiety symptoms at program termination when compared to admission, $t(47) = 4.25$, $p < .01$, $d = .57$, indicative of a medium effect size. These findings illustrate an improvement over time of about 57% of a standard deviation unit among participants completing the ten-week MBSR program. This outcome was consistent with previous analyses by Khoury et al. (2015) of MBSR that detected effect sizes falling within the medium range ($d = .55$) at post-test. The difference in mean scores from admission ($M = 35.8$, severe range) to termination ($M = 23.1$, moderate range) indicates a clinically significant degree of improvement among the severity or frequency of the symptoms associated with anxiety. Additional analyses suggested that age and number of sessions attended may influence the degree of improvement reported by participants. Statistically significant negative correlations were detected for age ($r = -.83$, $p < .01$) and number of sessions attended ($r = -.57$, $p < .01$), suggestive of large effect sizes. These findings indicate that older participants tended to report greater improvements in anxiety symptoms. Likewise, participants who attended a greater number of sessions tended to report larger decreases in anxiety symptoms.

These findings suggest that after ten weeks of MBSR programming, participants reported statistically significant decreases in anxiety symptoms that were consistent with findings from previous researchers and are within the limits of clinically relevant improvements in anxiety management. Additionally, the largest improvements tended to be experienced by older participants who attended most sessions. Taken together, these findings provide some preliminary support for mitigating the deleterious experiences of individuals coping with life following a natural disaster.

Displaying Findings

Relevant information depicting the amount of improvement, statistical significance, and effect size can be depicted in a table. Similar tables can be created to separate the same statistics by categorical variable.

	Pre-MBSR		Post-MBSR					
Outcome	*M*	*SD*	*M*	*SD*	*N*	*t*	*p*	*d*
Anxiety	35.80	24.30	23.10	19.30	48	4.25	< .01	.57

Relevant information depicting relationships between participant and treatment characteristics can be provided in a basic correlation matrix.

	Age	Number of Sessions
Change in HAM-A Scores	–.83	–.57
	$p < .01$	$p < .01$

Differences in raw scores between groups can be displayed using a bar graph:

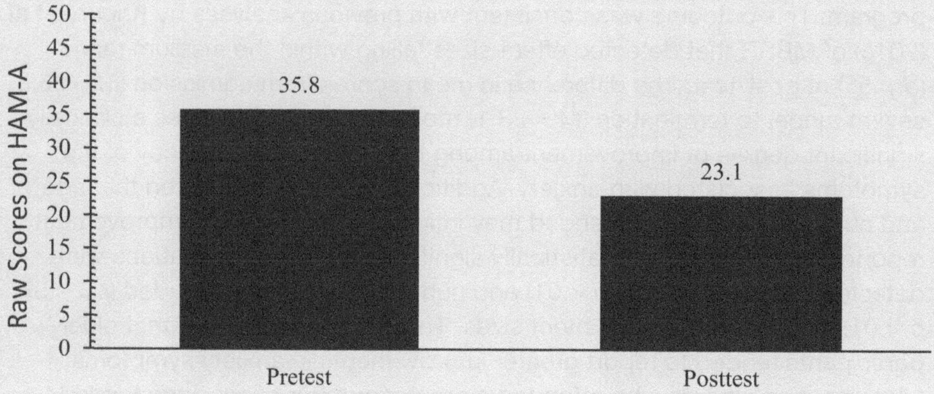

Figure 11.1 Visual Depiction of Differences in Raw Scores Between Groups

CHAPTER SUMMARY

This chapter presented foundational concepts and tools for implementing single-group designs. With this information, you are well-situated to clarify your purpose and begin developing your own project based on logically connected research/evaluation questions, design selection, analyses, and reporting practices. These concepts and tools were illustrated with a case example of an MBSR program delivered in a primary care setting to a unique population. By referencing the checklist presented in this chapter, you are equipped to begin evaluating programs that have potential to stimulate meaningful changes in your community. Through the use of the resources in this chapter, we encourage you to share these findings within your academic community, among stakeholders, and with relevant policymakers as applicable.

RESOURCES

- Linfield, K. J., & Kniffley, S. D. (2025). *Program evaluation: Methods and case studies* (10th ed.). Routledge.
- Marsden, E., & Torgerson, C. J. (2012). Single group, pre- and post-test research designs: Some methodological concerns. *Oxford Review of Education*, *38*, 583–616. https://doi.org/10.1080/03054985.2012.731208

- *National Center for Complimentary and Integrative Studies*, Pilot Studies: Common Uses and Misuses. www.nccih.nih.gov/grants/pilot-studies-common-uses-and-misuses
- *SAMHSA* Evidence-Based Practices Resource Center. www.samhsa.gov/libraries/evidence-based-practices-resource-center

REFERENCES

Appelbaum, M., Cooper, H., Kline, R. B., Mayo-Wilson, E., Nezu, A. M., & Rao, S. M. (2018). Journal article reporting standards for quantitative research in psychology: The APA publications and communications board task force report. *American Psychologist*, *73*, 3–25. https://doi.org/10.1037/amp0000151

Balkin, R. S., & Kleist, D. (2022). *Counseling research: A practitioner-scholar approach (2nd Ed.)*. American Counseling Association.

Blampied, N. M. (2022). Reliable change and the reliable change index: Still useful after all these years? *The Cognitive Behaviour Therapist. 15*, e50. https://doi.org/10.1017/S1754470X22000484

Khoury, B., Sharma, M., Rush, S. E., & Fournier, C. (2015). Mindfulness-based stress reduction for healthy individuals: A meta-analysis. *Journal of Psychosomatic Research*, *78*, 512–528. https://doi.org/10.1016/j.jpsychores.2015.03.009

Lenz, A. S. (2020). Estimating and reporting clinical significance in counseling research: Inferences based on percent improvement. *Measurement and Evaluation in Counseling and Development*, *53*(4), 289–296. https://doi.org/10.1080/07481756.2020.1784758

Lenz, A. S., Gonzales-Wong, C. D., & de Vries, S. (2024). Experimental designs. In C. J. Sheperis, J. S. Young, and M. H. Daniels (Eds), Counseling research: Quantitative, qualitative, and mixed methods (3rd ed., pp. 124–147). Pearson.

Levitt, H. M., Bamberg, M., Creswell, J. W., Frost, D. M., Josselton, R., & Suárez-Orozco, C. (2018). Journal article reporting standards for qualitative primary, qualitative meta-analytic, and mixed methods research in psychology: The APA publications and communications board task force report. *American Psychologist*, *73*, 26–46. https://doi.org/10.1037/amp0000151

Linfield, K. J., & Kniffley, S. D. (2025). *Program evaluation: Methods and case studies* (10th ed.). Routledge.

Matza, L. S., Morlock, R., Sexton, C., Malley, K., & Feltner, D. (2010). Identifying HAM-A cutoffs for mild, moderate, and severe generalized anxiety disorder. *International Journal of Methods in Psychiatric Research*, *19*(4), 223–232. https://doi.org/10.1002/mpr.323

CHAPTER 12

Comparing Differences between Groups

As you may have noticed in previous chapters, the methods we have discussed are unique in the ways they reveal information about impact and meaningfulness. As wonderful as these methods are, with the exception of some single-case research designs, the limitations to internal validity leave us unable to defend assertions of cause-and-effect associations between interventions, programs, and their outcomes. Yet stakeholders expect us to be able to defend claims of effectiveness when fulfilling our ethical and professional obligation to use evidence-informed practice. How can we be relatively confident that one intervention is more helpful than another? What kind of impact might we notice when we introduce a new program to our students? Given the administrative, monetary, and human resources that go into implementing new counseling interventions or restructuring existing programs, we need to find ways to go beyond conjecture to answer these questions.

BOX 12.1 CHAPTER LEARNING OUTCOMES

- Develop research questions consistent with use of between-group designs
- Design, plan, carry out, record, and analyze the results of quasi-experimental and experimental designs
- Communicate findings from between-group studies using a variety of methods
- Identify and critique data associated with experimental and quasi-experimental studies

Experimental and quasi-experimental research and evaluation designs allow us to compare outcomes between two or more groups of participants. We may use this class of strategies to strategically manipulate interventions, control for extraneous variables, and determine the degree to which an intervention or program has an intended outcome compared to no intervention or another intervention. Although you may have conjured up images of lab coats and Pavlov's pups when you read the word *experimental*, real-world comparison of the effectiveness of two different interventions or programs can be within your wheelhouse. With these tools at your disposal, you will be able to produce the types of evidence stakeholders request regarding interventions

DOI: 10.4324/9781003586210-14

and programs. From these findings, you will be able to communicate evidence with varied degrees of causal attributions, and your results may also generalize to clients in similar settings.

This chapter introduces you to essential activities associated with experimental and quasi-experimental research designs used to evaluate differences in outcomes between groups of participants. Unlike most other methods we have explored so far, well-developed between-group designs will allow you to make inferences about cause-and-effect relationships. Specific methods we cover in this chapter include quasi-experimental and experimental designs. We will apply elements of between-group designs to a case study of a counselor education program.

BOX 12.2 CASE STUDY

The program coordinator of a counselor education program in the northwestern United States has received feedback from multiple student cohorts requesting engagement in experiential counseling skill development activities earlier in their programs of study. Although some faculty members are in favor of introducing this instructional approach within early courses, other faculty members have insisted that the focus should remain on developing a strong understanding of foundational theories and concepts before meaningful skill development may occur. Thus, a debate has ensued surrounding the viability of early coursework as a platform for counseling skill development through an experiential training model.

As a scholar-practitioner, the program coordinator developed a strategy for evaluating this point objectively using an experimental between-groups design. Specifically, 40 newly admitted students were randomly assigned to one of two sections of an *Introduction to the Helping Profession* course upon their enrollment in the program. Both sections meet from 5pm to 8pm; however, one section is on Tuesdays, while the other is on Wednesdays. The coordinator met with the instructor of record for each course to control for class content; time dedicated to each topic; and other elements such as assignments, methods for evaluation, and ranges for grades. One course section received the department's traditional didactic-reflective strategy, while the other received an abbreviated didactic strategy with additional experiential, process-oriented components. Dependent variables were quality of empathic responding using the rating scale described by Lenz and Sangganjanavanich (2013), counseling student self-efficacy (Melchert et al., 1996), and final course grade. Prior to beginning the course, participants completed pre-intervention measures of empathic responding and self-efficacy; they completed post-intervention measures 15 weeks later just after final examinations. Finally, de-identified course grades were made available to the program coordinator following completion of the semester.

OVERVIEW OF BETWEEN-GROUPS DESIGNS

What Are Between-Groups Designs?

Between-groups designs are a class of research methods intended to support inferences about causes of changes in outcome variables following exposure to an intervention or program. As connoted from the term, between-groups designs involve two or more groups of participants, one of which receives a target intervention or program; the other group may receive no treatment, sometimes referred to as a control group, or they may receive an alternative intervention or program. The utility of between-group designs is grounded in the assumption that if two groups of participants are similar with respect to a trait or variable before introducing an intervention *and* we can account for influence of extraneous variables, then we can assume later differences were the result of exposure to the independent variable. Therefore, in between-groups studies, the independent variable is group affiliation (e.g., treatment versus no treatment) while the dependent variable remains the outcome that is intended to be influenced by the intervention or program. As you will see, these fundamental propositions guide our use and understanding of between-groups designs to inform clinical decision making and best practice.

Core Features of Between-Groups Designs

Between-group designs have several common characteristics: comparisons between groups, random assignment, manipulation of independent variables, control of extraneous variables, and systematic measurement of outcomes. These characteristics are essential for establishing the functional relationship at the heart of between-group designs (Montgomery, 2019).

Comparisons Between Groups

All between-groups studies feature comparisons across two or more groups. To attribute the relationships between group affiliation and the dependent variable, we need to be able to be sure the groups are similar before we introduce the intervention or program. It is also worth noting that comparisons in counseling research are not all created equal. Specifically, comparisons of a counseling intervention or program to nothing (e.g., wait list or no treatment) provide a differently valued type of evidence than comparisons to viable or standard-of-practice interventions. Certainly, if we already know the counseling relationship leads to more change than specific interventions, it does not make sense to compare those who participate in child-centered play therapy (CCPT) with those who did nothing; rather, we generate more compelling evidence by comparing those in the CCPT condition with those who see a professional counselor using the counselor's methodology of choice (i.e., treatment as usual).

Random Assignment of Participants

Random assignment of participants to an intervention or program condition is the cornerstone feature that distinguishes experimental designs from quasi-experimental ones. Whether randomly assigning participants as individuals or in meaningful blocks such as by school, classroom, or days in a clinic, the main goal is to fairly provide participants an equal chance for assignment to an intervention condition. This process promotes equal distribution of individual traits and characteristics within and between groups of participants. In some circumstances, it is not possible to use random assignment, thus the result is a quasi-experimental design. Although quasi-experimental designs are vulnerable to threats to internal validity, such as selection bias, history effects, and differential attrition, in some cases they may represent the most feasible approach to estimating the effects of an intervention or program (Handley et al., 2018).

Manipulation of Independent Variable(s)

Between-groups designs inherently involve manipulation of at least one independent variable such as the type of intervention or setting of programs. We manipulate independent variables across at least two levels, and we can also manipulate across additional levels. To continue the running example earlier, in a simple study, we might specify CCPT condition and wait list as the two levels of our independent variable. But we might also make things more complex by selecting three of more levels or the independent variable: CCPT, CCPT with parent consultation, treatment as usual, and wait list.

Control of Extraneous Variables

Every study is affected by some degree of external influence, which distorts our ability to observe the actual intervention or program effects. By controlling or accounting for extraneous variables, we can improve the probability that differences observed between groups of participants were a function of the intervention or program that they completed. For example, we may ensure participants are not engaged in additional services that may affect their response to our intervention, or we may keep teachers "blind" to which intervention group students are in to reduce the likelihood that they engage differently with students based on their expectations of outcomes.

Systematic Measurement of Outcomes

Our ability to compare outcomes between groups requires that we are careful when selecting outcomes and collecting data. At the very least, we must collect data before and after interventions (i.e., pre-test and post-test). However, we might decide to include follow-up assessments at meaningful intervals to see whether participants were able to maintain gains over time.

BOX 12.3 INDICATORS OF A QUALITY BETWEEN-GROUP DESIGN

- Description of the random assignment of participants to an intervention.
- Flow chart illustrating participant allocation to groups and related attrition
- Manipulation of independent variable(s).
- Control of extraneous variables.
- Systematic measurement of outcomes.
  - Description of the intervention program fidelity
  - Description of outcome measure features including sample-specific reliability estimates
- Reporting and interpretation of statistical, practical, and clinical significance estimates.
- Findings situated in the context of design limitations.
- Use of tables and visual depictions to support reporting of findings.

When Are Between-Groups Designs Indicated?

Between-group designs have some distinctive features that make them a valuable addition to your research and evaluation toolkit. As you have gathered by now, these designs are most useful when attempting to make defensible arguments regarding the degree to which an intervention or program produced a desired response. Use of between-group designs is indicated in three primary instances: (a) estimating differential performance of novel interventions or programs; (b) understanding performance in comparison to an existing standard; and (c) understanding interactions between interventions, outcomes, and other important variables. With these indications in mind, let's venture a bit more into how between-groups methods can be relevant for you. We provide examples of questions that correspond to each purpose using the case study as a framework. In each example, we italicize the distinguishing component that links the evaluation purpose to the question content.

Estimating Performance of Novel Interventions or Programs

Counselors develop interventions and programs with the expectation that they will make meaningful differences in participants' well-being. If we are developing a new intervention with the hope that it makes a difference for the average person's quality of life, we do not have an ethical requirement to ensure that both groups receive an intervention. In this case, individuals in one group may participate in the intervention, while those in the other group go about living their lives as they normally would. Ultimately, we can compare outcomes of waitlisted or untreated groups with those that received the intervention. If we observe differences in outcomes, we can conclude that these differences represent the influence of the intervention or program participants. We may ask questions like:

- Does a 15-week experiential, process-oriented class instruction intervention *lead to* improvements in empathic responding?

- Does a 15-week experiential, process-oriented class instruction intervention *cause* improvements in empathic responding and counseling student self-efficacy?

Differential Performance of an Intervention or Program Compared to an Existing Standard

In most cases, professional counselors already have an established standard of treatment for use with their client population. Thus, it does not make sense to compare a new or innovative program with nothing, and it may not be ethical to ask those who are already struggling with a condition for which there is effective treatment to do nothing. It makes more sense to compare a novel or innovative approach to the existing standard. If both interventions are supposed to be effective, we become most interested in the differential effect of one treatment compared to the other. We may ask questions like:

- Is there a *statistically significant difference* in empathic responding *between students* who receive didactic-reflective pedagogy versus those who receive experiential, process-oriented class instruction?
- What is the *practical significance of differences* in *course grades* between students who receive didactic-reflective pedagogy versus those who receive experiential, process-oriented class instruction?

Understanding Interactions between Interventions, Outcomes, and Other Important Variables

So far, both indications for between-groups studies have been associated with answering the question "what works?" This information can be very useful in guiding stakeholder decision making. Nevertheless, we can make the most informed decisions when we understand not just what works, but for whom and under which circumstances (APA, 2021; APA Presidential Task Force on Evidence-Based Practice, 2006; Nielsen & Miraglia, 2017; Wampold et al., 2002). Fortunately, advances in descriptive and statistical approaches for evaluating outcomes of between-groups studies allow us to detect nuanced interactions such as gender, age, amount of intervention, and program setting with outcomes. We may ask questions like:

- Is experiential, process-oriented class instruction *more effective than* didactic-reflective pedagogy for improving counseling student self-efficacy, but only for older students?
- Is experiential, process-oriented class instruction *more effective than* didactic-reflective pedagogy for improving empathic responding, but only when self-efficacy is high to begin with?

With these questions in mind, you are ready to begin conceptualizing a between-groups study through identifying the purpose, developing related questions, and selecting the design that suits your project.

TYPES OF BETWEEN-GROUPS DESIGNS

Applied researchers and program evaluators who are interested in approximating causal relationships using between-groups designs have several options. In this section, we introduce you to three approaches in order of their increasing degrees of complexity and internal validity: (a) quasi-experimental designs, (b) post-test-only designs, and (c) experimental designs. Each type of design has its merits, limitations, and methods for controlling limitations (see Table 12.1).

Quasi-Experimental Designs

Core Features

Quasi-experiments involve comparison between groups, manipulation of independent variables, control of extraneous variables, and systematic measurement of outcomes. Quasi-experiments are distinct from experiments in that they do not feature random assignment of participants to groups. Researchers collect data concurrently in many quasi-experimental designs, but sequential data collection (e.g., comparing to historical data) may be a reasonable option in some scenarios.

Intended Uses and Design Considerations

Quasi-experimental designs allow evaluators to compare participant outcomes in one program or intervention against another condition in which data are collected concurrently *or* against an existing standard that was historically implemented, often referred to as treatment as usual (TAU). For concurrent quasi-experimental designs, for example, we might assign some participants to clinicians with family systems training and others to clinicians certified to offer a new dialectical behavior therapy (DBT) intervention. In a sequential quasi-experimental design, Lenz and Del Conte (2018) compared a novel DBT intervention for adolescents to historical performance data for a family systems approach within the same treatment setting. Their analysis found that each approach was associated with clinically relevant changes but also had some unique influences on client well-being and functioning. In a quasi-experimental comparison by Lothes and Hall (2025, DBT was delivered in two different treatment settings-intensive outpatient and partial hospital programs-which served as the quasi-manipulation of the independent

TABLE 12.1 Assessment Intervals and Design Considerations for Types of Between-Groups Designs

	Assessment intervals			Design considerations
Design type	Pre-test	Post-test	Follow-up	
Quasi-experiment	✓	✓	Maybe	No random assignment; concurrent or sequential assessment
Post-test Only	⊘	✓	Maybe	Requires random assignment
Experimental	✓	✓	Maybe	Requires random assignment

variable. In each case, these quasi-experimental designs provided an impetus for clinicians and administrators to weigh the value of DBT-based interventions for supporting therapeutic outcomes within the broader population of treatment-seeking individuals.

Although sequential approaches are convenient and sometimes the only viable option a researcher or evaluator has, they are not without their limitations. Specifically, you will have to be mindful about whether observed treatment effects may be influenced by outside events or contaminated by other interventions. For example, if we collect data concurrently, we can be reasonably certain that anything that might happen during that intervention (e.g., an act of violence in the community) affects both groups equally. If we collect data sequentially, we have no way of knowing how an external event affected overall results.

Additionally, a key strategy for maintaining a degree of experimental control in quasi-experimental designs is assuring that the observations are independent. To secure independence, we need assurance that sequenced data are reasonably distanced in time from the point of intervention crossover so that observations across groups are not related in any meaningful way. Another design element that may strengthen causal inferences is the inclusion of measures that theoretically should not change (e.g., personality traits) during the intervention or program. When data show expected patterns (e.g., meaningful changes in targeted outcomes and stability in unrelated variables), we gain confidence in the intervention's impact and are better able to defend causal inferences when presenting results to colleagues, stakeholders, and policymakers.

Data Analysis and Interpretation

Analysis of experimental designs is based on approaches that lead to statistical inferences and support null hypothesis testing while accounting for as much nonrandom error as possible. When we analyze quasi-experiments, we work to improve precision by reducing the influence of extraneous variables. Most analyses can be accomplished through the use of *t*-tests (two groups) or one-way analysis of variance (ANOVA; three or more groups) when inspecting a single outcome. Similarly, we can use multivariate analysis of variance (MANOVA) procedures when looking at several outcomes that are theoretically or statistically related in meaningful ways. Lastly, each statistical procedure has extensions that allow us to identify and control for sources of variation (e.g., participant age or pre-test scores) in our findings. Finally, analysis of covariance (ANCOVA) and multivariate analysis of covariance (MANCOVA) strategies allow researchers to adjust expression of outcome measurement by accounting for the influence of extraneous variables in our statistical models. In the end, we can interpret data using bar graphs and line graphs that portray data trends across groups.

Post-Test-Only Experimental Designs

Core Features

Post-test-only experimental designs feature the experimental control that emerges from randomization of participants to treatment group. In this specific type of design, researchers only assess outcomes after participants complete the intervention or program.

Intended Uses and Design Considerations

Post-test-only experimental designs can help us make inferences about terminal effects of an intervention when it is not viable to collect pre-test data at the outset of the project. In our case study, one of our outcome variables is course grade. Given the nature of the sample, a pre-test assessment of course grade is not practical. Post-test-only designs can be useful when an outcome is associated with whether participants met a meaningful criterion (e.g., secured employment within three months of program completion).

Although this design has the upside of being associated with randomization, which promotes equal dispersion of participant differences within and between groups, we are still limited by the absence of a baseline assessment to which we can contrast post-test values. However, as with other post-test-only designs (see Chapter 11), this strategy can be defensible when outcomes are concrete and have some degree of intrinsic meaning.

Data Analysis and Interpretation

Analysis of post-test-only experimental designs can range from relatively simple visual analyses to statistically based approaches. Visual analyses often rely on bar graphs or frequency distributions of outcomes that portray the amounts of performance associated with each intervention or program. When possible, it is more defensible to use statistical inferences.

When we have two groups, we can evaluate statistical and practical significance using an independent samples *t*-test and effect size such as Cohen's *d* or Hedge's *g*. When we are evaluating contrasts across three or more groups, we can determine statistical significance using ANOVA or MANOVA procedures paired with an effect size such as eta squared (η^2). As with other analyses, we will need to use some combination of visual and statistical analyses to extrapolate nuances from projects with three or more groups.

Experimental Designs

Core Features

Considered the *gold standard* of research, experimental designs, sometimes called randomized control trials or RCTs, feature random assignment of participants to treatment groups, assessment of outcomes prior to and following completion of a program or intervention, strategic manipulation of the independent variable, and strategies for controlling for extraneous variables. In experimental designs, researchers assess outcome variables in identical ways during a similar interval of time. Using pre-test scores alongside post-test scores helps us to be transparent regarding the equivalence of groups at the outset of the project, and it allows us to interpret the degree of change experienced by participants.

Intended Uses and Design Considerations

If you want to be able to make causal inferences, you are in the right place! Experimental designs are intended to control the influence of non-intervention or program-related variables that may affect a study's outcome so that the most plausible explanation for changes over time is the influence of your intervention or program. Although experimental designs account for similarities between groups at pre-test measurement intervals, they are still susceptible to testing effects wherein participants become aware of how progress is being measured and what may constitute success. Ideally, a large enough sample allows these effects to dissipate across participants; however, without more complex designs such as the Solomon four-group design, this is just a limitation you can note when discussing your results.

Data Analysis and Interpretation

Analysis of experimental designs is largely based on approaches that lead to statistical inferences and support null hypothesis testing. Statistical inferences can be garnered with two groups using an independent samples *t*-test paired with the Cohen's *d* or Hedge's *g* effect size. When evaluating contrasts across three or more groups, we can determine statistical significance using ANOVA, MANOVA, or MANCOVA procedures combined with an effect size such as η^2. In these latter instances, we will need to use post-hoc analyses (e.g., Tukey's HSD, Scheffé's test) to identify where the statistically significant differences between groups are occurring. As with other between-groups designs, we can interpret these findings using bar graphs and line graphs that depict changes across groups and time.

Putting Findings into Context

Between-groups designs offer you an opportunity to situate your unique findings in terms of their statistical, practical, and clinical significance *and* to make causal attributions about what may have led to these outcomes. As a result, your findings have the potential to inform applied practices in your settings. With those responsibilities in mind, it is important to develop impact statements, interpret effect sizes, estimate clinical significance, and shape a summative conceptualization regarding the efficacy of your intervention or program. Box 12.4 depicts a six-step guide you can use to put your findings into context. You can modify the capitalized components to fit your project. As with other templates, this template cannot fully breathe life into your findings: that task is yours.

BOX 12.4 BASIC FRAMEWORK PUTTING BETWEEN-GROUPS DESIGN FINDINGS INTO CONTEXT

Step 1: Characterize the general impact of your findings

The results of our analyses indicated MINIMAL/MODERATE/MIXED/STRONG support for differences in OUTCOME VARIABLE between participants who completed the INTERVENTION/PROGRAM NAME versus the INTERVENTION/PROGRAM NAME within SETTING NAME.

Step 2: Report the findings of your statistical significance test and practical significance estimates

Findings from INDEPENDENT SAMPLES *t*-TEST/ANOVA/MANOVA/ANCOVA/MANCOVA suggested that participants REPORTED/DID NOT REPORT statistically significant differences in OUTCOME VARIABLE at POST-TEST/FOLLOW-UP when compared to PRE-TEST/ADMISSION, $t/F(\text{df}) = t/F$-VALUE, $p = p$-VALUE, *EFFECT SIZE* = ES VALUE indicative of a SMALL/MEDIUM/LARGE effect size.

Step 3: Interpret the meaning of your effect size

For d-family effect sizes: These findings illustrate that participants in the GROUP NAME reported an INCREASE/DECREASE in scores for OUTCOME VARIABLE of *d*-FAMILY VALUE CONVERTED TO PERCENTAGE standard deviation units when compared to participants in the GROUP NAME.
For r-family effect sizes: These findings illustrate that differences between groups of participant accounted for *r*-FAMILY VALUE CONVERTED TO PROPORTIONS OF VARIANCE of change within observed scores.

Step 4: Compare your findings to previous studies

This outcome WAS/WAS NOT consistent with previous studies of INTERVENTION that detected effect sizes ranging within the SMALL/MEDIUM/LARGE range.

Step 5: Situate your findings into the clinical/educational context

The differences in mean scores for POST-TEST/TERMINATION/FOLLOW-UP of VALUE INDICATES/DOES NOT INDICATE A CLINICALLY/AN EDUCATIONALLY significant degree of difference between scores representing OUTCOME VARIABLE.

Step 6: Develop a summative statement about your findings

Constructively integrate all of this information through your uniquely informed lens to make a conservative, even-handed summative statement about the differential performance of the interventions/programs for participants.

Developing General Impact Statements

We should be cautious when using causal language in impact statements associated with between-groups studies. Although we can make cause-and-effect attributions between interventions and outcomes, limitations to our designs will affect how well we can defend those attributions. The more we have controlled for the influence of threats to validity in designing our evaluation (e.g., by randomizing participants, using fidelity checks, collecting data at multiple points in time), the more we will be able to communicate our results with confidence. Still, we must own the limitations of our design and our findings. In so doing, we provide an honest, even-handed representation that does not overstate importance to colleagues, stakeholders, and policymakers. As with findings from single-group designs, we may conceptualize results of projects across a continuum ranging from no evidence to strong evidence for differences between programs and interventions; we may also characterize findings as comprising minimal, moderate, mixed, or strong support.

Interpreting Significance

Following a general statement of impact, we should substantiate our conclusions with some metrics that can be communicated with clarity across professionals. Between-groups designs are well-suited for reporting results of null hypothesis statistical testing (*p*-values), estimates of effect size, and clinical significance. We can infer statistical significance from statistical significance testing for all studies with *p*-values less than.05. We can infer practical significance between scores for two groups from interpreting *d*-family effect sizes such as Hedge's *g*, which are conceptualized as units of standard deviation and interpreted as small (g =.20), medium (g =.50), or large (g =.80) associations (Ellis, 2010). Alternatively, for studies comparing three or more groups, *r*-family effect sizes such as η^2 depict the amount of change in outcomes associated with participant groups and are interpreted as small (η^2=.02), medium (η^2 =.13), or large (η^2 =.26) associations (Richardson, 2011). Finally, we can infer clinical significance by comparing differences in mean scores from pre-test, post-test, or follow-up data and referencing how they relate to relevant indicators of success such as reliable change index, shifts between categories of symptom severity (e.g., from severe to mild distress), or use of non-technical metrics such as percent improvement (Blampied, 2022; Kendall, 1999; Lenz, 2021).

Shaping Summative Findings

Between-groups designs often yield a lot of data by outcome, so summative statements are important for helping others understand what the take-home message may be for them. This statement should be brief, a sentence or two, and account for the strengths and limitations of your project within its ecological context. Although you can interpret statistical, practical, and clinical significance with reference to the conventions inherent in *p*-values, effect sizes, and clinical benchmarks we noted earlier, this statement is stronger if you are able to connect the statistical to the human dimensions in ways that are plainly spoken and succinct.

DISPLAYING RESULTS

Results of between-groups designs are similar to those used with single-group designs, but we modify the presentation to allow contrasts across groups of participants. To display results, we recommend using line charts with descriptive statistics tables. Each of these strategies is well-suited for communicating results to colleagues, stakeholders, or policymakers in transparent ways. The case study illustrates one way to present the results of a between-groups evaluation design.

BOX 12.5 CASE STUDY REVISITED

Using our case study as an example, the program coordinator decides to complete an experimental between-groups design to determine if transition to an experiential, process-oriented approach to student development is supported by student-level data. This section will provide a brief application of chapter content to illustrate between-group principles and practices you can replicate in your work.

Purposes of Study

- Understanding performance of an intervention in comparison to an existing standard.

Related Questions Guiding the Evaluation

- Are there statistically significant differences in empathic responding, counseling student self-efficacy, and course grades between students who receive didactic-reflective pedagogy versus those who receive experiential, process-oriented class instruction?
- What is the practical significance of differences in empathic responding, counseling student self-efficacy, and course grades between students who receive didactic-reflective pedagogy versus those who receive experiential, process-oriented class instruction?

Selected Single-Group Design

- Experimental design with mixed pre-test and post-test (empathic responding, counseling student self-efficacy) and post-test-only (grades) features.

Putting Findings into Context

Empathic responding. The results of our analyses indicated moderate support for differences in empathic responding between participants who completed the didactic-reflective pedagogy versus those who received experiential, process-oriented class instruction within their introductory coursework. Findings from an independent samples *t*-test suggested that participants reported statistically significant differences in empathic responding at post-test when compared to pre-test, $t(38) = 2.31$, $p = .04$, $g = .66$ indicative of a medium effect size. These findings illustrate that participants in the experiential, process-oriented group reported an increase in scores for empathic responding of 66% of a standard deviation when compared to participants in the didactic-reflective pedagogy group. This outcome was consistent with previous studies of experiential training for counseling students that detected effect sizes ranging within the medium and large ranges. The differences in mean scores for post-test empathy measures of.45 indicate a clinically significant degree of difference between scores representing quality of empathic responding.

Counseling student self-efficacy. The results of our analyses indicated strong support for differences in counseling student self-efficacy between participants who completed the didactic-reflective pedagogy versus those who received experiential, process-oriented class instruction within their introductory coursework. Findings from an independent samples *t*-test suggested that participants reported statistically significant differences in self-efficacy at post-test when compared to pre-test, $t(38) = 3.01$, $p < .01$, $g = .93$, indicative of a large effect size. These findings illustrate that participants in the experiential, process-oriented group reported an increase in scores for self-efficacy of 93% of a standard deviation when compared to participants in the didactic-reflective pedagogy group. This outcome was consistent with previous studies of experiential training for counseling students that detected effect sizes ranging within the medium and large ranges. The differences in mean scores for post-test empathy measures of 1.60 do not indicate an educationally significant degree of difference between scores representing the amount of self-efficacy.

Grades. The results of our analyses indicated no support for differences in grades between participants who completed the didactic-reflective pedagogy versus those who received experiential, process-oriented class instruction within their introductory coursework. Findings from an independent samples *t*-test suggested that participants did not report statistically significant differences in grades at post-test when compared to pre-test, $t(38) = .27$, $p = .78$, $g = .01$. These findings illustrate that participants in the experiential, process-oriented group reported an increase in grades of 1% of a standard deviation when compared to participants in the didactic-reflective pedagogy group. This outcome was consistent with previous studies of experiential training for counseling students that detected effect sizes ranging within the small range. The differences in mean scores for post-test empathy measures of.05 do not indicate an educationally significant degree of difference between grades.

Taken together, these findings suggest that engagement in experiential process-oriented class instruction was associated with clinically relevant changes in empathic responding when compared to didactic-reflective pedagogy. Although changes in self-efficacy were statistically and practically relevant, it is reasonable that the changes associated with this single class were not educationally significant. Finally, these findings suggest that neither instructional strategy was associated with differences in student achievement as measured by course grades.

Displaying Findings

Relevant information depicting the amount of differences between groups, statistical significance, and effect size can be depicted in a table.

	PRE-TEST		POST-TEST				
	D-R	**E-P**	**D-R**	**E-P**	***T***	***p***	***g* [95% CI]**
EMPATHY	1.25 (.44)	1.35 (.48)	1.80 (.61)	2.25 (.71)	−2.13	.04	.66 [.09, .88]
CSES	75.75 (1.40)	75.45 (1.70)	79.20 (1.67)	81.80 (3.48)	−3.01	< .01	.93 [−.08, 1.77]
GRADE			89.50 (3.29)	89.55 (3.70)	.27	.78	.01 [−1.09, 1.07]

Figure 12.1 Differences in raw scores over time between groups can be displayed using a bar graph

Using Line Charts

We can use line charts to display data trends across groups of participants over time at pre-test, post-test, and/or follow-up intervals. In quasi-experimental and experimental designs, the values of scores will be situated on the Y-axis (vertical) and the groups as markers on the X-axis (horizontal). These charts can be helpful visual aids for portraying the influence of interventions and will support statements about clinical significance. You can easily generate and edit line charts in most word processing and data management programs.

Bar Graphs

Although line charts are preferred for projects with measurements across time, bar graphs are the visual display of choice for post-test-only designs. These bar graphs readily depict the final data point of your project with score values on the Y-axis (vertical) and groups as markers on the X-axis (horizontal).

Using Descriptive Statistics Tables

For between-groups projects, it is standard to include sample size, means, standard deviations, and effect sizes. Tables should reflect a balance between including all data necessary for critical consideration of your findings with parsimonious, self-evident presentation. As a rule, if your table only requires a few columns, it may not be necessary. Although tables should reflect the text of your scientific or evaluation report, readers should be able to easily understand the table on its own.

CHAPTER SUMMARY

This chapter presented you with introductory concepts and tools to implement between-groups designs. When putting this chapter's contents into action, you will be poised to determine your project's purpose and begin designing a strategy that connects research or evaluation questions, design selection, analyses, and reporting practices. These concepts and tools were illustrated with a case example of an applied research project evaluating teaching strategies in a counselor education program. By referencing the content in this chapter, you are prepared to begin researching and evaluating projects with a degree of certainty regarding cause-and-effect attributions. Through the use of the resources in this chapter, we encourage you to share findings within your academic community, among stakeholders, and with relevant policymakers.

RESOURCES

- Linfield, K. J., & Kniffley, S. D. (2025). *Program evaluation: Methods and case studies* (10th ed.). Routledge.
- Montgomery, D. C. (2019). *Design and analysis of experiments* (10th ed.). Wiley.
- *Patient-Centered Outcomes Research Institute*, PCORI Methodology Standards. www.pcori.org/research-related-projects/about-our-research/research-methodology/pcori-methodology-standards

REFERENCES

American Psychological Association. (2021). *Professional practice guidelines for evidence-based psychological practice in health care*. www.apa.org/about/policy/psychological-practice-health-care.pdf

APA Presidential Task Force on Evidence-Based Practice (2006). Evidence-based practice in psychology. *American Psychologist*, *61*(4), 272–285. https://doi.org/10.1037/0003-066X.61.4.271

Ellis, P. D. (2010). *The essential guide to effect sizes: Statistical power, meta-analysis, and the interpretation of research results*. Cambridge University Press.

Handley, M. A., Lyles, C. R., McCulloch, C., & Cattamanchi, A. (2018). Selecting and improving quasi-experimental designs in effectiveness and implementation research. *Annual Review of Public Health*, *39*, 5–25. https://doi.org/10.1146/annurev-publhealth-040617-014128

Kendall, P. C. (1999). Clinical significance. *Journal of Consulting and Clinical Psychology*, *67*(3), 283–284. https://doi.org/10.1037/0022-006X.67.3.283

Lenz, A. S., & Del Conte, G. (2018). Efficacy of DBT-A among adolescents in a partial hospitalization program. *Journal of Counseling and Development*, *96*, 15–26. https://doi.org/10.1002/jcad.12174

Lenz, A. S., & Sangganjanavanich, V. F. (2013). Evidence for the utility of a photovoice task as an empathic skill acquisition strategy among counselors in training. *Journal of Humanistic Counseling*, *52*, 39–53. https://doi.org/10.1002/j.2161–1939.2013.00031.x

Lenz, A. S. (2021). Clinical significance in counseling outcome research and program evaluation. *Counseling Outcome Research and Evaluation*, *12*(1), 1–3. https://doi.org/10.1080/21501378.2021.1877097

Melchert, T. P., Hays, V. L., Wiljanen, L. M., & Kolocek, A. K. (1996). Testing models of counselor development with a measure of counseling self-efficacy. *Journal of Counseling & Development*, *74(6)*, 640–644. https://doi.org/10.1002/j.1556-6676.1996.tb02304.x

Lothes, J., & Hall, M. (2025). Utilizing dialectical behavioral therapy in a partial hospital and intensive outpatient program: Outcomes on patient's mindfulness, clinical ratings, and PTSD. *Counseling Outcome Research and Evaluation*, *16*(2), 186–204. https://doi.org/10.1080/21501378.2024.2437990

Montgomery, D. C. (2019). *Design and analysis of experiments* (10th ed.). Wiley.

Nielsen, K., & Miraglia, M. (2017). What works for whom in which circumstances? On the need to move beyond the "what works?" question in organizational intervention research. *Human Relations*, *70*, 40–62. https://doi.org/10.1177/0018726716670226

Richardson, J. T. E. (2011). Eta squared and partial eta squared as measures of effect size in educational research. *Educational Research Review*, *6*, 135–147. https://doi.org/10.1016/j.edurev.2010.12.001

Wampold, B. E., Lichtenberg, J., & Waehler, C. A. (2002). Principles of empirically supported interventions in counseling psychology. *The Counseling Psychologist*, *30*, 197–217. https://doi.org/10.1177/0011000002302001

CHAPTER 13

Understanding Lived Experiences

As professional counselors, we hold individual uniqueness and experience in high regard and understand the power of story, experience, context, and nuance in lived experience. Although scientists have historically valued numbers and statistical control, there is growing appreciation for and publication of rigorous, systematic qualitative inquiries in peer-reviewed journals. Certainly, the incorporation of qualitative perspectives is essential in applied research and program evaluation. As a service provider, you may value knowing that the number of referrals for aggressive behavior decreased (quantitative), but you likely also want to understand *why* and *how* these referrals decreased (qualitative). Even our most effective programs may have limited impact if our target populations do not view them as relevant, culturally responsive, and meaningful. There are just some things numbers cannot tell us.

This chapter introduces you to essential activities associated with implementing qualitative methodologies in applied research and program evaluation. This chapter opens with a general overview of qualitative methods and a summary of six classic qualitative designs used in published research. Next, we attend to processes for conducting qualitative inquiry, with special attention to the use of semi-structured interviews, focus groups, and document analysis in real-world counseling settings. The chapter concludes with attention to qualitative data analysis and reporting considerations unique to qualitative evaluation of interventions and programs.

BOX 13.1 CHAPTER LEARNING OUTCOMES

- Develop research questions consistent with use of qualitative methodology
- Articulate key features of different types of qualitative research designs
- Understand when qualitative methods may be appropriate for use in applied research and program evaluation endeavors
- Develop procedures for conducting semi-structured interviews, focus groups, and document analysis
- Identify common methods of analyzing qualitative data
- Critique studies using qualitative methodology

DOI: 10.4324/9781003586210-15

BOX 13.2 CASE STUDY

Youth Matters is a community-based nonprofit agency that is nearing completion of year one of an after-school program for children in an urban, high-needs area in which community members have expressed concerns related to ongoing gang and drug activity. The program is primarily funded by donors and was launched in recognition of a high number of children who were either unsupervised or supervised by older siblings while their parents worked in the afternoons and early evenings. Children participate in the program on school grounds. During the afternoon, children have a nutritious snack, participate in a brief social-emotional learning curriculum, have the opportunity for help with homework, and have time for play. The program also offers several service-learning opportunities for older youth to support the program, and it provides parenting skills and career development resources for parents. As the program nears completion of the first year and the agency prepares to launch a funding campaign, donors requested participant feedback regarding the program.

OVERVIEW OF QUALITATIVE RESEARCH DESIGNS

What Are Qualitative Designs?

A quick review of the literature will show you that there are dozens of highly nuanced definitions related to qualitative designs or inquiries. These definitions are often philosophical in nature with strong attention to ways of knowing about the complicated lived experiences of humans. Most designs in this text focus on the use of numbers to capture thoughts, feelings, behaviors, and changes associated with participation in an intervention or program. Those quantitative methods focus on knowing through numbers. We use qualitative research to focus on understanding experience and meaning through words. Of course, this is a gross oversimplification of a highly nuanced and often debated process.

Although specific characteristics of qualitative design will depend on the nature of the qualitative inquiry in focus, four core characteristics are common across qualitative designs (Tisdell et al., 2025, pp. 19–22):

- Focus on meaning and understanding
- Researcher as primary instrument
- An inductive process
- Rich description

Table 13.1 includes a comparison of the characteristics of qualitative and quantitative research.

TABLE 13.1 Comparison of Characteristics of Qualitative and Quantitative Research

Point of comparison	Qualitative research	Quantitative research
Focus of research	Quality (nature, essence)	Quantity (how much, how many)
Philosophical roots	Phenomenology, symbolic interactionism, constructivism	Positivism, logical empiricism, realism
Associated phrases	Fieldwork, ethnographic, naturalistic, grounded, constructivist	Experimental, empirical, statistical
Goal of investigation	Understanding, description, discovery, meaning, hypothesis generating	Prediction, control, description, confirmation, hypothesis testing
Design characteristics	Flexible, evolving, emergent	Predetermined, structured
Sample	Small, nonrandom, purposeful, theoretical	Large, random, representative
Data collection	Researcher as primary instrument, interviews, observations, documents	Inanimate instruments (scales, tests, surveys, questionnaires, computers)
Primary mode of analysis	Inductive, constant comparative method	Deductive, statistical
Findings	Comprehensive, holistic, expansive, richly descriptive	Precise, numerical

(Tisdell et al., 2025, p. 24)

When Are Qualitative Designs Indicated?

We have already established that qualitative designs are particularly useful for understanding experiences, processes, and meaning-making. It makes sense that we use these designs when we want to understand those things that numbers cannot tell us. From a program development and evaluation standpoint, qualitative designs hold special promise for needs assessments, process evaluations, and giving context to quantitative findings. Qualitative methods can help us answer questions related to what, why, and how. Slight distinctions in questions answered will depend on the purpose of the inquiry and the specific nature of the framework. After describing each indication for qualitative design, we think back to the opening case study to provide examples of corresponding questions.

Needs Assessment

In Chapter 8, we discussed needs assessment as a process for gathering data from a variety of sources to better understand opportunities to better serve our stakeholders. Qualitative exploration of needs is particularly important when we are not certain of a starting point or need to generate a more nuanced understanding of a general starting point. For example, these designs are particularly well-suited to understanding individuals' (e.g., potential consumers, consumers, staff, or experts) perceptions of needs or barriers as expressed in open-ended survey responses, semi-structured interviews, or focus groups. We might ask:

- What do parents and teachers perceive as the most important elements in a community-based after-school program?
- What do key stakeholders identify as the greatest unmet needs of the population participating in a community-based after-school program?

Process Evaluation

Qualitative designs are also well-suited for complex questions regarding how and why a program works (or doesn't work). When focused on consumers, qualitative designs may help us understand what keeps them engaged, what aspects of a program are most meaningful, what aspects of a program are confusing or frustrating, and how the intervention or program affected their lives. When focused on staff members, qualitative designs may help us understand insights into what is working and not working, observations about participant response, and obstacles or barriers to implementing programs as intended. In all, qualitative designs are often indicated as part of process evaluations. We might ask questions such as:

- How do students experience relationships with staff within the community-based after-school program?
- What aspects of the community-based after-school program do parents and guardians perceive as particularly impactful and meaningful for their students?
- What obstacles do staff members encounter when attempting to deliver the structured peer relationships curriculum within the community-based after-school program?

Giving Context to Quantitative Findings

Finally, qualitative designs may be useful as part of mixed-methods evaluations. We may utilize qualitative data to support, contrast, or illuminate quantitative findings. Such an inquiry may give context and richness to data, illuminating specific takeaway skills or changes and adding a human touch to what may otherwise fall flat. Certainly, we may be encouraged by a quantitative finding that 80% of participants reported greater relationship satisfaction after taking part in an enrichment program for couples. However, that number tells us little about what changed, how those changes affected quality of life, or how support from program staff influenced the outcome. Qualitative findings may round out quantitative findings in ways that are more deeply meaningful for all involved. Sample questions are:

- How do youth experience changes in holistic wellness after participating in the community-based after-school program?

- What changes do parents or guardians experience in their children as a result of participating in the community-based after-school program?

Classic Types of Qualitative Research Designs

Researchers may build upon a number of philosophical frameworks when designing and implementing qualitative research designs. Although we believe working within these hallmark designs is very important when generating research for publication, the classics may be less useful from a program development and evaluation standpoint. Although we understand you are not likely to use a specific qualitative framework to navigate your duties as a counselor, we expect you will encounter references to these frameworks as you use literature to support your practice. Thus, we present a very quick tour through six classic approaches to qualitative inquiry. For each, we highlight philosophical foundations, key features, intended uses, and a corresponding research question. We also suggest sources you may find useful for understanding the approach in greater depth.

Generic, Basic, or Descriptive

Although not always explicitly named, much qualitative research falls under what is often referred to interchangeably as generic, basic, or descriptive qualitative research. These approaches are characterized by a focus on "(1) how people interpret their experiences, (2) how they construct their worlds, and (3) what meaning they attribute to their experiences" (Tisdell et al., 2025, p. 29). Researchers using generic qualitative designs typically do not align with the specific assumptions or procedures of a distinct qualitative tradition explored below. Instead, they may blend elements from multiple traditions or prioritize pragmatic alignment with their research context. From a basic qualitative perspective, a researcher may ask: How do participants and caregivers describe the most helpful elements and impacts of the community-based-after-school program? Researchers often choose generic approaches for their flexibility, adaptability when working with community partners, and potential for innovation (Waalkes et al., 2024). For more information on generic qualitative research, consult Kostere and Kostere (2022) and Waalkes et al. (2024).

Phenomenology

Phenomenology is both a philosophy and a research method. At its core, phenomenology is focused on meaning-making related to lived experiences, often working to distill experiences into an "essence." Phenomenological researchers most often use in-depth interviews with individuals who have experienced common events or phenomena. Researchers work to uncover individual participants' experiences and meaning-making process in depth. Then, researchers work across cases to uncover shared elements of these experiences. From a phenomenological perspective, a researcher may ask: *What is the lived experience of adolescents who have witnessed violence in their community?* For more information on phenomenology, consult Husserl (1970), Moustakas (1994), and Smith et al. (2022).

Grounded Theory

Grounded theory is focused on using data to build a substantive theory about a process or phenomenon. Grounded theory designs most often use semi-structured interviews as a primary data source; however, they can also include observation and document review. Researchers engage in a process of constant comparative analysis to understand units of meaning within and across cases, ultimately leading to the identification of categories (groups of units) and creation of a theory that explains relationships and processes among categories. From a grounded theory perspective, a researcher may ask: *What is the theory that explains the process of navigating home, school, and community for adolescents who have witnessed violence in their community?* For more information on grounded theory, consult Charmaz (2024), Corbin and Strauss (2015), and Glaser and Strauss (1967).

Narrative Inquiry

Narrative inquiry is focused on using the art of story to illustrate meaning and experience. Given the focus on story, narrative designs use oral and written word as primary data sources. This often includes the use of semi-structured interviews but may also incorporate experiences conveyed in autobiographical writings, images, or videos. The research process includes collecting stories and experiences, analyzing for themes, and constructing a common shared story. From a narrative inquiry perspective, a researcher may ask: *How do adolescents who have witnessed violence in their community navigate home, school, and community?* For more information on narrative inquiry, consult Clandinin (2022) and Riessman (2008).

Ethnography

Grounded in the study of culture, ethnography focuses on understanding cultural groups or phenomena. Ethnographic methods involve immersion in a site and feature a heavy focus on prolonged observation and engagement. In traditional ethnographic methods, anthropologists and sociologists are immersed in fieldwork, often for months or years at a time. During these times, they observe individuals and interactions, making notes of artifacts (e.g., photos, documents, items used in everyday living or working). In addition to observations, researchers interview community members in hopes of uncovering greater cultural meaning while making sense of observations. Ethnography may involve the study of just one individual, a small group, or a community as a whole. From an ethnographic perspective, a researcher may ask: *What are the social and cultural rules of engagement among adolescents who live in an area with known gang activity?* For more information on ethnography, consult Denzin (2014), Fetterman (2019), and LeCompte and Schensul (2010).

Qualitative Case Study

Case studies apply very well to program evaluation because they are focused on understanding one program or unit well, often from multiple perspectives. The unit of analysis in case study research is a "bounded system" researchers examine in its own context. A bounded system is clearly defined in scope or boundaries, leading the case to be specific and distinct. The bounded system may refer to a specific setting (e.g., one clinic or school), group of individuals (e.g., clients or students enrolled in a program, service providers in an organization), or a program (e.g., bundle of interventions offered over a specific period of time), or an organization. Case study research involves the triangulation of multiple data sources within the bounded case. For example, a researcher conducting a case study on an after-school program may conduct observations, review records, interview program staff, and conduct focus groups with parents and children. Some types of case studies even incorporate quantitative data as part of the overall exploration. Then, the analysis focuses on tying data sources together to describe the case and central themes. From a case study perspective, a researcher might ask: *How does the community-based after-school program enhance quality of life for adolescents who have experienced violence in their community*? For more information on case studies, consult Stake (1995) and Yin (2018).

QUALITATIVE EVALUATION PROCESS

Although there is great depth in the six traditional approaches to qualitative research, you will need advanced preparation in order to utilize them for research and publication purposes. Counselors working in schools and agencies will rarely have the time and logistical resources to carry out a traditional qualitative inquiry. In the interest of practicality, we focus this section on specific steps for using qualitative data in the context of program evaluation.

Determining the Purpose and Focus of the Inquiry

As with all applied research and program evaluation, the first step is to determine the specific purpose and focus of the inquiry. Determining the purpose and focus of the inquiry forces you to specify what you are focused on understanding (i.e., individual, program, agency, school, policy, group of consumers) and what you would like to understand (i.e., experience or phenomenon). We must also consider *why* we want to answer these questions and *how* we will use them in developing, evaluating, and improving our interventions and programs.

Identifying Key Informants and Data Sources

With purpose and focus in mind, we are ready to identify key informants and data sources. This step involves thinking through how we can best access the type of information we need to answer our questions. In some cases, we may decide that *people* can best help us answer our questions. We may wish to hear from potential consumers, active consumers, staff, or experts. So we must design a sampling plan that corresponds to the purpose of our inquiry. As presented in Chapter 4, this sampling plan should be purposive and may include a wide range of strategies, including identifying typical cases, working to hear from deviant cases (i.e., someone who had an outcome very different from others), or engaging in maximum variation sampling to secure a broad range of perspectives.

Although most qualitative methods involve using interviews with people as a primary source of data, we may also find other sources to answer our inquiry. In some cases, we may use school or agency records, reports, and other written information as data sources. For example, rather than interviewing new clients about their needs, we might decide to review intake records over the last six months to better understand why and how people presented to an agency.

In qualitative work, the researcher is the primary data collection tool. Inherent in deciding key informants and data sources is also deciding who should be responsible for collecting data. Ideally, this should be someone with interviewing expertise, strong interpersonal skills, and familiarity with the population of focus. Given power differentials and emotional ties involved in many therapeutic relationships, we caution against having counselors solicit interview data from their clients. Such a practice may confound the relationship and may limit the trustworthiness of the information received.

Data Collection Procedures

After we determine data sources, we are ready to determine specific methods for gathering data. As inferred previously, this may include use of phone, video, or in-person semi-structured interviews; focus groups; observations; responses to open-ended survey questions; and review of existing documents such as client files or agency records. If using interviews or focus groups, we must create an interview guide (or I-guide) and make decisions about how to carry out and document interviews. Because we believe you are most likely to use interviews, focus groups, and document review in your work, we cover considerations for each next.

Semi-Structured Interviews

Semi-structured interviews (SSIs) are individual interviews that are often conversational in nature, involve both open-ended and closed-ended questions, and include follow-up probes or prompts to elicit deeper understanding (Adams, 2015). SSIs are most appropriate when we want to understand the independent thoughts of individuals, are concerned that informants may not be candid in front of others, want one-on-one time with administrative staff for formative evaluation, or are "examining uncharted territory" (p. 494). More specifically, use SSIs when you need to:

- Seek individual perspectives.
- Identify individual narratives.
- Seek personal and sensitive information.
- Collect detailed, in-depth information.
- Describe complex issues or processes.
- Access geographically dispersed participants. (Hennick, 2014, p. 28)

Adams (2015) provided an overview of considerations for designing SSIs, noting that protocols are always a work in progress and may change over time to reflect lessons learned or emerging themes. Design considerations include optimal timing (i.e., less than one hour), careful selection of topics, and careful ordering of questions. For example, you may wish to open the I-guide with customary pleasantries and a few questions to break the ice. Then, interviews should progress in terms of depth and relevance. It may be helpful to open with closed-ended questions that use a yes/no or rating system and follow up with questions designed to understand nuances related to the interviewee's position. In addition, we might sequence questions so positive questions come first, followed by invitations to explore drawbacks, disadvantages, and potentially negative information. Finally, you may wish to save potentially embarrassing or sensitive questions for the end of the interview when, presumably, you will have built trust and rapport.

When conducting SSIs, it is important to help participants understand why they were selected for the interview, how you will use their information, and how you will protect their privacy. Interviewers should be careful to use nondirective listening skills, demonstrating acceptance of both person and message, reflecting understanding, and clarifying unclear statements. Interviewers must decide when and how to probe contributions while also keeping an eye on the larger purpose and process of the interview. At the conclusion of the interview, it may be helpful to provide a summary of major points of conversation, remind participants how their information will be used to improve interventions and programs, and recap how you will protect their privacy when using information they provided.

Focus Groups

Commonly used in the corporate world, focus groups involve gathering information via an interactive small-group process. Focus groups may be used to assess needs and assets, design interventions, evaluate policy options, pilot-test data collection instruments, understand qualitative findings, and monitor and evaluate agency options (Krueger & Casey, 2015, pp. 507–508). Focus group interviewers use carefully developed questions and processes with the intent of generating a range of opinions. Rather than push a group to come to consensus, skilled facilitators help group members articulate their thoughts and share contrasting opinions. More specifically, you may use focus groups when you need to:

- Capture a range of views and experiences.
- Discuss or explain issues.
- Explore new issues.
- Identify social and community norms.
- Seek broad community-level information.
- Observe group interactions. (Hennick, 2014, p. 28)

As with other qualitative methods, we must first start with a sampling plan. Given the nature of focus groups, it is important that participants be relatively homogenous in terms of role (e.g., all staff members with similar amounts of power or all potential consumers). An ideal size for a focus group is six to eight participants; however, you may conduct focus groups with as few as five and as many as ten participants (Hennick, 2014). Focus groups also require development of an I-guide with a target length of 60 to 90 minutes. As with other interview protocols, it is important to put questions in an order that elicits multiple opinions, rich perspectives, and conversations among participants about those perspectives (Hennick, 2014; Krueger & Casey, 2015). See Box 13.3 for a sample I-guide focused on a generic program.

BOX 13.3 SAMPLE I-GUIDE FOCUSED ON FORMATIVE PROGRAM PARTICIPATION (KRUEGER & CASEY, 2015, P. 518)

- Tell us how you participated in the program.
- What did you like the best about the program? (What has been most helpful to you?)
- What did you like the least about the program? (What was least helpful to you?)
- What are the important accomplishments of the program?
- What are the biggest weaknesses of the program?
- What should be changed?
- What should be continued and kept the same?
- What other advice do you have about the program?

As with semi-structured interviewing, it is important to attend to process skills while facilitating focus groups. This includes drawing out participation from multiple contributors, inviting contrasting opinions, and remaining supportively neutral so we do not influence the overall outcome or content. The focus group interviewer has the added responsibility of managing group dynamics, ideally facilitating discussion among participants rather than using a moderator–participant–moderator–participant volley. As with interviews, it is often helpful to close a focus group by summarizing major points of conversation, helping participants understand how you will protect their privacy, and noting how their contributions will be helpful in program development or evaluation.

Document Review

Document review is one final data collection source that may be particularly useful within your work setting. You likely already have access to a number of documents containing qualitative data that may be useful for program development and evaluation. These documents may help you understand common themes in needs, experiences, or program engagement without requiring additional investment in rigorous interview processes.

Consider, for example, how a review of the following documents might help you understand the individuals you serve, their needs, and your programs better:

- Client records, including intake reports, case notes, and periodic assessments.
- Student records, including attendance, grades, standardized test scores, disciplinary referrals, and IEP/504 reports.
- Supervision notes for staff members in their first two years of service.
- Session reflection forms gathered weekly as part of a closing group counseling ritual.
- Incident reports completed within a group home or residential facility.

As with interviews, we must decide how we will access the information we seek to understand. For example, we may have a reason to explore all records entered during a specific period, only records with a specific outcome (e.g., suspension from school, progression to a higher level of care, successful completion of program), or a random selection of records.

Data Management Strategy

As you have likely noted by now, qualitative data are rich, complex, and messy. Thus, they require an active data management strategy. Although recording and transcription are hallmark features of qualitative research, they are not always feasible or necessary in evaluation work (Adams, 2015; Royse et al., 2006). Rather, you may need to truncate some classic methods to make them realistic for use in real-world settings. For example, Royse et al. (2006) suggested "using consensually developed domains to structure the interviews, analyses, and findings; substituting note-taking for verbatim transcriptions; identifying themes based on the domains rather than indirectly via open coding" (p. 104).

Thus, you will need to determine whether to record interviews or rely exclusively on a note-taking system. Although we believe recording is a good idea (even if one does not transcribe), you may decide to forego recording based on privacy concerns. In this case, you will need to develop a documentation strategy that allows you to capture overall responses and key quotes while also staying engaged in the interview. For example, you might use a copy of the interview guide with space to write key phrases and quotes under each question.

When conducting focus groups, you might have participants generate ideas on a white board or butcher-block paper, later taking a picture of the lists generated for analysis. Given the complexity of focus groups, it would be a good idea to include a co-facilitating note-taker to record responses, freeing one person to attend solely to group facilitation.

Finally, when using document review, you will need to decide whether to analyze records as a whole or utilize a shorthand note-taking strategy; for example, rather than relocate entire file cabinets into your office, you might complete a one- to two-page worksheet for each document reviewed, then work from those notes for overall analysis.

Trustworthiness Protections

Given the unique role of the researcher and the subjective nature of data explored in qualitative methods, there is a need to take active steps to ensure the trustworthiness of one's approach. In other words, we need to provide evidence that the information accurately captures participants' experiences and that conclusions generated were done so with rigor and credibility. An American Psychological Association Taskforce conducted a comprehensive review of trustworthiness as a concept and provided a report regarding how qualitative researchers can attend to methodological integrity within their work (Levitt et al., 2017). In the end, they suggested a number of data collection and analysis procedures that ensure fidelity to subject and utility in achieving goals. You may find researchers enacting these concepts by using strategies such as prolonged engagement, negative case analysis, triangulation of data sources, triangulation of coders, audit trails, peer debriefing, and member checks.

Although formal trustworthiness principles and resulting strategies are important for traditional qualitative research, they are less feasible for implementation in program development and evaluation settings. Lub (2015) connected traditional principles regarding trustworthiness in qualitative research to validity in qualitative evaluation. In the end, it is important to consider safeguards we can build into our designs so stakeholders can trust that our findings reflect participant contributions. Box 13.4 includes some ideas for boosting the trustworthiness of your work.

BOX 13.4 TRUSTWORTHINESS STEPS IN QUALITATIVE EVALUATIONS

- Prior to engaging in data collection and analysis, take some time to write about your experiences and expectations related to the topics of focus; being transparent about your expectations will help you note when your bias may creep into questioning and analysis.
- Although we value self-exploration and examination related to our work, do not take the lead on evaluating your own program; rather, switch off with a colleague so that the evaluator can provide more of an "arm's-length" perspective.
- Collaborate with one to two colleagues on data analysis, making sure to come to a consensus regarding your overall findings; if this is not possible, have a peer at least "audit" your findings by reviewing all original documents and your analysis.

Ethical Protections

Finally, preview all proposed procedures to ensure you have embedded adequate ethical protections (see Chapter 6). In particular, you will need to ensure participants do not feel coerced to participate and are able to offer their contributions freely, without fear of retaliation or loss of esteem. Some contributions may be personally identifiable, so work to ensure you have adequate privacy protections in place, perhaps masking specific stories or examples or using individual interviews rather than focus groups for sensitive topics.

QUALITATIVE DATA ANALYSIS

Procedures used for qualitative data analysis will match classic frameworks, and these frameworks rarely provide a clear step-by-step method for analysis. We realize that may not be helpful to you. In this section, we provide overviews of two primary data analysis frameworks you may find helpful: reflexive thematic analysis and consensual qualitative research (CQR). We review both frameworks here, and we close the section by noting several practical tools for data analysis.

Thematic Analysis

Thematic analysis is a foundational method for qualitative analysis that helps researchers organize and describe data in detail and is applicable across a broad range of methodological frameworks (Braun & Clarke, 2022). Braun and Clarke proposed a six-step guide for conducting thematic analysis, as illustrated in Table 13.2. This

TABLE 13.2 Phases of Thematic Analysis

Phase	Description of the process
1. Familiarizing yourself with your data	Transcribing data (if necessary), reading and re-reading the data, noting down initial ideas.
2. Generating initial codes	Coding interesting features of the data in a systematic fashion across the entire dataset, collating data relevant to each code.
3. Searching for themes	Collating codes into potential themes, gathering all data relevant to each potential theme.
4. Reviewing themes	Checking if the themes work in relation to the coded extracts (Level 1) and the entire dataset (Level 2), generating a thematic "map" of the analysis.
5. Defining and naming themes	Ongoing analysis to refine the specifics of each theme and the overall story the analysis tells, generating clear definitions and names for each theme.
6. Producing the report	The final opportunity for analysis. Selection of vivid, compelling extract examples, final analysis of selected extracts, relating back of the analysis to the research question and literature, and producing a scholarly report of the analysis.

(Braun & Clarke, 2006, p. 87)

process involves an iterative process of connecting individual pieces of data within transcripts or documents to codes, connecting codes to themes, connecting themes to each other, and supporting overall analysis with the use of specific pieces of data. Please refer to the original source for detailed guidance regarding each step and discussions of criteria for good thematic analysis.

Consensual Qualitative Research

CQR is a method for qualitative research analysis that focuses on "use of multiple researchers, the process of reaching consensus, and a systematic way of examining the representativeness of results across cases" (Hill et al., 1997, p. 519). Hill and colleagues initially articulated eight key components and three steps for CQR. Key components are:

1. Data are gathered using open-ended questions in order not to constrain the responses of the participants.
2. The method relies on words to describe phenomena rather than using numbers.
3. A small number of cases are studied intensively.
4. The context of the whole case is used to understand the specific parts of the experience.
5. The process is inductive, with conclusions being built from the data rather than imposing and testing an *a priori* structure or theory.
6. All judgments are made by a primary team of three to five researchers so that a variety of opinions are available about each decision. Consensus is used so that the best possible construction is developed for all of the data.
7. One or two auditors are used to check the consensus judgments to ensure that the primary team does not overlook important data.
8. The primary team continually goes back to the raw data to make sure that their results and conclusions are accurate and based on the data. (p. 522)

The three general steps of CQR are:

1. Responses to open-ended questions from questionnaires or interviews for each individual case are divided into domains (i.e., topic areas).
2. Core ideas (i.e., abstracts or brief summaries) are constructed for all the material within each domain for each individual case.
3. A cross-analysis, which involves developing categories to describe consistencies in the core ideas within domains across cases, is conducted. (p. 523)

Since initially proposing this methodology, Hill and colleagues have continued to develop and refine these procedures. Several sources include detailed instructions for applying the method (Hill et al., 2005; Hill & Knox, 2021; Hill et al., 1997).

BOX 13.5 CHECKLIST OF INDICATORS OF A QUALITY QUALITATIVE DESIGN

- Purpose and focus of the qualitative inquiry are well defined and logically connected.
- There is a logical connection between the purpose of study/evaluation, related research/evaluation questions, and analytic strategy.
- Key informants and data sources are appropriate to purpose and focus of the inquiry.
- Data collection procedures are clearly described and appropriate to the purpose and focus of the inquiry.
- Trustworthiness protections are clearly described.
- Ethical protections are clearly described.
- Process for qualitative data analysis is clearly described.
- Findings are supported with direct quotations or illustrative stories.
- As appropriate, author provides sense of frequency, prevalence, and weight/intensity of findings.
- Tables and visual depictions support reporting of findings.

Data Analysis Tools

If you find yourself engaging in qualitative analysis, you will quickly note the need for a data analysis and management strategy. Traditionally, researchers have used software systems such as NVIVO (at up to $2000/license!); however, there are a number of free or open-source software options to use. We have had success using Dedoose (www.dedoose.com), a proprietary system that works on a subscription basis to allow individual and team analysis with prices beginning at $17.95 per month. However, depending on the size of your qualitative dataset, you may not need to use software at all. Many qualitative researchers are able to manage the coding process using simple Excel or Google Sheets documents for naming codes, highlighting themes and categories in different colors, associating supporting data or quotes, and organizing into themes. Some researchers are beginning to lean on artificial intelligence for qualitative data analysis. Although this may be tempting and even appropriate in some circumstances, it is important to recognize and consider questions of data ownership, data privacy, and limitations of using inhuman tools for understanding the human condition (Davison et al., 2024).

REPORTING FINDINGS

As with any applied research and program evaluation, the impact of our hard work is often tied to the manner in which we report our findings. Chapter 17 includes practical ways you can organize reports and present findings to partners. In this section, we attend to several practical tips and standards for presenting qualitative findings. Key considerations include transparency in method, clarity of themes and categories, and using data to support assertions.

As part of any presentation of findings, it is important to begin with a description of the purpose and focus of your inquiry. Then focus on how you collected and analyzed your data. This should include descriptions of recruitment or selection processes, participant roles and demographic characteristics, individuals involved in the process, data collection methods, and data analysis methods. For example, you might note that you conducted three 75-minute focus groups in which a total of 15 potential consumers participated, providing readers with a sense of who the potential consumers were, how you found them, and what you asked them to do. You might also note who served as facilitators, their qualifications for doing so, and their connection to the overall programs evaluated. Finally, you will note steps taken to analyze data, safeguard trustworthiness, and ensure ethical protections.

As you report findings, it will be important to provide clear descriptions of themes and categories derived from the data. In some instances, it will be helpful to provide a table in which you name all themes and categories and a definition for readers. Participant voice is critical for giving life to the data and substantiating our analysis and interpretation. We recommend supporting each theme or category with at least two to three exemplar quotes from participants. If participants present varying opinions or experiences, it is important to capture that variation in the quotations. In some instances, it may be helpful to use pictures or diagrams to demonstrate relationships between themes and categories.

Depending on the nature of your questions and methodology, it may be appropriate to note frequency (number of mentions), prevalence (number of participants speaking to the idea), or weight/intensity (energy around the idea) of your data. In some cases, themes and categories will emerge across participants. In other cases, just a few participants may speak to an area; however, they may do so with intensity, or you may begin to notice a pattern that warrants further attention (e.g., if only women or people of color speak to a theme). Refer to Chapter 17 for additional tips on presenting results and writing for impact.

BOX 13.6 CASE STUDY REVISITED

As the first part of an evaluation plan, the program director selected one week for family feedback and asked each family member to respond to a satisfaction survey when picking up their child. Although numbers were positive and helpful for providing general context, the numbers provided little direction regarding opportunities for growth. The program director decided to use qualitative methods to hear from parents about their experiences within the program. This section provides a brief application of chapter content to illustrate the use of qualitative data to support program evaluation.

Purpose of Needs Assessment

- Understand parents' experiences during the first year of the Youth Matters After-School Program.
- Utilize findings to support ongoing development of the program.

Related Questions Guiding the Evaluation

- What did parents like best and least about the Youth Matters After-School Program?
- What changes do parents recommend for further development of the Youth Matters After-School Program?

Overview of Data Sources

All parents were invited to participate in a focus group held at 6:00 pm (the most common pickup time). Parents who agreed to participate in the focus group were provided a meal in one room while their children engaged in a meal and special supervised activity in another room. The program held a total of three focus groups which lasted 55 to 65 minutes in length and included five to seven participants each. A counselor employed with Youth Matters but not directly involved in program operations facilitated each focus group using an I-guide based on Box 13.3. To facilitate conversation regarding the most and least valuable aspects of the program, the facilitator asked parents to brainstorm ideas on a poster board. Then, they invited participants to comment on the items by elaborating on their thoughts and providing examples.

Putting Findings into Context

Focus group participants (n = 18) provided valuable insights into elements of the Youth Matters After-School Program. Across groups, participants generated a number of best-liked features; participants most often discussed:

- Provided a safe place for their children, *consensus* (e.g., "I don't have to worry" and "He's not out running the streets with his brother.").
- Homework assistance, *consensus* (e.g., "She used to *fight* homework every night, but now I don't have to do that battle" and "His grades went up because they do his homework here.").
- Staff relationships, *common* (e.g., "The workers know his name and my name" and "They are always happy to see her, even when she talks back.").

Participants generated a number of least-liked features; they most often discussed:

- Parent workshops, *common* (e.g., "Just because I can't afford a fancy program doesn't mean I don't know how to take care of my child" and "They want me to reward my child for doing what he's supposed to do. I know best how to discipline him.").
- Early closures, *common* (e.g., "They close early a whole lot. That makes it real hard at work" and "I don't always get the message when they close early.").

Parents sometimes disagreed regarding most- and least-liked features:

- Nutrition (e.g., "My child won't eat the foods they serve, and he's always hungry" vs. "They don't pay the bills or do the shopping, but they tell her the foods I give her aren't healthy" vs. "I like that he gets to try new kinds of food here.").
- Communication (e.g., "The daily reports help me know how he's doing" vs. "I don't think they even think about what they put on the daily reports. It's always the same.").

Finally, parents made several suggestions regarding ways to enhance the program:

- Parent engagement, *common* (e.g., "They think they know how we need to eat, discipline, and act, but they don't ask us" and "They keep doing these workshops, but nobody asked us what we want to learn").
- Communication, *common* (e.g., "Give us more notice if closing early" and "Tell specific things my child is doing right").

CHAPTER SUMMARY

This chapter included a definition and overview of qualitative research designs, questions amenable to qualitative designs, and resources for understanding six classic approaches to qualitative research. Then, we turned attention to practical steps for utilizing qualitative frameworks within program evaluation. In particular, we outlined considerations for use of semi-structured interviews, focus groups, and document reviews. We also provided resources related to two frameworks for analyzing qualitative data: thematic analysis and CQR. The chapter concluded with unique considerations for reporting qualitative program evaluation activities and findings. A case study illustrated how qualitative frameworks may be helpful in designing and evaluating a community-based after-school program for children.

RESOURCES

- Administration on Children, Youth & Families, *Qualitative Research Methods in Program Evaluation: Considerations for Federal Staff*. https://acf.gov/sites/default/files/documents/opre/qualitative.pdf
- Braun, V., & Clarke, V. (2022). *Thematic analysis: A practical guide*. Sage.
- Hill, C. E., & Knox, S. (2021). *Essentials of consensual qualitative research*. American Psychological Association.

- National Defense Research Institute, *Data Collection Methods: Semi-structured Interviews and Focus Groups*, www.rand.org/pubs/technical_reports/TR718.html

REFERENCES

Adams, W. C. (2015). Conducting semi-structured interviews. In *Handbook of practical program evaluation* (4th ed., pp. 492–505). Wiley.

Braun, V., & Clarke, V. (2006). Using thematic analysis in psychology. *Qualitative Research in Psychology*, *3*(2), 77–101. https://doi.org/10.1191/1478088706qp063oa

Braun, V., & Clarke, V. (2022). *Thematic analysis: A practical guide*. Sage.

Charmaz, K. (2024). *Constructing grounded theory* (3rd ed.). Sage.

Clandinin, D. J. (2022). *Engaging in narrative inquiry* (2nd ed.). Routledge.

Corbin, J., & Strauss, A. (2015). *Basics of qualitative research: Techniques and procedures for developing grounded theory* (4th ed.). Sage.

Davison, R. M., Chughtai, H., Nielsen, P., Marabelli, M., Iannacci, F., van Offenbeek, M., Tarafdar, M., Trenz, M., Techatassanasoontorn, A. A., Díaz Andrade, A., & Panteli, N. (2024). The ethics of using generative AI for qualitative data analysis. *Information Systems Journal*, *34*(5), 1433–1439. https://doi.org/10.1111/isj.12504

Denzin, N. K. (2014). *Interpretive autoethnography (2nd ed.)*. Sage.

Fetterman, D. M. (2019). *Ethnography: Step-by-step* (4th ed.). Sage.

Glaser, B. G., & Strauss, A. (1967). *The discovery of grounded theory: Strategies for qualitative research*. Aldine.

Hennick, M. M. (2014). *Focus group discussions: Understanding qualitative research*. Oxford University Press.

Hill, C. B., Knox, S., Thompson, B. J., Williams, E. N., Hess, S. A., & Ladany, N. (2005). Consensual qualitative research: An update. *Journal of Counseling Psychology*, *52*(2), 196–205. https://doi.org/10.1037/0022-0167.52.2.196

Hill, C. E., Thompson, B. J., & Williams, E. N. (1997). A guide to conducting consensual qualitative research. *Counseling Psychologist*, *25*(4), 517–572.

Hill, C. E., & Knox, S. (2021). *Essentials of consensual qualitative research*. American Psychological Association.

Husserl, E. (1970). *The crisis of European sciences and transcendental phenomenology*. North University Press.

Kostere, S., & Kostere, K. (2022). *The generic qualitative approach to a dissertation in the social sciences: A step by step guide*. Routledge.

Krueger, R. A., & Casey, M. A. (2015). Focus group interviewing. In *Handbook of practical program evaluation* (4th ed.). Wiley.

LeCompte, M. D., & Schensul, J. J. (2010). *Designing and conducting ethnographic research: An introduction* (2nd ed.). AltaMira.

Levitt, H. M., Motulsky, S. L., Wertz, F. J., Morrow, S. L., & Ponterotto, J. G. (2017). Recommendations for designing and reviewing qualitative research in psychology: Promoting methodological integrity. *Qualitative Psychology*, *4*(1), 2–22. http://dx.doi.org.proxy.lib.utk.edu:90/10.1037/qup0000082

Lub, V. (2015). Validity in qualitative evaluation: Linking purposes, paradigms, and perspectives. *International Journal of Qualitative Methods*, *14*(5), 1–8. https://doi.org/10.1177/1609406915621406

Moustakas, C. (1994). *Phenomenological research methods*. Sage.

Riessman, C. K. (2008). *Narrative methods for the human sciences*. Sage.

Royse, D., Thyer, B. A., Padgett, D. K., & Logan, T. K. (2006). *Program evaluation: An introduction* (4th ed.). Thompson.

Smith, J. A., Flowers, P., & Larkin, M. (2022). *Interpretive phenomenological analysis: Theory, method and research (2nd ed.)*. Sage.

Stake, R. E. (1995). *The art of case study research*. Sage.

Tisdell, E. J., Merriam, S. B., & Stuckey-Peyrot, H. L. (2025). *Qualitative research: A guide to design and implementation* (5th ed.). Jossey-Bass.

Waalkes, P. L., DeCinco, D. A., Somerville, T., Phelps-Pineda, M. M., Flynn, S. V., & LeBlanc, J. (2024). *Counselor Education and Supervision*, *63*(4), 392–404. https://doi.org/10.1002/ceas.12316

Yin, R. K. (2018). *Case study research and applications: Design and methods* (6th ed.). Sage.

CHAPTER 14

Combining Findings across Studies or Sites

To this point, everything we have identified and discussed has been on the singular: one evaluation, one research project, one group of interest holders or participants. To be sure, we can pick up a lot of inspiring and useful information from the results of a single study or evaluation. Yet stakeholders rarely make sweeping policy and funding decisions based on the results of a single activity. Likewise, it may be irresponsible to make comparisons between studies without using a rigorously systematic and even-handed approach that accounts for the limitations of individual studies such as sampling biases, measurement error, and conflicting results. With a little effort, it is possible to combine findings across research articles or program sites to depict not only what works but also who it works for, how, and under what circumstances.

This chapter introduces you to the essential activities associated with combining findings across studies or sites using meta-analysis. Specific methods covered in this chapter include mean effects meta-analysis, subgroup analysis, and meta-regression. Elements of each method will be applied to a case study of a school evaluating the impact of a cyberbullying prevention program.

BOX 14.1 CHAPTER LEARNING OUTCOMES

- Develop research questions consistent with the use of meta-analysis
- Design, plan, carry out, record, and analyze the results of meta-analysis
- Communicate findings from meta-analysis studies using a variety of methods
- Identify and critique data associated with meta-analyses

BOX 14.2 CASE STUDY

A large, private school is interested in investing significant funding, administrative resources, and human resources into the implementation of the

DOI: 10.4324/9781003586210-16

Let Me Know (LMK) cyberbullying prevention program for middle school and high school students. The school board wants their investments to be data-driven to maximize the probability that their curriculum choice is a prudent one. However, the program is relatively new, and the evidence provided by the program retailer seems too good to be true. In response, the school board has contracted you to help them understand the general effectiveness of the program and answer some questions related to the characteristics of their student body who are associated with grades 6–12, tend to be from various socioeconomic backgrounds, and report Asian American, Black, Hispanic/Latine, and White identities. You decide that a meta-analytic design may provide you with the most even-handed strategy for providing the school board answers to their questions about the effectiveness of the LMK program and its overall fit for their student body.

OVERVIEW OF META-ANALYTIC DESIGNS

What Are Meta-Analytic Designs?

Meta-analytic designs, or meta-analyses, feature systematic approaches to identifying studies within published and unpublished literature with similar purposes, methods, participants, and outcomes and combining their results into a single quantitative estimate of effectiveness. Meta-analyses can be completed with all quantitative designs described so far in this text: correlational studies, single-case research designs, single-group designs, and between-groups designs. Additionally, advances in statistical formulae have provided opportunities to combine a wide variety of outcomes related to intervention or program effectiveness, risk, and costs in ways that account for influences of publication bias, sample size, and sampling error. Thus, a well-designed meta-analysis provides an even-handed representation of the state of the research evidence and has the potential to guide decision making about local practices or broader policies.

Core Features of Meta-Analyses

All meta-analyses feature some common procedures and elements. Namely, these tend to be associated with systematic ways of identifying and extracting relevant information from studies, as well as ways data are expressed and interpreted. All meta-analyses include a predetermined set of **inclusion and exclusion criteria** which include types of studies, variables, interventions, outcomes, and participant characteristics within a specific range of publication dates. Additionally, you will need to establish some **information sources** for identifying eligible studies across databases (e.g. PsycINFO, Medline), specific journals (e.g., *Journal of Counseling & Development*, *Counseling Outcome Research and Evaluation*), repositories (The Campbell Collaboration Library), and consultation with topical experts.

Once you have identified studies, you will need to develop a strategy for **study selection** and **data collection** to ensure that only the data relevant to answering your research questions are extracted, coded and compiled into a data management platform with an acceptable degree of completeness. Data management systems include systems that you may already be familiar with such as Microsoft Excel or Google Sheets, more specialized free software such as JASP or R, and fee-based programs including RevMan and Comprehensive Meta-Analysis. The basic categories that you may find helpful include bibliographic data, statistics needed to compute effect sizes, and descriptive statistics that support understanding who the mean effect best represents (Borenstein et al., 2021; Erford et al., 2010; Lenz, 2022). Coding of studies is particularly important because errors in the dataset will lead to inaccurate findings about combined effectiveness and implications. For this reason, we suggest formalizing procedures using a coding guide and employing multiple coders. These steps will help you increase consistency and accuracy, estimate the degree of agreement between coders, and support internal validity for your project.

With the data from individual studies accounted for, you will be poised to select a **method of synthesis** to combine study outcomes into an average outcome referred to as the *mean effect size*. The mean effect size depicts the *magnitude* and *direction* of effects associated with variables, interventions, or programs. Although the mean effect size provides helpful information about the average effect, it does not reveal much about the accuracy of your estimation, and thus how much confidence can be attributed to the results. To address this issue, all meta-analyses include reporting of **confidence intervals** for individual and mean effect sizes (Borenstein et al., 2021; Erford et al., 2010). Confidence intervals (CI), typically reported as a probability (e.g., 95% CI), represent a range with lower and upper limits that represent the accuracy or precision of your mean effect. Taken together, through a series of systematic steps, you will be able to identify, code, and analyze the results of many published studies or program outcomes into a single effect size describing the average effectiveness associated with an intervention-outcome association or how strong relationships are between variables.

When Are Meta-Analytic Designs Indicated?

As you can imagine, a lot of intention, time, and effort go into completing a meta-analysis. Decisions related to the usefulness of an intervention and statements regarding the nature of relationships between variables cannot be inferred from the results of a single study (Borenstein et al., 2021). Meta-analyses are indicated in at least a few cases. First, meta-analyses provide summaries of existing research literature and thus serve to characterize the context around a phenomenon, population, intervention, or program. Relatedly, this context provides a platform to plan new studies by identifying which questions and hypotheses appear to be resolved and which are ambiguous or unknown. Second, meta-analyses can provide an opportunity to understand which outcome measures, treatment settings, participant characteristics, and intervention features tend to be associated with the strongest findings. Third, statistical procedures in meta-analyses allow researchers to predict what types of effects could be observed in future studies or projects. Together, stakeholders can use this information to make informed decisions about policy development, identification of best practices, and allocation of resources.

BOX 14.3 INDICATORS OF A META-ANALYTIC DESIGN

- Well-defined purpose statement.
- Inclusion/exclusion criteria clearly depict variables included, eligible study designs, target population, and study setting.
- Search strategy features multiple sources to locate studies.
- Reporting of the study and sample characteristics.
- Reporting and interpretation of mean effect size and related confidence intervals.
- Reporting and interpretation of heterogeneity estimates.
- Reporting and interpretation of publication bias estimates.
- Findings situated in context.
- Tables and visual depictions support reporting of findings.

What Types of Questions Can Be Answered Using Meta-Analytic Designs?

Meta-analysts are poised to answer three types of research questions: (a) those related to the mean effect across eligible studies, (b) those related to the participant and study characteristics that influence the mean effect, and (c) those related to predicting effect sizes that could be expected from future studies.

Mean Effect Associated with an Intervention or Program

Meta-analyses provide a great way to answer questions about the average effect associated with an intervention or program. In a way, this represents a singular statement about the status of empirical support for a topic of interest. Put another way, when someone asks a general question such as, "*What does the literature say about the effectiveness of cyberbullying prevention programs?*" discussing the mean effect is a good starting place for a reply.

When developing these questions, the *mean treatment effect* refers to combining results of studies that compare the results of one deliberate intervention to another. Alternatively, the term *mean effect size* refers to synthesizing the relationships between two variables. Examples of questions related to mean treatment effect and mean effect size include:

- *What is the mean treatment effect* of a cyberbullying prevention program for increasing intention to intervene among adolescents when compared to alternative psychoeducational approaches?
- *What is the mean effect size* associated with school climate and intention to intervene among adolescents who have participated in a cyberbullying prevention program?

Relationships of Participant and Study Characteristics Associated With Mean Effect

The second category of research question answered by meta-analysts relates to understanding relationships between characteristics of individual studies and mean effects. These questions are grounded in your understanding of population, intervention, outcome, and contextual features. From this informed perspective, you can develop a hypothesis regarding variables that may contribute to heterogeneity in your sample of studies. For example, McKibben et al. (2023) hypothesized that age of participants and attachment type would be influential variables related to relationship between attachment style and ratings of working alliance with supervisors. McKibben et al. proposed these factors *a priori* based on previous literature and clinical experience, each of which should be considered as you develop your own hypotheses. Similarly, when investigating the effectiveness of mental health apps to support treatment for depression, Luo et al. (2025) believed that the frequency of use and type of app would predict the size of treatment outcome. Luo et al. found that only one of those factors—frequency of use—predicted intervention success. Stated plainly, participants' consistency in app use, regardless of the mental health app used, predicted reductions in depression symptoms. Examples of questions relating participant and study characteristics to the mean effect size for our working example include:

- To what degree is *participant age associated with* increased intention to intervene among adolescents completing a cyberbullying prevention program?
- What are the *differences between* treatment effects *associated with* face-to-face or web-based approaches to a cyberbullying prevention program?

Predicting Future Effects for Similar Studies

Meta-analyses are often completed to inform present decision making and best practices. Ironically, decision making in the present is often based on evidence from the past alone, without accounting for reasonable projections about what could be expected in the future. Thus, our third type of research questions for meta-analyses helps round out the utility of the method. Using some modest statistical modeling procedures, you can answer the critical question related to what the projected range of treatment effects or effect sizes may look like in the future based on everything that we know from the past. Although previous research questions for meta-analyses have great value in moving practice forward, predictions of future effects have a clinical value that is transparent, straightforward, and easily interpreted (Borenstein, 2022; Migliavaca et al., 2022). Examples of predicting future effects for similar studies include:

- *What is the predicted mean treatment effect* in similar studies of a cyberbullying prevention program for increasing intention to intervene among adolescents?
- *What is the predicted mean effect size* in similar studies of associations between school climate and intention to intervene among adolescents who have participated in a cyberbullying prevention program?

TYPES OF META-ANALYTIC METHODS

All meta-analyses share some common methodological steps related to (a) computing mean treatment effects, (b) explaining the differences between study effects, (c) differentiating performance based on participant and study characteristics that moderate treatment effects, (d) addressing the effects of publication bias, and (e) predicting future effects for similar studies. A complete review of all procedures inherent with these activities is beyond the scope of this chapter; however, many plainly spoken resources are available (See Erford et al., 2010; Lipsey & Wilson, 2001). To promote practicality and accessibility of content, our discussions about meta-analytic procedures will be focused on completing basic analyses for evaluating mean treatment effects of studies that compared the results of one intervention to another.

Computing Mean Effects and Precision

You may be having some anxiety thinking about what computing the mean treatment effect size for a meta-analysis looks like and questioning your ability to make that happen. We promise the basics are doable if you stick with us for a minute. The effects of individual (primary) studies can be misleading because of sample size, bias, and error. Relatedly, effect sizes can be biased or unbiased due to those misleading characteristics (Erford et al., 2010; Lenz, 2022). A biased effect size such as Cohen's *d*qn001.tif that is used with a small sample study (e.g., $N = 16$) has more sampling error than one with a larger sample with less error (e.g., $N = 116$), yet would result in the same mean effect size. Therefore, meta-analysts use unbiased effect sizes such as Hedge's *g* that provide statistical adjustments that make depictions of effect more *fair*. Similarly, meta-analysts control for each study's influence on the mean effect size formula by weighting their unique effect sizes before adding them all up $\left(\Sigma\left[w_i ES\right]\right)$, and dividing by the sum weights $\left(\Sigma w_i\right)$ See? You made it! Well, almost.

Although the mean treatment effect provides useful information about the magnitude and direction of treatment effects, this estimate is out of context without some reference to its precision. More precise estimates are more defensible. Therefore, meta-analysts compute and report confidence intervals surrounding their individual and mean treatment effects (Borenstein et al., 2021; Erford et al., 2010). Confidence intervals are grounded in the standard error estimates of an effect size $(SE = \sqrt{\frac{n_1 + n_2}{n_1 n_2}} + \frac{g^2}{2(n_1 + n_2)})$. This value is multiplied by ± 1.96 to establish boundaries for a 95% confidence interval or ± 2.58 for a 99% confidence interval. Researchers in counseling and related health care professions tend to reference 95% confidence intervals as a standard of practice, but high-stakes decisions may want to rest upon the precision offered through 99% confidence intervals. Long story short, if you know the means and standard deviations for intervention and comparison groups, you can make remaining computations using pencil and paper or simple data management programs such as Excel.

When interpreting *d*-family effect sizes (e.g., Cohen's *d*, Hedge's *g*), the resulting metrics are conceptualized using some standard practices. First, you can reference accepted conventions for characterizing the size of effect such as those presented by

Lipsey and Wilson (1993) as small (.30), medium (.50), or large (.67). Next, convert and report your metric in terms of standard deviation units. For example, an effect size of.50 represents half a standard deviation of change. Similarly, an effect size of 1.50 is equivalent to one and a half standard deviation units. Finally, place your effect size value within the unique clinical or educational context.

Confidence intervals are subjected to the same processes, but they are representative of the range of mean effects represented in your data. Thus, an *observed mean treatment effect* of.50 with a 95% confidence interval ranging from.40 to.60 could be interpreted with 95% confidence that the *probable mean treatment effect* lies between.40 and.60. Generally speaking, the greater the confidence interval value, the wider the range of potential treatment effects.

Estimating Heterogeneity

Mean treatment effects represent weighted average outcomes reported within a sample of individual studies. You can assume that many studies reported results that were different from one another. Some of those variations are *actual differences*, and others are *spurious differences* related to non-random error (Borenstein et al., 2021). Therefore, meta-analysts compute and report estimates of heterogeneity that represent variation in outcomes between studies due to non-random error rather than actual differences. When there is minimal variation among studies, results are regarded as homogeneous and suggest that results are not influenced by differences in participant or study characteristics. Alternatively, sizable variation among studies suggests heterogeneity; heterogeneity indicates the need for secondary analyses evaluating the influence of participant or study characteristics.

Two routine approaches for approximating the degree of heterogeneity among a sample of studies are inspection of Cochran's Q and the Inconsistency Index (I^2). Both Q and I^2 have general guidelines to identify and estimate the degree of heterogeneity. First, researchers inspect Q values. When Q values are statistically significant and greater than degrees of freedom (number of studies in analysis minus 1), it is probable that heterogeneity exists (Borenstein et al., 2021; Erford et al., 2010). Next, you can inspect I^2 values to understand how much heterogeneity is present within your estimate of the mean treatment effect. I^2 values of 25%, 50%, and 75% represent small, medium, and large amounts of heterogeneity (Borenstein et al., 2017). Therefore, when Q is greater than degrees of freedom and statistically significant and I^2 is greater than 50%, it is likely that random error may be affecting your mean treatment effect, and you should explore moderators associated with differential outcomes (Borenstein et al., 2021; Lipsey & Wilson, 2001).

Differentiating Performance Based on Characteristics

When the distribution of effect sizes within your sample of studies is homogeneous, it can be inferred that differences in the outcomes represent true variations rather than random error. By contrast, when heterogeneity is present, we need to explain the participant and sample characteristics that may contribute to random error within the mean treatment effect. Moderator analyses can help depict for whom, how, and under what circumstances interventions and programs are most suited. Two approaches to exploring moderators of the mean treatment effect include subgroup analyses and meta-regression. Each account for heterogeneity within your sample of studies.

Subgroup analyses are used to explore differences between mean treatment effects by categorical subgroups within your sample of studies. This practice is similar to the analysis of variance (ANOVA) procedures used in between-groups studies and provides an estimate of statistically significant differences between groups. Some common categories researchers investigate include study setting, reasons for referral, and treatment modality.

Meta-regression can be used with continuous variables such as participant age, number of sessions, or number of providers delivering treatment. Meta-regression procedures are interpreted similarly to those practices described in Chapter 9 wherein an R^2 value estimates the proportion of variance within the mean treatment effect size that can be explained by predictor variables. Within predictive models, individual predictors (e.g., participant age, number of sessions, or baseline values of the dependent variable) can be inspected for statistical significance and unique contributions to the overall model.

Addressing the Effects of Publication Bias

All meta-analyses depict estimates based on what has been reported by others. Although results will represent a statistically accurate combination of outcomes, outcomes themselves may be influenced by the tendency for studies reporting high effect sizes to be published. This *publication bias* may skew findings in ways that artificially inflate the magnitude and importance of interventions or relationships between variables (Page et al., 2021).

There are three tools to help identify evidence of publication bias on the mean treatment effect. These tools help us understand how robust the findings are against the potential presence of the *file drawer effect*—a key source of publication bias wherein studies with positive, affirming findings tend to be published more than those with negative or null results. First, evidence of publication bias can be evaluated using funnel plots that situate individual study effect sizes on the X-axis and their related standard errors on the Y-axis (see Figure 14.1). In the absence of bias, plotted studies are symmetrically distributed around the center line representing the mean treatment effect; asymmetrical plots may suggest some degree of bias. Next, Duval and Tweedie's (2000) trim and fill procedure provides an estimate of the impact of publication bias by replacing (i.e., filling in) the missing studies that created asymmetry in a funnel plot and recomputing the mean treatment effect with these theoretically missing studies included. As a result, you can have an idea of the number of missing studies and how their inclusion would influence the mean effect (Shi & Lin, 2019). Finally, *Fail Safe N* (N_f) can be used to determine the number of unpublished studies with null findings that would be required to invalidate your observed mean effect size. Although there are no benchmarks for this value, a strikingly low N_f should be cause for concern that an observed effect was an artifact of publication bias.

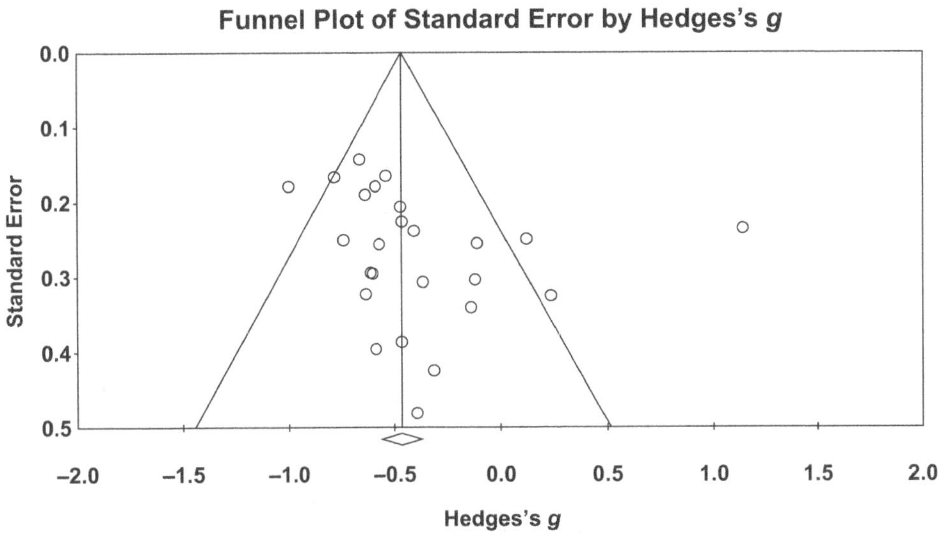

Figure 14.1 Funnel Plot of Effect Sizes by Standard Errors

Predicting Future Effects for Similar Studies

Effect sizes and confidence intervals will provide you with some important information for stakeholders, but stakeholders will likely also want to know what kind of results they might expect at their site. To achieve this task, meta-analysts compute and report prediction intervals that contain the range of most probable values for treatment effects in future settings that are similar to those in your sample of studies. Comparison of these values with clinically relevant thresholds may help you speculate about potential benefits versus risks.

Interpreting prediction intervals is much like confidence intervals: There is a range with a lower limit and an upper limit. For example, a mean treatment effect of.50 with a prediction interval of.25 to.75 would indicate that future studies with similar samples and participants could be expected to yield effect sizes as small as 25% of a standard deviation, as large as 75% of a standard deviation, or anywhere in between. The prediction interval does not reveal *what* effect sizes would be in future studies, but rather *where* along a continuum they could be expected to fall.

PUTTING FINDINGS INTO CONTEXT

Putting meta-analytic findings into context involves some common assumptions and strategies. First, findings do not represent how effective a treatment is. Rather, findings reflect how strong a treatment fared against some other treatment in studies you were able to find and use. Despite the potential for a very large aggregate sample size that results when combining studies, there is a boundary to the generalization of findings. Relatedly, findings only apply to samples represented within your sample of studies.

Using our case study as an example, findings based on results with boys may be less relevant when attempting to depict the effectiveness of the LMK program with girls. Finally, no matter how small or large they are, effect sizes are meaningless outside of their clinical or educational context. With these assumptions in mind, you can use the six-step guide depicted in Box 14.4 as a guide to reporting findings in context. As the title suggests, these domains are the basic reporting domains and do not account for more complex analyses. As with other guidelines, you can modify words in all caps to suit your results, but only you can breathe life into your narrative and portray findings in a way that honors your stakeholders' needs.

BOX 14.4 BASIC FRAMEWORK FOR REPORTING META-ANALYTIC FINDINGS IN CONTEXT

Step 1: Describe results of your meta-analyses, including mean treatment effect, confidence interval, and statistical significance

The VALUE effect sizes included in the analysis of INTERVENTION versus COMPARISON for INCREASING/DECREASING DEPENDENT VARIABLE (*N* = VALUE) yielded a mean effect size of VALUE (CI95 = LOWER LIMIT, UPPER LIMIT), *p* =/</>. VALUE, suggesting that the null hypothesis related to superiority of INTERVENTION can be ACCEPTED/REJECTED.

Step 2: Provide an interpretation of your effect size metric for the model

Interpretation of the mean effect size value suggests that participants completing INTERVENTION experienced VALUE% of a standard deviation of change among scores representing DEPENDENT VARIABLE, indicative of a SMALL/MEDIUM/LARGE effect size.

Step 3: Report and interpret the values for your prediction intervals

This analysis resulted in a prediction interval ranging from VALUE to VALUE, suggesting that the range of true effects in future studies with similar samples may be as small as VALUE% of a standard deviation or as large as VALUE% of a standard deviation.

Step 4: Report and interpret estimates of heterogeneity among your sample of effect sizes

The effect size distribution within the sample of studies WAS/WAS NOT heterogeneous Q(VALUE) = VALUE, *p* =/</>. VALUE and I^2 = VALUE, indicating that about VALUE% of the observed differences in effect sizes reflect actual differences; thus, exploration of moderating variables WAS/WAS NOT warranted.

Step 5: Report and interpret estimates of publication bias

The funnel plot of effect size-standard error combinations illustrated a SYMMETRICAL/ASYMMETRICAL pattern of studies surrounding the mean effect. This sample yielded a N_f of VALUE, indicating that VALUE unpublished studies with an effect size of zero would need to be identified for the test of null hypothesis to exceed.05.

Step 6: Provide a summative statement integrating your findings meaningfully

Constructively integrate all of this information through your uniquely informed lens to make a conservative, even-handed summative statement about the usefulness of your analyses for understanding the criterion of interest.

DISPLAYING RESULTS

Although there are several strategies for displaying findings of meta-analyses, the two hallmarks are summary tables and forest plots. With these resources, you will be able to assemble large amounts of data, yet present findings in a way that is transparent and readily understood by stakeholders and other professionals.

Summary Tables

Summary tables tend to illustrate characteristics for individual studies that characterize their most prominent features, which is helpful for placing them into context with one another while also providing information that is relevant to moderator analyses. A sample header for these tables is depicted in Table 14.1. This includes an abbreviated study identifier, objective of study, sample size, mean participant age, description of participant ethnic identities, length of treatment, outcome measures, and brief description of significant results. This information will help you characterize your sample of studies and detail information that may be helpful for moderator analyses.

Forest Plots

Meta-analysts display their findings in a type of visual aid called a *forest plot* which is part table, part figure, and an all-around helpful tool for demonstrating the dispersion of effect sizes and your mean treatment effect. All forest plots will include some common information for each study: the study identifier, effect size, confidence interval, and *p*-values. Summary data are provided for the mean treatment effect, confidence interval, statistical significance, and prediction interval. As displayed in the forest plot included within our case study (see Box 14.5), individual study effect sizes

TABLE 14.1 Example of Headings for Summary Table of Study Characteristics

Study ID	Study objective	N	Age	Participant characteristics	Length of treatment	Outcome measures	Significant Outcomes

are represented on a scale using a marker (line, square, circle) with confidence intervals indicated by whiskers on either side of the marker. Mean effect sizes and confidence interval are indicated by a diamond spanning the range of values, with a horizontal line through the mean treatment depicting the range covered by your prediction interval. This figure helps stakeholders *see the forest for the trees* and consider results from statistical and visual perspectives.

BOX 14.5 CASE STUDY REVISITED

Using our case study as an example, a meta-analysis was completed to identify the general effectiveness of the *Let Me Know* (LMK) program for increasing intention to intervene among adolescent girls. This section will provide a brief application of chapter content to illustrate meta-analytic principles and practices that can be simulated in your projects.

Purposes of Evaluation

- Mean treatment effect associated with the LMK program.
- Predicting future effects for similar studies.

Related Questions Guiding the Evaluation

- *What is the mean treatment effect* of the LMK program for increasing intention to intervene among adolescents when compared to alternative psychoeducational approaches?
- *What is the predicted mean treatment effect* in a local application of the LMK program for increasing intention to intervene among adolescents when compared to alternative psychoeducational approaches?

Selected Meta-Analytic Design

- Database searches for trials of the LMK program compared to other psychoeducational interventions that reported findings related to intention to intervene with adolescent girls.
- Coding bibliographic data, effect size data, and information depicting participant and study characteristics.

Putting Findings Into Context

The five effect sizes included in the analysis of LMK versus alternative psychoeducational programs for increasing intention to intervene (N = 3,472) yielded a mean effect size of.64 (CI95 =.53,.74), p <.01, suggesting that the null hypothesis related to superiority of LMK can be rejected. Interpretation of the mean effect size value suggests that participants completing LMK experienced 64% of a standard deviation of change among scores representing intention to intervene when witnessing cyberbullying, indicative of a medium effect size. This analysis resulted in a prediction interval ranging from.32 to.93, suggesting that the range of true effects in future studies with similar samples may be as small as 32% of a standard deviation or as large as 93% of a standard deviation. The effect size distribution within the sample of studies was not heterogeneous $Q(4) = 7.75$, p =.11, and I^2 = 46%, indicating that about 46% of the observed differences in effect sizes reflects actual differences; thus, exploration of moderating variables was not warranted. The funnel plot of effect size-standard error combinations illustrated an asymmetrical pattern of studies surrounding the mean effect, with more studies to the right (therapeutic side) of the mean effect. This sample yielded a N_f of 372, indicating that 372 unpublished studies with an effect size of zero would need to be identified for the test of null hypothesis to exceed.05. Taken together, these findings suggest that within the universe of studies included herein, LMK was a superior treatment that may result in small to large effects within future studies completed with similar samples.

Displaying Findings

Data representing participant and methodological features for included studies can be presented using a summary table

Study ID	N	Age	Participant characteristics	Weeks of treatment	Significant outcomes
Study 1	602	15.2	Girls (345 African American; 220 Caucasian; 22 Hispanic; 15 other) attending a private school.	30	Increased intention to intervene; lower disciplinary referrals
Study 2	846	15.7	Girls (231 African American; 505 Caucasian; 87 Hispanic; 23 other) attending a private school.	30	Increased intention to intervene; increased empathy

Study ID	N	Age	Participant characteristics	Weeks of treatment	Significant outcomes
Study 3	545	16.8	Girls (24 African American; 500 Caucasian; 11 Hispanic) attending a private school.	26	Increased intention to intervene
Study 4	798	14.3	Girls (235 African American; 97 Caucasian; 274 Hispanic; 192 other) attending a private school.	28	Increased intention to intervene; increased school climate
Study 5	681	12.6	Girls (489 African American; 30 Caucasian; 47 Hispanic; 115 other) attending a private school.	10	Increased intention to intervene; increased empathy

Data representing effect sizes, confidence intervals, and prediction intervals can be reported and illustrated using a forest plot.

Effect Sizes, 95% Confidence Intervals, and p-Values for Studies Evaluating the Let Me Know (LMK) Program for Increasing Intention to Intervene When Compared to Alternative Psychoeducation Approaches

Study	Effect Size and 95% CI	*p*
Study 1	.73 [.56, .89]	< .01
Study 2	.71 [.54, .87]	< .01
Study 3	.67 [.50, .83]	< .01
Study 4	.64 [.48, .81]	< .01
Study 5	.44 [.28, .60]	< .01
Mean Effect Size	.64 [.53, .74]	< .01
Prediction Interval	[.32, .93]	

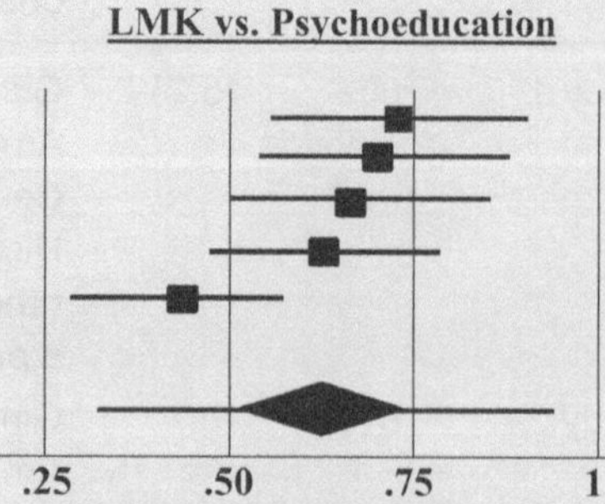

Figure 14.2 Forest Plot Depicting Effect Sizes, Confidence Intervals, and Prediction Intervals

Note: Larger effect size values indicate greater treatment outcomes favoring LMK versus alternative psychoeducational approaches.

CHAPTER SUMMARY

This chapter provided a brief overview of the basic, foundational activities associated with implementing meta-analytic designs. With the information provided herein and the use of the many resources available, you will be well-positioned to combine the results of existing studies. Although these activities may be beyond the scope of your interests or clinical activities, we have good news! The information in this chapter will support you when interpreting findings of published meta-analyses to inform local best practices and policy decisions.

RESOURCES

- Borenstein, M. (2019). *Common mistakes in meta-analysis and how to avoid them*. Biostat.
- Borenstein, M., Hedges, L. V., Higgins, J. P., & Rothstein, H. (2021). *Introduction to meta-analysis* (2nd ed.). Wiley.
- *The Campbell Collaboration*, Online library of systematic reviews and meta-analyses for social, behavioral, and educational outcomes. https://campbellcollaboration.org
- *The Cochrane Collaboration*, Online library of systematic reviews and meta-analyses for health-related outcomes. www.cochranelibrary.com
- Erford, B. T., Savin-Murphy, J. A., & Butler, C. (2010). Conducting a meta-analysis of counseling outcome research: Twelve steps and practical procedures. *Counseling Outcome Research and Evaluation*, *1*, 19–43. https://doi.org/10.1177/2150137809356682
- Preferred Reporting Items for Systematic Reviews and Meta-Analyses (PRISMA) website. www.prisma-statement.org

REFERENCES

Borenstein, M. (2022). In a meta-analysis, the I-squared statistic does not tell us how much the effect size varies. *Journal of Clinical Epidemiology*, *152*, 281–284. https://doi.org/10.1016/j.jclinepi.2022.10.003

Borenstein, M., Hedges, L. V., Higgins, J. P., & Rothstein, H. (2021). *Introduction to meta-analysis (2nd ed.)*. Wiley.

Borenstein, M., Higgins, J. P. T., Hedges, L. V., & Rothstein, H. R. (2017). Basics of meta-analysis: I^2 is not an absolute measure of heterogeneity. *Research Synthesis Methods*, 8, 5–18. https://doi.org/10.1002/jrsm.1230

Duval, S. J., & Tweedie, R. L. (2000). Trim and fill: A simple funnel-plot-based method of testing and adjusting for publication bias in meta-analysis. *Biometrics*, *56*, 455–463. https://doi.org/10.1111/j.0006-341X.2000.00455.x

Erford, B. T., Savin-Murphy, J. A., & Butler, C. (2010). Conducting a meta-analysis of counseling outcome research: Twelve steps and practical procedures. *Counseling Outcome Research and Evaluation*, *1*, 19–43. https://doi-org/10.1177/2150137809356682

Lenz, A. S. (2022). Synthesizing quantitative research results using meta-analysis. In R. S. Balkin & D. Kleist (Eds.), *Counseling research: A scholar-practitioner approach to research in the counseling profession (2nd ed.;* pp. 187–212). American Counseling Association.

Lipsey, M., & Wilson, D. (2001). *Practical meta-analysis*. Sage.

Lipsey, M. W., & Wilson, D. (1993). The efficacy of psychological, educational, and behavioral treatment: Confirmation from meta-analysis. *American Psychologist*, *48*, 1181–1209. https://doi.org/10.1037/0003–066X.48.12.1181

Luo, Y., Stice, B. L., & Lenz, A. S. (2025). Mental health apps for depression: A meta-analysis. *Journal of Counseling & Development*, 103, 25–38. https://doi.org/10.1002/jcad.12535

McKibben, W. B., Lenz, A. S., & Sheperis, D. (2023). A meta-analysis of supervisee attachment style and the supervisory relationship. *Journal of Counseling & Development*, *101*, 323–333. https://doi.org/10.1002/jcad.12476

Migliavaca, C. B., Stein, C., Colpani, V., Barker, T. H., Zielgelmann, P. K., Munn, Z., & Falaigna, M. (2022). Meta-analysis of prevalence: I^2 statistic and how to deal with heterogeneity. *Research Synthesis Methods*, *13*(3), 363–367. https://doi.org/ 10.1002/jrsm.1547

Page, M. J., Sterne, J. A. C., Higgins, J. P.T., & Egger, M. (2021). Investigating and dealing with publication bias and other reporting biases in meta-analyses of health research: A review. *Research Synthesis Methods*, *12*, 248–259. https://doi.org/10.1002/jrsm.1468

Shi, L., & Lin, L. (2019). The trim-and-fill method for publication bias: Practical guidelines and recommendations based on a large database of meta-analyses. *Medicine*, *98*(23), e15987. https://doi.org/10.1097/MD.0000000000015987

PART III
Putting Evaluation Practice into Motion

CHAPTER **15**

Selecting Assessment Measures

Wherever we work, we will have some degree of responsibility for producing evidence that our services result in positive and meaningful change for our clients, students, and communities. Some settings will provide us with standardized metrics to use across individuals served. In other settings, we may be responsible for planning the intervention and programs, complete with assessment measures to determine effectiveness. At still other times, we will customize assessment practices for individual consumers.

In Chapter 4, we provided some exploration regarding the purpose of process and outcome measures and the role that measures play methodologically. In Chapter 5, we attended to methodological and statistical concepts such as reliability of test scores and validity for the specific test use. These are important foundations. This brief chapter will help you identify, evaluate, and select assessment measures that are both affordable and practical for your unique needs. We start the chapter assuming you have already completed coursework in assessment and testing, thus leaving you prepared to dig into this material in a practical way. If you have not had formal preparation in assessment and testing, you will need to complete appropriate training before you can select, administer, and interpret assessment results; this chapter may be more helpful after that step.

We open the chapter by discussing situations in which we will need assessment measures. Then, we step through the process of evaluating assessment measures with careful attention to objectives, psychometrics, and practicality. Once we have that foundation, we will provide some practical tips for locating existing measures. We conclude the chapter with a few cautions regarding developing your own measures for outcome evaluation purposes.

BOX 15.1 CHAPTER LEARNING OUTCOMES

- Name situations in which you may need to select or develop outcome measures
- Evaluate existing measures for use in your programs and practices
- Identify existing measures appropriate to your population and setting
- Understand the risks and benefits of creating your own assessment measures

DOI: 10.4324/9781003586210-18

WHEN ARE ASSESSMENT MEASURES USED?

As you have learned in prior assessment training, there are a variety of reasons we may look to assessment measures in counseling practice. Some measures, such as those described in Chapter 8, will help you understand need within the population served. Other measures may help you understand a specific client's needs or experiences. These measures may screen for a wide variety of concerns or be diagnostic in nature, helping you determine whether a mental disorder is present and, if so, the severity of that disorder. Measures can also assess well-being, wellness, and assets unique to our professional counseling identity. Needs assessment, screening, and diagnostic measures may be helpful for planning large-scale programs and deciding appropriate services for a specific client.

A second primary purpose of assessment measures is to assess change. When we assess at the beginning of a counseling relationship, we understand a client's baseline or starting point. Then, assessments over time can help us understand changes (or lack thereof) that guide the counseling process and generate information about the effectiveness of our services. There is mounting evidence that providing both client and counselor with feedback from outcome measures may affect overall persistence in treatment and outcome of services, especially for those who are less on track toward positive outcomes at the beginning (Delgadillo et al., 2022; Gondek et al., 2016). In short, actively assessing outcomes and discussing them appear to foster change.

Finally, we utilize data from outcome measures to advocate for interventions and programs. Those in managed care settings may need to use initial assessments and periodic updates to certify clients for care and advocate for continued resources. Those who rely on grant or donor funding may need to show their programs are working in order to unlock additional resources. Likewise, school counselors are called upon to show that the services they offer make a difference in their schools; these data can even be used to make the argument for additional personnel and expansion of services.

Across these scenarios, selecting appropriate assessment measures is vital to planning services, understanding the impact of services, and advocating for clients and programs. In the following section, we turn our attention to procedures for evaluating existing measures.

EVALUATING EXISTING MEASURES

As you identify indicators and formal measures for inclusion in your process and outcome assessment efforts, it is important that you evaluate their appropriateness for your specific context. Most importantly, the purpose of the measure must match your objectives. In addition, the measure should have strong evidence of validity appropriate to the population of focus, be sensitive to change (if using for outcomes), and be feasible to implement.

The checklist in this chapter includes central concepts and questions you should ask yourself when determining whether a measure is appropriate for you. This information should be readily accessible in a test manual, or other publications designed to accompany the measure. If you are unable to locate this information even after contacting the publisher, you should view the measure with a great deal of caution. In other words, a lack of psychometric data and guidelines for instrument use is a *big red flag*. Finally, Box 15.2 reminds us of the importance of attending to culture when we select assessment instruments.

BOX 15.2 MULTICULTURAL ASSESSMENT STANDARDS

Mental health professionals are ethically responsible for ensuring appropriate attention to culture when selecting, administering, and interpreting assessment instruments. The Association for Assessment and Research in Counseling published *AARC Standards for Multicultural Assessments* (2018) to help practitioners consider aspects of social and cultural diversity in the assessment process. You may access these standards via https://aarc-counseling.org/standards/.

BOX 15.3 CHECKLIST FOR EVALUATING ASSESSMENT MEASURES

- **Objective –** What is the objective or focus for this client or program? To what degree does the purpose of this measure match the objectives of my service or program? Do those I work with typically begin services with scores that would allow me to assess change using this specific instrument? In the end, will this measure help me know what I really want to know about my program or service?
- **Population –** What are the age and cultural characteristics for whom this measure was developed? How does the intended population align with the age and cultural characteristics of those I serve?
- **Reliability –** What does the author report as the internal consistency reliability of test scores for similar populations or uses? Generally speaking, we would like to see reliabilities in mid.80s or higher. See Chapter 5 for a discussion of this concept.
- **Validity –** What evidence does the author provide regarding test score validity of the measure matched to my specific need? Specifically, what evidence is available based on test content, internal structure, response processes, convergence and divergence with other variables, and consequential validity? See Chapter 5 for a discussion of these concepts.
- **Repeated measures and sensitivity to change –** How often can the instrument be re-administered? How well does this timeline match my assessment needs? How sensitive is the instrument to change? Does the

author provide a reliable change index or other indicators to help interpret data within my program?

- **Cost** – How much does this instrument cost to administer and score compared to similar candidates? Is this feasible within the context of my organization?
- **Training** – What special training or credentials are required for administering this measure? Is this feasible within the context of my organization?
- **Time** – How long does each assessment take to administer and score? How well does this match the available time resources of clients and service providers in my setting?
- **Reading level** – At what reading level is this instrument written? How does that compare to the educational profiles of those I serve?
- **Alternative administrations** – What types of alternative administrations (e.g., translation, oral administration, completion by another informant) does this measure allow? To what degree are these administrations important and feasible in my service setting?
- **Cultural responsiveness** – Assuming this instrument was developed and normed for my population in general, how well does this instrument fit the populations I serve? Does it appear to be culturally responsive? Are there items that may be confusing or culturally insensitive to the populations I serve? Is the measure written in a way that is accessible to consumers?
- **Overall assessment** – Given all the strengths and limitations noted, how well will this assessment meet both the needs of my organization and the needs of the clients or students I serve?

IDENTIFYING EXISTING MEASURES

Now that you understand *why* we may use assessment measures to evaluate practice and you have refreshed on *how* we evaluate their usefulness to us, it is time to focus our attention on identifying measures. Before we delve into resources you will want to consult time and again, we would like to remind you that not all interventions and programs will require assessment instruments as the outcome measures. In many cases, however, you will also need to have some data you glean from assessment instruments or protocols. Most traditional assessment textbooks will send you to classic resources. A number of books or searchable databases are available to help you locate assessment instruments.

- Buros offers ***Tests in Print*** (Anderson et al., 2022), which costs $325 and "contains descriptive information on approximately 2,300 testing instruments. Detailed descriptions of each test include data on test purpose, target population, scores, administration time, publication date(s), author(s), and pricing" (Buros Center for Testing, n.d.). This book is available in most academic libraries.

- Educational Testing Service (ETS) ***Test Collection at ETS***, a database of over 25,000 tests, which the publisher boasts is "the largest compilation of such materials in the world" ("The Test Collection at ETS," n.d.). Users can search the open-access database to identify potential instruments, complete with information regarding how to access them.
- ***Health and Psychosocial Instruments*** (HaPI) includes over 200,000 records regarding 50,000 measurement tools used across a variety of health and mental health disciplines. HAPI is a database available for searching at many academic libraries.
- American Psychological Association's ***PsychTESTS*** includes over 79,000 records of instruments relevant to the social and behavioral sciences. This resource is available as a database subscription at many academic libraries.

Another classic source is the ***Mental Measurements Yearbook*** (MMY; Carlson et al., 2021). The MMY "includes timely, consumer-oriented test reviews, providing evaluative information to promote and encourage informed test selection" (Buros Center for Testing, n.d.). The MMY is interdisciplinary in nature, including attention to education, psychology, law, health care, counseling, and management. Currently in its twenty-first edition, the MMY is produced every three years, costs approximately $210, and is available in many academic libraries. The publisher's website includes a list of the tests reviewed in the manual and offers an option to purchase individual reviews. This resource provides a rich foundation on which to build, and reviews within the yearbook tend to be comprehensive, complete with attention to an overview of expected costs. Still, you can expect most measures to be commercial in nature.

Did you get overwhelmed just reading that? Certainly, there are many rich academic resources that nerds—um, we mean assessment professionals—like us tend to love. At the same time, we realize you may not be a specialist, you likely work in a setting that does not have richness of database access or budget for securing instruments, and you might just need some help culling through the tens of thousands of entries to find an instrument that helps you know if youth who participate in your program are better off when they leave than when they started. In short, if you are to use outcome measures at all, you need a real-world strategy for finding, reviewing, and implementing them.

Using a systematic process, Beidas et al. (2015, p. 4) identified 29 adult and 20 youth measures that were:

> (a) of importance for stakeholders in that they meet the needs for outcome assessment, a growing reality and requirement in many public systems, (b) are low burden to administer because they have fewer than 50 items, (c) are broadly applicable because they are appropriate for high prevalence conditions, (d) are sensitive to change when intended to be used as progress monitoring instruments, and (e) measure actionable constructs such as symptoms of a mental health disorder that are amenable to change through treatment.

This open-access article, listed in the resources section, is an excellent starting place for considering instruments that may be relevant to your practice. The authors categorize focus areas into those that most readily apply to mental health practice: anxiety, depression, disruptive behavior disorders, eating disorders, mania, overall mental health, personality disorders, suicidality, and trauma. The article includes an overview of the instrument; appropriateness for screening, diagnosis, and/or outcome evaluation; and a link to the outcome measure itself.

You may find other journal articles helpful for narrowing the scope of outcome measures to use in your practice. For example, Deighton et al. (2014) identified and reviewed 11 mental health and well-being outcome measures for youth, including several open-access and several commercial instruments. Whipple and Lambert (2011) also provided attention to outcome measures in mental health practice with attention to the process of feedback and measures developed for this purpose. Finally, Miglietta et al. (2018) provided a systematic review of scales for assessing satisfaction with mental health care, thus providing you with a starting place for identifying satisfaction measures.

The following list includes some go-to places to identify other free or low-cost measures you may find helpful:

- **National Institutes of Health (NIH) Patient-Reported Outcomes Measurement Information System (PROMIS)**. The set of hundreds of PROMIS measures was developed with federal funding and "evaluates and monitors physical, mental, and social health in adults and children" (HealthMeasures, 2023). Adult measures relevant for mental health professionals include (but are not limited to) those focused on anxiety, depression, alcohol, anger, life satisfaction, psychosocial illness impact, and ability to participate in social roles and activities. Youth measures relevant for mental health professionals include (but are not limited to) anxiety, depression, anger, life satisfaction, psychological stress experiences, peer relationships, and family relationships. These measures, including many in Spanish and other languages, are free and publicly available via www.healthmeasures.net.
- **American Psychiatric Association (APA) DSM-5-TR Online Assessment Measures**. When it launched the DSM-5, the APA also launched a website in which they provided "patient assessment measures . . . developed to be administered at the initial patient interview and to monitor treatment progress." These items are free to the public and may be used for general screening (Level 1 measures), to support diagnosis (Level 2 measures), and to measure severity (disorder-specific severity measures). The APA also endorsed and provided access to the World Health Organization Disability Assessment Schedule (WHODAS) 2.0. The measures are available via www.psychiatry.org/psychiatrists/practice/dsm/educational-resources/assessment-measures. It is important to note that the APA varied greatly in the nature of development and psychometric information provided for these instruments. You may find Schmit and Balkin (2014) a helpful resource for evaluating the usefulness of these measures in your practice.
- **The Joint Commission Behavioral Healthcare Instruments Listing**. Available via https://manual.jointcommission.org/BHCInstruments/WebHome includes a

searchable list of outcome measurement tools that may be of interest to behavioral healthcare providers. Each profile includes a URL, information about restrictions or costs, and an overview of instrument attributes. Many of the instruments are free to use with permission and appropriate training.

We hope these tools provide a strong starting place for identifying real-world options for your program and practice evaluation efforts. Regardless of where and how you locate your outcome measures, you are ethically responsible for ensuring that you select strong instruments that are appropriate for the population you serve. In addition, you are ethically responsible for ensuring that you are qualified to administer and interpret the assessment tools you select. If you have not yet completed a course on assessment and testing in counseling, you will learn more about Level A, B, and C instruments and licensure regulations specific to administration in your state.

CREATING UNIQUE MEASURES

By now you may be thinking that selecting assessment measures seems like an arduous task. You may be tempted to just create a scale or a few items that ask consumers exactly what you want to know. Easy and straightforward, right? Not so fast.

Instrument construction is (or should be) a highly scientific process we do not take lightly. In the previous section, we asked you to consider psychometric information such as norming, validity for specific use, test score reliability, sensitivity to change, reading level, and cultural appropriateness. Most practitioners will not have the specialized training and the kind of time it would take to develop a new instrument. When we create new instruments without time or training, we run the risk of not really knowing what we are assessing and making inaccurate conclusions about the effectiveness of our interventions and programs. Using home-brewed assessment instruments (i.e., locally developed measures without established validity evidence) also dilutes our advocacy power, as outside funders often expect us to use instruments with validity evidence.

Before creating your own assessment measures, be sure to invest time in locating a previously validated, well-accepted instrument. If you are unable to locate such an instrument, you may find it helpful to consult with other professionals in the field or contact a faculty member at a university who has specialty expertise in your area; they may be happy to lend support in identifying appropriate instruments.

Those warnings delivered, it is not *always* inappropriate to design our own program measures or indicators. For example, you may want to develop a few quantitative or qualitative survey questions (see Chapter 8) as part of your school or agency's process assessment to help you understand how best to support your clients and students. Alternatively, you may have identified some very specific behaviors your program is dedicated to impacting (e.g., engagement in self-injurious behavior, number of days drinking, talking to a trusted friend when stressed), which might be assessed via simple yes/no responses. And, finally, some programs designed to increase knowledge regarding a particular topic may be appropriate to assess with brief quizzes taken before, after, and at follow-up. Although we prefer you use established instruments, you may choose not to for some very good reasons.

CHAPTER SUMMARY

This chapter included a summary regarding situations in which you may find yourself needing to use assessment measures. After reviewing practical guidelines for evaluating the appropriateness of assessment measures to your unique practice setting, we provided you with an overview of real-world, go-to outcome measures relevant to mental health professionals. Finally, we warned you regarding the risks of creating your own assessment measures without a comprehensive development process to ensure evidence of test score validity. Together, these sections should provide you with a strong starting place for identifying, selecting, and utilizing outcome measures with individual clients and in larger programs.

REFERENCES

Anderson, N., Schlueter, J. E., Carlson, J. F., & Geisinger, K. F. (Eds.). (2022). *Tests in print X*. Buros Center for Testing.

Beidas, R. S., Stewart, R. E., Walsh, L., Lucas, S., Downey, M. M., Jackson, K., . . . Mandell, D. S. (2015). Free, brief, and validated: Standardized instruments for low-resource mental health settings. *Cognitive and Behavioral Practice*, *22*(*1*), 5–19. https://doi.org/10.1016/j.cbpra.2014.02.002

Buros Center for Testing. (n.d.). *Mental measurements yearbook*. https://buros.org/test-reviews-information/mental-measurements-yearbook/

Buros Center for Testing (n.d.). *Tests in print X*. www.nebraskapress.unl.edu/buros-center-for-testing/9780910674690/tests-in-print-x/

Carlson, J. F., Geisinger, K. F., & Jonson, J. L. (Eds.). (2021). *The twenty-first mental measurements yearbook*. Buros Center for Testing.

Deighton, J., Croudace, T., Fonagy, P., Brown, J., Patalay, P., & Wolpert, M. (2014). Measuring mental health and wellbeing outcomes for children and adolescents to inform practice and policy: A review of child self-report measures. *Child and Adolescent Psychiatry and Mental Health*, *8*(*1*), 14. https://doi.org/10.1186/1753-2000-8-14

Delgadillo, J., Deisenhofer, A.-K., Probst, T., Shimokawa, K., Lambert, M. J., & Kleinstäuber, M. (2022). Progress feedback narrows the gap between more and less effective therapists: A therapist effects meta-analysis of clinical trials. *Journal of Consulting & Clinical Psychology*, *90*(7), 559–567. https://doi.org/10.1037/ccp0000747

Gondek, D., Edbrooke-Childs, J., Fink, E., Deighton, J., & Wolpert, M. (2016). Feedback from outcome measures and treatment effectiveness, treatment efficiency, and collaborative practice: A systematic review. *Administration and Policy in Mental Health*, *43*, 325–343. https://doi.org/10.1007/s10488-015-0710-5

HealthMeasures. (2023). *PROMIS*. www.healthmeasures.net/explore-measurement-systems/promis

Miglietta, E., Belessiotis-Richards, C., Ruggeri, M., & Priebe, S. (2018). Scales for assessing patient satisfaction with mental health care: A systematic review. *Journal of Psychiatric Research*, *100*, 33–46. https://doi.org/10.1016/j.jpsychires.2018.02.014

Schmit, E. L., & Balkin, R. S. (2014). Evaluating emerging measures in the DSM-5 for counseling practice. *The Professional Counselor*, *4*(3), 216–231. https://doi.org/10.15241/els.4.3.216

The Test Collection at ETS. (n.d.). www.ets.org/test-collection.html

Whipple, J. L., & Lambert, M. J. (2011). Outcome measures for practice. *Annual Review of Clinical Psychology*, 7, 87–111. https://doi.org/10.1146/annurev-clinpsy-040510-143938

CHAPTER 16

Managing and Protecting Data

By this point you likely have a strong understanding of *what* types of information you may need to collect as part of your evaluation strategy, and you probably have a good idea of *how* you can obtain that data. For your evaluation to be effective, you will need to have a clear data management plan.

I (Casey) once worked with a nonprofit agency where the staff provided strong, culturally responsive, evidence-based services. This staff was meticulous about collecting client satisfaction surveys and outcome assessments the first week of every month. When I offered to help analyze the data for an upcoming grant application, the point person looked relieved and said she would forward the data that day. The next morning, I received a medium-sized box on my doorstep. Inside that box were hundreds of single-page satisfaction surveys and de-identified outcome surveys. As experienced as I was, I was lost. Certainly, the hardworking counselors at the agency were lost as well.

This chapter will provide you with some clear and practical guidelines for managing and protecting data in a variety of mental health service settings. We discuss different levels or types of data you may encounter, including options for tracking that information. Then, we provide guidance regarding elements of a strong data management plan. Finally, we attend to practical strategies for housing aggregate data, enhancing compliance, dealing with missing data, and protecting privacy in accordance with legal and ethical requirements.

BOX 16.1 CHAPTER LEARNING OUTCOMES

- Understand options for individual and aggregate-level data collection
- Create a data management plan
- Take steps to protect privacy as part of the data management plan

LEVELS OF DATA

Before we discuss how to create a data management plan, it is important to consider the different data counselors may use in school or agency practice. The types and levels

DOI: 10.4324/9781003586210-19

of data you access—and how you store them—will depend on the nature of your evaluation activity. In this section, we attend to individual-level data, system-level data, and data from special studies or activities.

Individual-Level Data

Regardless of your setting, you will likely be called on to demonstrate effectiveness with individual clients, students, families, or units served. For clarity, we refer to these as individual-level data. From a purely clinical standpoint, you may use individual-level data to better understand needs and progress for one service unit. For example, if you are working with a client who is showing disruptive behavior, you may want to know the level of disruptive behavior at the beginning of your work together and periodically throughout your counseling process, thus allowing you to tailor your approach to the client. If you are working with a program for which reduction of disruptive behavior is a primary objective, you will need to be able to gather this information for all clients enrolled in the program so that you can examine in aggregate, perhaps reporting average reductions in disruptive behaviors at certain points in the program *and* indicating the proportion of clients who benefited from the program.

Your options for utilizing individual-level data will depend on the complexity of your site, the nature of record-keeping at your site, and the format of the program or process you are evaluating. If your site still utilizes paper files, you might create an assessment summary sheet to be placed in a prominent location within the file. A summary sheet, as illustrated in Figure 16.1, might include spaces to enter dates of assessments, number of sessions completed, and assessment scores. By keeping this summary sheet in an easily accessible location, you are cued to stay on track with planned assessments, have an easy way to store information, and can readily find information when it is time to use the data.

If your site uses an electronic health record (EHR), the system should be able to cue, record, and report periodic assessments. In some cases, the assessment measures

Sample Summary Sheet

Client ___________________ Service/Program __________

Date	# Sessions	Indicator/Scale 1	Indicator/Scale 2	Indicator/Scale 3

Figure 16.1 Sample Summary Sheet

are already configured into the system. You will need to work with site administrators to ensure the system is set up in such a way that allows you to enter progress measures and generate reports about those measures over time.

Regardless of whether you keep paper or electronic records, you will need to have a plan for gathering data for analysis. This plan should be practical and feasible, and it must be done in compliance with the Family Educational Rights and Privacy Act (FERPA) and/or Health Insurance Portability and Accountability Act (HIPAA) protections relevant to your specific setting. One option for compiling data is to keep all assessments in files until a designated time (e.g., each quarter, end of each program cycle) during which a staff person runs an EHR report or pulls all files, locates reports, and enters results into a database. This option consolidates the recording activity to several times per year and may be a good option for small programs or agencies; however, it may lead to an "out of sight, out of mind" mentality in which staff forget about their data collection responsibilities.

Another option is to have counselors or designated staff members enter assessment results into a database designed to be continually updated. This option allows for a living and always-updated database, thus increasing the chances of using data for continuous quality improvement. This is a particularly good option for programs that run synchronously, thus allowing for batch entry of pre-test, mid-course, and post-test data. For programs that do not run on a set schedule, however, the frequency of updates or needing to go to a separate data collection location may be a hassle for already overloaded counselors.

System-Level Data

You will likely also need to access system-level data about the populations you serve as a whole or about your workplace operations. For example, school counselors may assess systemic impact of their work with attention to attendance, Grade Point Average (GPA), college applications, or disciplinary referrals. Those in hospital settings may have routine data regarding readmission and follow-up rates. In addition, many organizations track referrals, time to service, number of individuals served, and nature of services rendered as a regular part of process assessment. These system-level data may not be part of individual client files; however, they play an important role in understanding the overall functioning of a service location.

You will most likely gain access to system-level data by contacting administrators at your site and asking them about specific data points that may be of use to you for evaluation purposes. In some cases, system-level access will allow you to pull specific information about clients or students who participated in your programs in ways that allow reliable and accurate reporting of individual-level data (e.g., GPA, disciplinary action) you are also gathering.

Data from Special Studies or Activities

Finally, you may find yourself working with data from special studies or activities. For instance, results of satisfaction surveys or needs assessments are often collected anonymously; thus, they may not be part of the individual client or student record. Rather, there will need to be a system (beyond keeping them in a big box in the closet!) in place to store and access these data in a way that protects privacy. Depending on the nature of the program and sensitivity of information shared, someone other than the service provider may need to tally or aggregate feedback for reporting purposes.

Similarly, data from needs assessments or focus groups may be an important part of program development and evaluation. These data are rarely part of the clinical record or systems-level data, yet they need to be maintained in a manner that protects privacy and enhances utility. Chapter 6 is focused on ethical and legal considerations and includes some additional considerations for ensuring appropriate privacy for participants.

BOX 16.2 PRIVACY CONSIDERATIONS

Consumer- and system-level data are frequently used for program evaluation and quality improvement practices. In fact, ethical codes require counselors to routinely evaluate their practice and ensure the effectiveness of services. These same ethical codes—as well as state and federal law—also have stringent expectations for maintaining privacy. All data management plans must include methods for ensuring consumer privacy. The specific steps you take will depend on the nature of your site and the nature of the data you are using for evaluation. The following include a few suggested options for ensuring privacy when managing data:

- Assign each client a unique identifier that is only found within the client file. Use this code in lieu of a client name or a code name composed of initials and birthdates (which may inadvertently identify a client) within database entries. Doing so will allow you to match individual to aggregate data over time.
- Do not include identifying information regarding clients (e.g., address, phone number, specific demographic information) within aggregate outcome databases.
- Utilize encrypted, password-protected databases on secure servers in keeping with HIPAA and/or FERPA regulations.
- Require all those who have access to database information to complete HIPAA and/or FERPA training regarding confidentiality and use of records.
- Collect and manage satisfaction surveys separate from the clinical record; although service providers should receive periodic, aggregate feedback regarding satisfaction surveys, be cautious about providing feedback from active clients, especially if you have promised the feedback will remain anonymous.

If using third-party survey collection software to collect process or outcome measures, ensure the software includes adequate privacy protections and/or limits requests for identifying information.

CREATING A DATA MANAGEMENT PLAN

A strong program evaluation plan will include attention to many of the components we have discussed thus far in this book. It will be difficult to decide how to manage data if we are uncertain about what data we are collecting in the first place! Before you create a data management plan, let's review the components that it helps to already have in place:

- Objectives—Program objectives should be named in a clear and direct manner.
- Measures—Each objective should have at least one associated measure or indicator.
- Administration—Each measure should have an administration plan indicating the timing of data collection and person responsible for data collection.

At this point, it is time to consider how we will aggregate the data in preparation for data analysis (see Chapters 8 to 14 for details). Box 16.3 includes some self-assessment questions you can ask to guide yourself through building the data management plan.

BOX 16.3 DATA MANAGEMENT PLANS

Your data management plan should answer the following questions:

- What data pieces must be maintained in order to complete this plan?
- Where and how will these data pieces be maintained prior to aggregation?
- Where and how will these data pieces be maintained after aggregation?
- How important is it for data pieces to be tied to unique cases?
- What is an appropriate timeline or schedule for aggregating data?
- Who is responsible for ensuring data are collected as planned?
- Who is responsible for ensuring data are aggregated as planned?
- Who should have access to the aggregate data?
- What privacy protections must I take to comply with ethical and legal requirements?

PRACTICAL CONSIDERATIONS

In addition to the logistical questions posed in Box 16.3, there are a number of practical considerations for managing data. In this brief section, we highlight some common challenges and tips for addressing them.

Software and Database Resources

As you read the earlier sections, you might have found yourself wondering how you would keep your data. Although more sophisticated options are available, a simple spreadsheet such as one created in Microsoft Excel or Google Sheets will suffice for tracking cases and even doing most data analysis. As is illustrated in our case study, you may keep a spreadsheet with a unique client identifier only housed in a file and the series of data collection points needed for analysis. As you add each case to the spreadsheet, you create a database that is ever-ready for analysis. In some work settings, it may be appropriate to share one file centrally, thus allowing individual clinicians or other staff members to enter data continuously. In other work settings, those who collect data may bring it to a staff person designated for interacting with the database.

In some instances, it may be safer to use survey collection tools as an initial point of data entry, then download results into one spreadsheet for analysis. For example, Google Forms, Qualtrics, and SurveyMonkey all offer data collection tools for which results can be easily downloaded and analyzed. Assuming privacy protections are followed, individual counselors may use a link to report results of measures for individual clients. A school or agency with access to tablets could have a satisfaction survey on a continuous loop, inviting individual clients to enter their responses while waiting for appointments a certain week each month. Alternatively, they could provide a paper copy of the assessment and/or email a link to the survey for completion.

Compliance

Compliance with data collection and analysis plans is a common, critical struggle in evaluation work. Counselors, clients, and students alike tend to be busy and are sometimes overwhelmed. This may result in incomplete collection plans or incomplete datasets. The success of the evaluation activity relies on active buy-in and compliance from key individuals and entities.

Staff are most likely to follow through with activities if they understand the purpose of the activity, understand how to do the activity, and can see how engaging in the activity will help them do their work. A staff member who understands that ongoing feedback about counseling outcomes enhances outcomes or who yields clinically relevant information in the process is more likely to make sure the assessments get done than someone who sees evaluation as just another administrative exercise. Additionally, the more you can build data collection into everyday activities (e.g., prompts on EHRs, pre-tests and post-tests gathered as part of group introduction and closing), the more likely you are to have strong compliance. Finally, when we "close the loop" (see Chapter 17) and the use results of evaluation to spur discussion and innovation, we illustrate that time contributing to the evaluation plan is time well spent. This enhances motivation to continue to engage with these activities. On the contrary, when we never see the results of our efforts or never use them to improve services, we are more likely to see these activities as not worthy of our time.

Likewise, consumers are most likely to engage in data collection activities if they understand why the information is collected, how it will be used, and how it will benefit them specifically. You can support this aim by using clear instructions and keeping instruments or collection tools as short and simple as possible. You may also find it helpful to explain how feedback or engagement in the assessment process has led to positive changes in the past.

Missing Data

Regardless of how well you design your data management plan and compliance protections, you are likely to encounter missing data in your work. After all, common wisdom tells us the mode number of counseling sessions completed is just one. We would be surprised if you do not encounter missing data as part of your data collection process.

Prior to analyzing data, we encourage you to examine missing data to determine whether you can identify any patterns in the data. For example, is there a particular counselor or set of counselors for whom data are missing? If so, might that tell you something about the importance of buy-in, staff training, or revision of procedures?

Similarly, can you discern a pattern in missing assessment data from clients? For example, do those who do not complete the data have something in common in terms of gender identity, culture, age, level of education, or concern? Is there a particular point at which data completion drops off, perhaps telling you something about a critical turning point in your program? Might something in this pattern help you revise the evaluation or data management plan in ways that boost participation and usable information?

BOX 16.4 CASE STUDY

In Chapter 11, we featured a case study involving a primary care clinic in a rural community that used a ten-week mindfulness-based stress reduction program for residents following a cancer diagnosis. Clients completed the Hamilton Anxiety Rating Scale (HAM-A) at the beginning of the program, one week after program completion, and six months later. In addition, program staff were interested in understanding potential interactions of the intervention with age, gender identity, and number of sessions completed.

In this case, the agency is interested in maintaining individual-level clinical data and examining outcome data in aggregate. The clinic maintained individual client files indicating dates and types of service contacts, intake assessment, case notes, and periodic assessments. In this case, the counselor decided to maintain all records as part of the client file, aggregating them into an Excel database at the end of the program. This allowed them to enter the scores into the database all at once, also noting the number of sessions attended and participant demographics. The counselor then used Excel to calculate HAM-A means and standard deviations for each administration, and she followed an online tutorial to compute *t*-test results in Excel. To keep client satisfaction data separate from clinical data, she created a survey using Qualtrics and requested responses via email.

CHAPTER SUMMARY

This chapter included an overview of types of individual-level, system-level, and special data you may be called upon to manage as part of an evaluation plan. Components of data management plans were outlined, and we suggested several options for dealing with unique data management struggles. The chapter ended with a case study illustrating a data management plan for an evaluation plan in a community agency and with a box focused on ensuring appropriate use of privacy protections in evaluation work.

CHAPTER 17

Closing the Loop and Sharing Findings

Throughout this book, we have focused on methodologies for planning and executing a variety of applied research and program evaluation activities. If we stop the process once we collect, manage, and analyze data, we have simply wasted *a lot* of precious time, energy, and resources. Rather, the entire point of this process is to help us use data to enhance counseling interventions and programs.

Focused on *closing the loop*, this chapter will help you understand how to engage in data-based, continuous quality improvement and share out findings with others. After revisiting the purpose of evaluation, we will focus on strategies for making data-based decisions within the context of program evaluation. This will include attention to modifying program activities based on data and assessing the impact of changes. The chapter also includes practical strategies for communicating program processes and findings to visible and nonvisible partners: those individuals, groups, or organizations affected by your outcomes. This chapter will help you with some foundational tools for designing reports that tell program stories about processes, outcomes, and individual experiences customized to your unique audience. Finally, we provide a guide to sharing your findings with other counseling professionals. Together, these processes will help you highlight your good work and advance the counseling profession.

BOX 17.1 CHAPTER LEARNING OUTCOMES

- Understand how to use data to improve interventions and programs
- Understand how to assess the impacts of changes
- Identify, describe, and develop common sections of an evaluation report
- Discuss the value of tables and figures for supplementing evaluation report narratives
- Identify opportunities for sharing program development and evaluation efforts with other counseling professionals

DOI: 10.4324/9781003586210-20

CLOSING THE LOOP

Revisiting the Purpose of Program Evaluation

In Chapter 3 you learned about the purposes of applied research and program evaluation. To recap, *applied research* is intended to investigate, describe, and generate solutions to everyday issues that affect development and well-being. You also learned about program evaluation as "a systematic method for collecting, analyzing, and using data to examine the effectiveness and efficiency of programs and, as importantly, to contribute to continuous program improvement" (Centers for Disease Control and Prevention, 2018, n.p.). We concluded that research projects are intended to *prove* something, and program evaluations are implemented to *improve* something.

Each of the program evaluation frameworks you learned about in Chapter 3 featured a final step in which one used findings to make decisions about programs. Certainly, it is hard to use data to improve something if the results of our efforts are simply tucked away in a report or folder. By taking this last step, we understand our interventions and programs in such a way that we can determine what is working, what is not working, and the next steps for improvement.

Throughout this book, we explored a variety of different types of data you may use as part of your program evaluation strategies. In an ideal setting, we are continuously using data to guide program decisions and implementation. Although there may be some situations in which we cannot adjust program delivery midstream, all interested parties are well served if there is immediacy to use our data. For example, if we find that over half of our clients are dropping out of a program at week three, would we want to cycle through an entire year before figuring out why and bolstering the program? Of course not! We would want to have that information as soon as possible so that we could do something different. At the most basic level, we tend to generate three types of evaluation data: needs assessment, process assessment, and outcome evaluation.

As discussed in Chapters 8 and 13, *needs assessment* data help us understand perceived and expressed needs, thus allowing us to develop counseling interventions and programs with these needs in mind. We can use needs assessment data to compare our service provision with needs expressed in our communities and schools. For example, we might compare characteristics of those we serve with those in our community, noting discrepancies that might indicate barriers to service. In a school setting, caregivers' or teachers' responses to a needs assessment survey may help us realize an unmet need within the student body. Once we have identified these discrepancies, we are able to develop new programs or make intentional program changes that are responsive to real people's real needs.

As discussed in Chapters 3 and 8, *process assessment* data involve consumer satisfaction with services, the number and nature of services offered, and the degree to which practitioners offer services as planned. By examining process assessment data, we can answer questions regarding whether we have implemented our programs as planned. This may illuminate opportunities to adjust programs or procedures to address gaps. For example, if we notice that clients of color drop out of a parenting education program at disproportionate rates, we may have to get curious and have a courageous conversation about why this might be happening. Such a conversation may help us realize our curriculum is not as culturally responsive as we thought *and* point to an opportunity for more focused professional development regarding multicultural considerations for our staff.

Finally, as discussed throughout this text, we generate *outcome evaluation data* regarding short-, medium-, and long-term impacts of our programs. Outcome evaluation allows us to understand the degree to which our program appears to have reached its objectives. If our clients and students are directly benefiting from programs, we can use this information with administrators, boards, and funders in ways that help us advocate for continued resources and program support. In addition, we might share these data with potential consumers, using findings to instill hope that engagement in the program is a good use of their limited resources. If, on the other hand, our programs are not as effective as we had hoped, we can use data to guide important explorations. For example, findings might help us identify specific areas where we are falling short and need to focus our attention. The data might also help us consider whether our program is long enough to result in substantial change, perhaps leading to a proposal to lengthen the program. And, finally, examination of outcome data may help us refocus efforts or energies, sometimes adjusting our benchmarks from idealistic to realistic.

Although we have addressed how we might use different types of findings to inform program decisions, it is important to consider all forms of data together. This is important for two reasons. First, if the outcome results show that a program is not effective, we need to understand *why* our program is not effective. If process assessment data indicate the program was indeed implemented with fidelity, we may conclude that the specific program is not serving our community's needs at this time. But what if process assessment data show us that counselors did not implement the intervention consistently, *or* outside factors such as weather cancellations disrupted program roll-out, *or* perhaps we did not use a measures appropriate to our population or sensitive enough to capture change? We might decide not to implement another round of data collection and exploration before drawing conclusions about the program. In our second example, outcome evaluation might find that a program is especially successful for the 30% of those who complete it. Exploration of process data can help us understand what happened to the 70% of participants who did not complete the program. This may result in administrative retention strategies (e.g., childcare, outreach) or program revisions that allow us to affect a greater proportion of consumers.

Determining Necessary and Recommended Changes

Just as counseling is both an art and a science, program evaluation is both an art and a science. In both cases, the central tension is how we allow science, data, and those things that appear objective to speak while also integrating clinical expertise, context, perspective, and those things that appear subjective. As was illustrated in the previous section, examination of program-related data should lead to a conversation in which we work to understand *why* and *how* we arrived at those findings. These conversations may be particularly difficult given our natural inclinations to defend those things we hold dear. Certainly, it may be hard to hear how an intervention or program we developed and implemented with the best of intentions simply does not reach the clients or students we serve.

After we have examined data and had conversations regarding potential reasons for our findings, we can begin determining necessary and recommended changes. First, we should consider the degree to which our findings and experiences appear consistent across time or are novel to a unique situation or context. There may be some situations in which we experience fluke results or bumps in the road. If we have strong reason to suspect our findings were idiosyncratic, we may continue implementing the program as planned, perhaps revisiting after another cycle or introducing an additional process assessment to help us understand more fully. When implemented in a planful, non-defensive manner, watchful waiting *is* an appropriate response to evaluation data. However, we should be cautious not to use watchful waiting to avoid confronting uncomfortable patterns or delay needed change.

When we identify a pattern of data or program issues that need more immediate attention, we can use what we have learned from our conversations to determine necessary and recommended changes. In this case, it may be helpful to hold a brainstorming session, using staff to generate as many potential solutions as possible. In addition, we may choose to return to the literature (see Chapter 7) in search of alternate evidence-based practices. We may consult with peer organizations to see how they address similar issues. We may even choose to implement another round of data collection, perhaps conducting focus groups or having collaborative conversations with key informants in search of solutions. By using several sources of data to determine which program changes may be necessary, we ensure our revisions have a strong grounding and probability of success.

At the end of the process, we may revisit program development and evaluation resources (see Chapter 3) to help us revise the program. From a quality improvement perspective, it is also important to document changes made and data-based reasons for the changes. Such documentation demonstrates engagement in the process and may be valuable to administrators and funders.

BOX 17.2 MAKING DIFFICULT DECISIONS

The American Counseling Association *Code of Ethics* (ACA, 2014) requires that counselors take action when they are aware of policies or procedures that "may limit the effectiveness of services provided" (D.1.h) and expressly states counselors' obligations to report unfavorable results (G.4.b). Although we primarily present applied research and program evaluation as an objective, scientific process, we know service delivery is more complicated than that. Presumably, we entered the counseling profession because we believe in the power of relationships and learning to promote healing, wellness, and optimal development. We would like to believe our efforts make a real difference to those we serve, and we are clearly invested in our programs and processes. Although this investment can serve as an important source of motivation and inspiration, it can present ethical dilemmas when we must make difficult decisions about valued programs and processes.

If we truly engage in program evaluation, we run the risk of uncovering unsavory findings. In some cases, the risks may primarily target our ego. Although we may get used to it as part of our process of becoming professional counselors, it is never easy to be observed or evaluated (if you doubt this, ask a few faculty members how they experience student evaluations of teaching!). To engage in meaningful program evaluation, we must be prepared to enter conversations about our tender spots, recognizing that even if our services are effective, there is *always* room for some sort of improvement.

In some cases, the risks of program evaluation go beyond ego and may even include livelihood. We may have legitimate concerns that funders will use unfavorable evaluation results to cut support for programs we see as vital to the mission of an organization, even if the program evaluation results do not support their effectiveness. Similarly, we may notice an agency working to identify target cut-points at which they discontinue clients for services, noting that they have likely reached the maximized benefit. Or we may become skeptical of efforts to quantify the effectiveness of individual and group delivery models, presumably in hopes of maximizing efficiency with group service models.

We believe it is essential to understand and face these risks and concerns directly. Refusing to collect data or ignoring what we find presents an ethical concern that can limit our growth mindset and ultimate success in the field. By planning and executing our programs with care, we create opportunities to truly understand our programs, use data to make them as effective as possible, and secure evidence to continue advocating for our clients and programs.

Demonstrating Impact of Changes

We titled this chapter in a way that reminds us of the importance of continuous program development and evaluation. Once we have created, evaluated, and revised programs, we are ready to begin another cycle of the process. In order to do so, it is important to revisit our program evaluation plans to consider which elements of our programs have changed. For example, have we changed interventions, objectives, or benchmarks? Is there a need for change in assessment methodology? Might we add a process assessment to help better understand whether and how we implemented the changes we planned (e.g., observations by trained peers, follow-up calls to those who discontinued the program, focus groups)? And, finally, when will we next examine data and facilitate conversations regarding the impact of changes?

By revising our evaluation plans to be responsive to program changes, we position ourselves to assess the impact of changes we have made. After a specified period, we may choose to use some of the applied research and program evaluation strategies discussed in this book to compare outcomes across groups. For example, we may explore the degree to which program participants met short-term outcomes before and after a program change, consumer satisfaction with services before and after the change, or the proportion of consumers completing the program before and after the change. When we converge these quantitative findings with qualitative indicators, observation, and clinical expertise, we can make a strong argument regarding the impact of changes on the overall service. Now that we better understand the purpose and process of closing the loop, we are ready to turn our attention to practical strategies for reporting the findings of our evaluations.

INTRODUCTION TO REPORTING EVALUATION FINDINGS

An evaluation report depicts key features of an evaluation project, including an overview of activities, key findings, and recommendations personalized to your audience. As a result, your reporting functions as a record for your project that nests its purpose, activities, and products across past, present, and future contexts. Within the pages and pictures of your reports, there lies great potential for interested parties to take actions that influence the development and well-being of communities. Despite the usefulness and support that a strongly prepared evaluation report can provide during the decision-making process, the Centers for Disease Control and Prevention (CDC, 2013) reported that nearly two-thirds of evaluation reports are not put into any reasonable form of action. This is likely due to several reasons, one of which is that the potential for key enhancements indicated in your document is just that—*potential*. With that perspective in mind, there are some key characteristics of evaluation reports that may help you convert potential into program-oriented action.

Characteristics of Strong Evaluation Reports

Several authors (CDC, 2013; Fitzpatrick et al., 2023; Linfield & Kniffley, 2025; Yarbrough et al., 2011) offered recommendations for strengthening the character of your evaluation report, including (a) reporting in accurate, even-handed ways; (b) accounting for your audience; (c) using pluralistic communication strategies; (d) timing your reports; (e) making appearance of documents and materials a priority; and (f) emphasizing social action and practical effects. We discuss each one in the following sections.

Reporting in Accurate, Even-Handed Ways

The components of evaluations are often tied together with the threads of time and passion. The best evaluations use plenty of both. Nevertheless, it is important to synthesize information, arrive at judgements, and present your findings with a sense of objective accuracy that is direct, plainly stated, and complete. Additionally, your reporting should be an even-handed presentation of facts that represent the program's story in ways that are fair, balanced, and without influence from personal biases.

Accounting for Your Audience

Every evaluation report should start with consideration of who you are going to address. Different audiences have diverse informational needs, and they may begin reading your commentary with different thoughts and feelings about the program and reporting process. Some funding agencies or partners will expect detailed descriptions of methodology and scrutinize details associated with design sensitivity and defensibility of conclusions based on analyses. Consumers may be solely interested in improvements and impact. Administrators and policy makers may want some details about program and evaluation features but focus more on costs and prudent utilization of resources. In each case, you will want to craft your report so that the content, language, and technical information match your audiences' needs and receptivity.

Using Multiple Communication Strategies

Different audiences may request different types of output from you. Some parties will prefer or require a formal report submitted to their office, which will be read by a staff member and summarized to them in a briefing. Others may request a series of one-to-one descriptions of your findings that are more informal in nature. Most frequently, you will be asked to present to small groups of varied composition. In all instances, you will want to be prepared to provide reports at varied levels of technical understanding, program knowledge, and use for your findings. Therefore, it is a good idea to use pluralistic strategies for communicating results.

Outside of a formal document, you may be able to provide one-page infographics or an interactive website that allows illustrations of key findings. Rather than relying on statistical jargon, we recommend tailoring representations of your output using easily understood graphs, charts, and figures. This will allow you to focus on engaging audiences in ways that go beyond the typical dry, scientific reporting toward a narrative, storytelling approach that communicates the overall message and facilitates learning.

Timing Your Reports

There is a tendency to think that the reporting for any project or program is done at its conclusion. However, reports can be either formative (i.e., used during program monitoring or development) or summative (i.e., final report at program completion) in nature, both of which are important for the vitality and usefulness of a program. You should consider setting a schedule that prompts providing routine reporting at intervals that match major points in your projects. Some reporting can be done informally through meetings, conference calls, and brief updates rather than submission of more formal reports. Such reports can be unscheduled or scheduled based on project needs. In all instances, you will want to document the date, timing, and nature of information provided to partners.

Prioritizing the Appearance of Documents and Materials

Whether providing a formal report or an informal infographic, make the appearance of your document and support materials a priority. Consider the experience of an administrator who just sat down to a two-hour program reporting meeting and sees a 50-page single-spaced document that has no major section breaks and features a cover page with a typo. Can you imagine how this would affect credibility and interest over the next two hours? Attend to the overall visual appearance of your document, use figures and graphics instead of lengthy text when reasonable, and break up the document into manageable, easy-to-navigate sections. When possible, use clear, self-explanatory supportive materials and avoid grainy figures, complicated tables, and complex figures.

Emphasizing Practical Effects and Social Implications

It can be easy to get caught in the minutia of your evaluation activities and reporting. However, most funders and community partners are interested in getting to points that answer those all-familiar questions: So what? Now what? Who can? and How will we know? Thus, it may be helpful to emphasize the practical, noticeable influence of a program rather than the lengthy provision of statistical details. For example, you might include a brief mention of statistical changes, highlight the portion of clients experiencing clinically significant changes, and then illustrate the impact using a sample quote from a client evaluation. Furthermore, including information about possible influence within the broader social impacts or implications can support decision making.

Although each report will respond to unique partner needs for information, these key characteristics represent some considerations to keep in mind when developing your reports. With these characteristics accounted for, it is time to outline the structure and content of your report.

Fundamental Components of Evaluation Reports

Evaluations often take a pluralistic look at multifaceted programs provided to complex subsets of diverse populations. Although there may be times when you report *all* outcomes and facets of a program, most reports will be defined by the nature of your community partners and their informational needs. For example, you may have a project with five evaluations, yet your audience is only interested in a few of them. Similarly, you may have collected a large amount of data as part of a broader initiative, yet your funder may only be concerned with outcomes related to a particular site, feature, or period of intervention of program delivery. Thus, it is critical to define the boundaries of your report in relation to your overall project.

With this scope in mind, you can begin preparing materials. Although no one set of headings or guidelines will suffice across all project reports, we have found that there are some fundamental components of evaluation reports that will get you started and serve you well. These components include (a) a cover page, (b) an executive summary, (c) an overview of the program and role of evaluation, (d) your evaluation methodology, (e) your findings and impact, (f) your conclusions and recommendations, and (g) appendices.

Cover Page

Your cover page set a strong first impression. It can be a good idea to keep it simple without too many colors or graphics, while also including the basics. Cover pages should include the project title and the evaluation term (e.g., interim, mid-cycle, or final). Next, you will want to identify the recipient of your report, name yourself or the team as those who prepared the content, and include the date of submission. Finally, include a suggested citation for the document for reference.

Executive Summary

The executive summary will provide readers with a brief description of the program, including why it was needed, how it was intended to meet the need, and what outcomes were anticipated. Next, link that content to activities by identifying the broad purpose for evaluation, the scope of your activities, and specific questions you intended to answer. Then, list key findings in an order that corresponds to evaluation questions. Finally, provide a glimpse into your conclusions and key recommendations. It can be tempting to give some aspects or findings of your evaluation more weight than the others within the report, but each domain should have about the same degree of text and presence in the executive summary.

Overview of Program and Role of Evaluation

An overview of the program will include a thesis statement identifying the broad local or societal issue the program was intended to address. Work to make a logical argument for how the program was intended to respond to the need and what short-term and long-term outcomes were expected from program activities (see Chapter 2). These descriptions would include information about frameworks and models the program was based upon, with identification of cultural, environmental, political, or social considerations that are important for putting the findings in context. This section should conclude with identification and description of partnerships, collaborators, and funding sources that were integral to program completion. Finally, you may want to mention what is known about program impact based on the results of any previous evaluations. With these details in place, you are poised to transition to where you fit into the picture.

The transition to describing your role as an evaluator should plainly state why the evaluation was completed, how results will support understanding about program impact, and ways findings may inform program development. Identify time frame, settings, and key personnel who contributed to the evaluation (e.g., name, title, and role). Finally, disclose any conflicts of interest that may affect the trustworthiness of your activities and related findings.

Evaluation Methodology

Now this is the part you have been waiting for, right? With the front-end material establishing the context and staffing of your program, it is time to transition to the evaluation methodology that was implemented. First, identify the evaluation questions that served as the impetus for subsequent activities. Second, describe the research design(s) you selected, with associated rationale for goodness of fit and suitability for meeting evaluation objectives (see Chapter 3). A critical part of this discussion is the identification of outcomes or criteria that were selected as the indicators of impact among those exposed to an intervention or program (see Chapters 2 and 15). Third, describe your sample with all pertinent characteristics required to portray an accurate depiction of the typical participant (e.g., age, gender, race, ethnicity, qualifying criteria). Fourth, include details related to data management, analyses, and interpretation. We recommend using a timeline to summarize all previous content. Finally, it is important to be transparent about any obstacles or limitations that occurred during the administration of the evaluation and provide an estimation regarding the degree to which these factors may have affected your findings.

Findings and Impact

There are many approaches to reporting your findings. For example, you may focus on reporting by outcome, site, or participant. We recommend reporting your findings by research question. Under each research question, provide a plainly spoken summary of findings, technical information, supportive tables/figures, and practical implications. Depending on your audience, it may be helpful to keep your headings under each research question informal, such as "Short Answer," "Technical Talk," and "How Does This Affect Participant Experiences?" This will probably be the longest, most thorough section of your report, but you may be aided in your efforts by developing a unified template for reporting that supports your writing and guides audience interpretation.

Conclusions and Recommendations

In the last section of your report, synthesize all previous content into a series of individual conclusions related to each research question and the program as a whole. This account will include strategies used to arrive at your conclusions, in addition to any considerations that require accounting. Based on these conclusions, offer a series of recommendations across three distinct categories: (a) recommendations related to program impact, (b) recommendations for enhancing sensitivity or ease of future evaluations, and (c) future directions and opportunities that appear to be indicated based upon your findings (i.e., Closing the Loop).

Appendices

In some cases, funders or sponsors may want to view or inspect materials or descriptions of resources in greater detail. You can use appendices to provide copies of consent forms, interview scripts, surveys, correspondences, timelines, and other related materials. Appendices can be made available in your document or electronically using resources such as external storage drives, weblinks, or QR codes.

As mentioned, these are not the only headings that may be relevant to evaluation reports, but they tend to be among the most utilized in both the evaluation literature (CDC, 2013; Fitzpatrick et al., 2023; Linfield & Kniffley, 2025; Yarbrough et al., 2011) and in our experiences. With your key characteristics and these fundamental components in place, you will be on the road to successful reporting.

BOX 17.3 CHECKLIST OF QUALITY INDICATORS OF A PROGRAM EVALUATION REPORT

- Visually appealing and free from basic spelling and typographical errors.
- Tailored to meet the information needs and engagement level of your audience.
- Reflects careful consideration of key characteristics.
- Provides a complete depiction of the project purpose and related evaluative activities.
- Includes cover page with clear details regarding focus of evaluation.
- Features executive summary with clear, succinct summary of program, activities, and findings.
- Provides details regarding evaluation methodology: research questions, designs, participants, and limitations.
- Clearly provides attention to findings and impact of the program, complete with summary of findings, technical information, supportive tables/figures, and practical implications.
- Addresses conclusions and recommendations related to program impact, evaluation, and future opportunities.

SHARING WITH OTHER PROFESSIONALS

Conference Presentations

Just as it is important to share results with those who have invested in your counseling programs, it is important to share promising practices with the broader community of professional counselors. Presenting your findings at a professional conference or meeting can be a relatively immediate strategy for information exchange with our professional communities. These opportunities range from meetings of local professional groups all the way to state, regional, and national conferences. Meetings also range in focus, size, and intended audience. For example, the American Counseling Association (ACA) Conference and Expo convenes thousands of professionals and includes hundreds of sessions that cut across dozens of specialty areas, while the American School Counselors Association (ASCA) convenes thousands of people who specialize in school settings. State branches of ACA or ASCA often provide accessible professional development and presentation opportunities. The Association for Assessment in Research and Counseling National Assessment and Research Conference is a more intimate group of professionals focused on issues related to assessment and research. The Smoky Mountain Counseling Association (a region of the Tennessee Counseling Association) hosts several dozen participants for monthly dinners focused on local counseling issues and topics.

Regardless of scope and topic, conference coordinators are always looking for quality submissions. Similarly, other counselors are eager to become familiar with information and strategies that will enhance their work. When sharing your findings at professional meetings, you will have opportunities to contribute your expertise to the benefit of others, receive outside feedback, and disseminate novel practices. As a result, you will be making meaningful contributions by sparking creativity as you help attendees think about their own efforts to promote development and well-being in their communities.

Exciting, right? The good news is that there are plenty of opportunities to make presentations at professional meetings. Once you have identified a professional group or meeting of interest, keep an eye out for a call for proposals. Generally, these will require you to provide information across common areas, including (a) a title, (b) a rationale why the presentation is of importance to attendees, (c) a brief synopsis of content, (d) learning objectives, and (e) an abstract for inclusion in the conference program if accepted. Many employers will support costs to attend and present at professional conferences as part of your ongoing professional development.

We recommend that you develop your proposal with the target audience in mind and fit your content to their needs. For example, content would be different for practicing counselors when compared to educators, supervisors, administrators, or policy makers. Similarly, if you are presenting to a group of youth practitioners, focusing on using an intervention for adolescents may be more relevant than presenting on that intervention across the lifespan.

Session content and dynamics should also account for the type of session you are presenting. Counseling conferences typically have three broad categories of presentations: instructional content sessions, conversational roundtables, and posters reporting findings of research projects and program evaluations. When you match proposal content, scope, and arc to the intended audience and type of session, your proposal will have a unified message, and a goodness of fit will shine through.

Flamez et al. (2017) suggested several guidelines to keep in mind when preparing to present. First, attendees do not need to know every aspect of your project, so stick to broad strokes and practical applications instead of getting bogged down in technical minutia or obscure details. This will allow the importance of your topic and your personality to stay at the forefront of your talk. Next, make sure your materials are parsimonious, easily understood, and minimally distracting. Attendees want to know about your topic, so limiting technical, audio, or visual barriers between them and your content can go a long way. Finally, it can be helpful to plan some talking points or processing prompts in the event that you run a little short of the scheduled time. Sometimes, these conversations can kindle new perspectives, professional conversations, and attendee collaborations that extend well beyond the conference dates.

BOX 17.4 CHECKLIST FOR PREPARING A CONFERENCE PRESENTATION OR POSTER

- Focus on main points, rather than minor details that may be irrelevant to attendees.
- Include key reporting elements discussed in this chapter.
- Keep materials parsimonious and easily understandable.
- Ensure visual materials are prepared in a way that will be accessible for a broad range of participants (e.g., minimum 24-point font on presentations and posters, careful use of color).
- Figures and tables should be self-explanatory.
- Provide a reference or resource list for further study.
- Prepare a few related discussion points for your attendees.
- Do at least one practice session to work out timing and flow.

Publications

Professional meetings present an excellent opportunity to share findings and connect with others. By definition, presentations are not permanent and are thus limited in their ability to influence broader swaths of counselors, educators, administrators, and policymakers. You may discover that publishing your findings provides ways to share findings with larger, more diverse audiences. Publishing findings lends them a certain degree of credibility, especially if vetted through peer review. In addition, publishers are motivated to get materials distributed and accessed to the widest reasonable audience. As a result, your findings may stimulate activities among related helping professionals and find their way into other disciplines. Although many options are available to you, we suggest three general sources for publications: (a) peer-reviewed journals, (b) agency reports, and (c) web-based document sharing.

Peer-Reviewed Journals

If you intend to submit a manuscript detailing procedures and findings for your intervention or program, we commend you. It is a bold endeavor to put your work out there with a sense of perpetuity. With some thoughtful preparation, attention to detail, and patience, you can be on the authorship end of an impactful article.

preparing a manuscript for publication, we recommend some key activities:

1. Identify a publication outlet that makes sense for your project in terms of journal scope, types of articles published, and reputation. This may include newsletters or journals published by state, regional, and national professional associations.
2. Acquaint yourself with the style of articles in the journal along with the specific author guidelines, which will give you information about writing style, title length, page numbers, and the submission process.
3. Consult with a mentor who is experienced in academic publishing; consider bringing on a co-author to support you in the academic writing and publication process.
4. Lead your document with a clear title and strong abstract that accurately depict your method, sample, interventions, variables of interest, and key outcomes. Reference the American Psychological Association *Journal Article Reporting Standards* (https://apastyle.apa.org/jars) for guidance on sections and information expected in most scientific journals.
5. Whether you are new to publishing or a seasoned veteran, invest in copyediting support as you prepare the body of your manuscript.
6. Prepare a cover letter to the editor describing your project, the details of the manuscript, and indicating your professional identity. When editors notice meritorious projects, they may be more inclined to work with practitioners to shape their writing into academic conventions through a supportive review process.
7. Steady yourself for the peer review experience. Reviews of your manuscript can take a few weeks or many months, and when the reviews are delivered, they can provide a large amount of feedback. The good news is that you likely know the answers to reviewer questions, and the process is principally intended to support your manuscript reaching its potential.

Agency Reports

Not every project needs to be published in a peer-reviewed journal. In some cases, the greatest impact can be associated with the publication of agency reports that are available to citizens, funders, and other interested parties. This has certainly been true within the fields of health inequity and social capital, where projects published as agency reports have influenced public policy and grant making within the United States (Grootaert & van Bastelaer, 2001; NASEM National Academies of Sciences, Engineering, & Medicine, 2017). Although some reports may originate from large national or international agencies, many more are engendered from smaller local mental health agencies, hospital systems, and school districts that serve counties and municipalities.

Agency reports do not adhere to the restrictive publication parameters of peer-reviewed publications and instead allow for greater explication and context building for your findings in ways reminiscent of the evaluation reports described in this chapter. In many cases, agency reports are made available through open access means simply by linking a summary document to a website; in other cases, they are more formally published and distributed (see Grootaert & van Bastelaer, 2001; NASEM, 2017). In all cases, they are intended to inform local practices and the public policies that guide them.

Web-Based Document Sharing

The internet has provided many options for web-based document sharing. Sites such as researchgate.net, academia.edu, and scholarlyhub.org provide platforms for researchers and project managers across the globe to share findings, discuss implications, and network toward related collaborations. These sites offer a global network of informational consumers and have the advantage of requiring little more than a registration email address to get started.

The upside of web-based document sharing is that documents are readily available if you own the copyright to your material and have consent to disseminate your findings using this platform ahead of time. By contrast, these sites may not be an optimal sharing space when a publisher owns the copyright to your data or an employer views the material as proprietary or confidential. Yet if you are sharing incremental reports, tables of key findings, or datasets with the broader community, these sites may be a great place to receive feedback, disseminate findings to broader audiences, and link with collaborators.

University and Organizational Partnerships

A final source for sharing findings and maximizing impact comes from synergistic partnerships between universities and organizations. These partnerships offer a reciprocal pipeline of information between current and future generations of service providers and can have remarkable implications for innovative practices. Partnerships can be cultivated through several avenues, including existing university–organizational networks, established internship or service agreements, and indicators of need from local media sources. At their height, such enterprises can inform university curricula with information that reflects the state of practice in your local community. In the best situations, these partnerships prompt a feedback loop wherein agencies inform the university curriculum, whose related innovations make their way back into our communities.

CHAPTER SUMMARY

This chapter included an overview of the importance of "closing the loop" in program development and evaluation. We outlined types of data that may be helpful for understanding our programs in deeper ways and discussed methods for having conversations that lead to program changes. By engaging in continuous quality improvement, we situate ourselves to maximize program impact and advocate for optimally effective interventions and programs. Next, we provided some introductory tools for developing and delivering evaluation reports that report findings and share the narrative of program processes, outcomes, and individual experiences. These guidelines will help you shape reports for your unique audience, situating your findings within the scope of your evaluation audience. Finally, we provided a brief discussion about sources for sharing the findings of projects with professionals in your community and beyond. Ultimately, you will need to identify what your sharing priorities are: Local or broad? General or specific? Meant for counselors, administrators/policy makers, interdisciplinary professionals united for a common purpose? With these answers in mind, you can put a plan in motion for presenting at an upcoming conference, publishing in a journal or related venue, or establishing a university–organizational partnership.

RESOURCES

- Montrosse-Moorhead, B., & Griffith, J. C. (2017). Toward the development of reporting standards for evaluations. *American Journal of Evaluation*, *38*, 577–602. https://doi.org/10.1177/1098214017699275
- APA *Journal Article Reporting Standards (JARS)*. https://apastyle.apa.org/jars
- *Program Evaluation and Reporting System (PEARS)*. https://extension.missouri.edu/programs/mu-extension-way/program-evaluation-and-reporting-system-pears
- *Standards for Quality Improvement Reporting Excellence (SQUIRE 2.0)*. www.squire-statement.org/
- Torres, R. T., Preskill, H., & Piontek, M. E. (2018). *Evaluation strategies for communicating and reporting: Enhancing learning in organizations* (2nd ed.). Sage.

REFERENCES

American Counseling Association. (2014). *Code of ethics*. www.counseling.org/ethics

Centers for Disease Control and Prevention. (2013). *Evaluation reporting: A guide to help ensure use of evaluation findings*. U.S. Department of Health and Human Services.

Centers for Disease Control and Prevention. (2018). www.cdc.gov

Fitzpatrick, J. L., Sanders, J. R., Worthen, B. R., & Wingate, L.A. (2023). *Program evaluation: Alternative approaches and practical guidelines* (5th ed.). Pearson.

Flamez, B., Lenz, A. S., Balkin, R. S., & Smith, R. L. (2017). *A counselor's guide to the dissertation process: Where to start and how to finish*. Wiley.

Grootaert, C., & van Bastelaer, T. (2001). *Understanding and measuring social capital: A synthesis of findings and recommendations from the social capital initiative*. The World Bank.

Linfield, K. J., & Kniffley, S.D. (2025). *Program evaluation: Methods and case studies* (10th ed.). Routledge.

National Academies of Sciences, Engineering, and Medicine. (2017). *Communities in action: Pathways to health equity*. The National Academies Press.

Yarbrough, D. B., Shulha, L. M., Hopson, R. K., & Caruthers, F. A. (2011). *The program evaluation standards: A guide for evaluators and evaluation users* (3rd ed.). Sage.

Index

A

B

C

D

E

N

O

Q

R

S